OSTEOSARCOMA - BIOLOGY, BEHAVIOR AND MECHANISMS

Edited by **Kanya Honoki**
and **Kurt Richard Weiss**

Osteosarcoma - Biology, Behavior and Mechanisms
http://dx.doi.org/10.5772/62700
Edited by Kanya Honoki and Kurt Richard Weiss

Contributors

Joseph Blattman, Danielle M Lussier, Nicole T Appel, John L Johnson, Alvin J Beitz, Branden Smeester, Branden Moriarity, Marie-Francoise Heymann, Dominique Heymann, Matthew Broadhead, Saumiyar Sivaji, Peter Choong, Zsolt Balogh, Daris Ferrari, Laura Moneghini, Federico Biglioli, Fabiana Allevi, Gaetano Bulfamante, Lor Randall, Matthew G Cable, Norio Yamamoto, Hiroyuki Tsuchiya, Alexander Leandros Lazarides, William Eward, Allison Putterman, Cindy A. Eward, Mitchell Fourman, Adel Mahjoub, Kurt Richard Weiss, Jared Anthony Crasto, Jon Mandell, Tadashi Kondo, Zhang Yan, Qing Mai, Yu Zhang, Xiaowen Zhang, Chunyuan Xie, Takahiro Ochiya, Yutaka Nezu, Tomoyuki Saito, Akira Kawai, Kosuke Matsuo, Kanya Honoki

Published by InTech

Janeza Trdine 9, 51000 Rijeka, Croatia

Publishing Process Manager Martina Usljebrka
Technical Editor SPi Global
Cover InTech Design team

First published April, 2017
Printed in Croatia
Legal deposit, Croatia: National and University Library in Zagreb

Additional hard copies can be obtained from orders@intechopen.com

Osteosarcoma - Biology, Behavior and Mechanisms, Edited by Kanya Honoki and Kurt Richard Weiss
p. cm.
Print ISBN 978-953-51-3095-6
Online ISBN 978-953-51-3096-3

Meet the editors

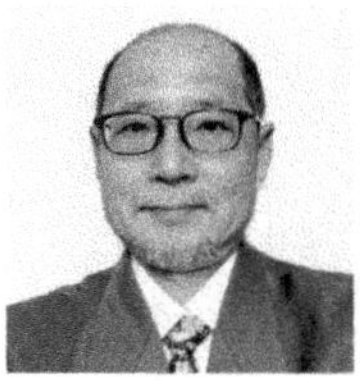

Dr. Kanya Honoki is an associate professor and the chief of musculoskeletal oncology unit in the Department of Orthopedic Surgery, Arthroplasty and Regenerative Medicine at Nara Medical University, Japan. After acquisition of his PhD degree at Nara Medical University, he finished his postdoctoral fellowship at Jefferson Medical College. He has devoted his effort, energy, and passion into the field of orthopedic oncology, especially both basic and clinical pathogenesis of the disease progression in sarcomas. Dr. Honoki is also engaged in the research of cancer and stem cell biology and regenerative and restorative medicine. He is an active member of American and European Association for Cancer Research and International Society for Stem Cell Research, Japanese Cancer Association, and Japanese Orthopedic Association and has numerous publications in these areas.

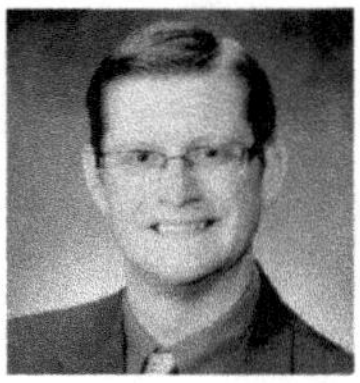

Dr. Kurt R. Weiss is an assistant professor in the University of Pittsburgh School of Medicine Department of Orthopaedic Surgery, Division of Musculoskeletal Oncology. Dr. Weiss attended Jefferson Medical College in Philadelphia. He performed his orthopedic surgery residency at the University of Pittsburgh and his musculoskeletal oncology fellowship at the University of Toronto. Dr. Weiss also directs the Musculoskeletal Oncology Research Center. As a bone cancer survivor, he brings passion and enthusiasm to the laboratory, clinic, and operating room. He is a member of the Musculoskeletal Tumor Society, the American Association for Cancer Research, and the Connective Tissue Oncology Society. He is an author of over 40 journal articles and book chapters on musculoskeletal oncology-related topics.

Contents

Preface

In 2016, a very impressive report was published describing that osteosarcoma is the oldest malignant neoplasm in humans evidenced by the fossil record, dating back 1.7 million years to the Homo ergaster era. Since then, we have accumulated great knowledge of its biology and behavior from tissue and cells to the molecular level. We have also developed many therapeutic weapons against this disease including limb-sparing surgery with megaprostheses and intensive chemotherapy with multiple cytotoxic agents. As a result, the prognosis of osteosarcoma dramatically improved in the 1980s. However, in spite of our continuous efforts to uncover the mechanisms and pathophysiology involved with disease progression including molecular pathways and microenvironment interactions, the prognosis of osteosarcoma has now remained unchanged for several decades. This is especially the case for patients with relapsed and/or metastatic disease, whose outlook remains poor. Osteosarcoma's very complex biology is accompanied by tremendous genetic instability and intratumoral heterogeneity. These mysteries must be solved in order to improve the prognosis of osteosarcoma.

This book aims to delve into current advances of basic and clinical science in osteosarcoma to guide the future directions of research and clinical practice. The book consists of 13 chapters including Chapter I that introduces the recent progress and issues to be discussed in osteosarcoma research. Upon this comprehensive overview, Chapters II to VII describe advances of the basic sciences that could be translated into the clinical arena in the near future. Chapters II and III focus on the molecular pathways that could reveal potential therapeutic targets such as phosphatase and tensin homolog (PTEN) and phosphoinositide 3-kinase (PI3K), as well as aldehyde dehydrogenase (ALDH), epidermal growth factor (EGFR), and insulin-like growth factor-1 receptor (IGF-1R). Chapters IV and V focus on the interaction between osteosarcoma cells and their microenvironment, including the role of mesenchymal stem cells. Chapters VI and VII describe the emerging field of cancer immune therapy and checkpoint inhibition. Chapters VIII to X include topics in the basic sciences that are potentially close to translation into the clinical setting. Chapter VIII describes the biology of one of the most prominent and challenging clinical symptoms: pain. The chapter describes novel strategies to combat pain from the view of its molecular mechanisms. Chapters IX and X discuss the identification of possible therapeutic biomarkers and targets of osteosarcoma through microRNAs and omics approaches. Chapters XI and XII include the clinical issues particular to the treatment of osteosarcomas of the extremities and jaw. Chapter XI proposes a novel technique using frozen autograft by liquid nitrogen for joint preserving surgery, and Chapter XII describes the unique biology of osteosarcoma of the jaw and its treatment strategy. Chapter XIII is a highlight of this book and presents a review of the comparative oncology of canine osteosarcoma as a human counterpart.

We believe that the information in this book will lead to further inspiration, ideas, and novel insights into the field of osteosarcoma research. Our hope is that the knowledge inspired by these pages will be returned to our patients.

Acknowledgments

I thank all contributors for their efforts dedicated to this book, especially Dr. Kurt R. Weiss who shared his time with me to complete this project. Ms. Martina Usljebrka supported the entire editing process of this book. I also appreciate all the authors for their contributions to write these chapters using their precious time and massive efforts. Finally, I thank my family and colleagues for their devoted cooperation and also appreciate my patients and their families who always straighten me up. —Kanya Honoki

I wish to acknowledge first and foremost Ms. Martina Usljebrka of InTech, whose tireless support has kept the preparation of this work moving forward. I thank Dr. Rashmi Agarwal for her editorial assistance, which has been invaluable. My family, clinical partners, and scientific team have all sacrificed so that I could be involved with this project, and I appreciate all of their patience and generosity. Finally, it is with heartfelt thanks and sincere admiration that I acknowledge Professor Kanya Honoki for allowing me to be his partner on this adventure. The opportunity to work with such a wise and inspiring teacher has been a reward unto itself and an honor greater than I deserve. —Kurt R. Weiss

Kanya Honoki, MD, PhD, MMed Sci
Associate Professor
Nara Medical University
Department of Orthopedic Surgery
Kashihara, Nara, Japan

Kurt Richard Weiss, MD
Assistant Professor
University of Pittsburgh School of Medicine
Department of Orthopaedic Surgery, Division of Musculoskeletal Oncology
Director, Musculoskeletal Oncology Research Center
Pittsburgh, USA

Section 1

Introduction

Chapter 1

Introductory Chapter: From Chaos to Cosmos – Toward Precision Medicine in Osteosarcoma

Kanya Honoki and Kurt Richard Weiss

Additional information is available at the end of the chapter

http://dx.doi.org/10.5772/67265

In 2016, a very impressive report was published describing that osteosarcoma (OS) is the earliest human cancer in the fossil record, dating back 1.7 million years to the Homo ergaster era [1]. This demonstrated that OS is the oldest recognized malignant neoplasm with concrete (no pun intended) evidence. In general, OS is the most common malignant bone tumor and mostly affects children, adolescents, and young adults. OS shows significant genetic instability, resulting in a very complex biology with multifaceted cellular and molecular mechanisms and behaviors. This is the main reason why treatment options are still limited and the prognosis has remained unchanged for several decades, despite significant improvements in the 1980s through advancements in systemic chemotherapy and definitive surgery [2]. The prognosis for patients with relapsed and/or metastatic disease is still quite poor.

The concept of "toward precision medicine" was proposed in 2011 to bring about a new treatment paradigm in which clinicians, researchers, patients, policymakers, the pharmaceutical industry, and health care systems work together to improve human health at all levels—disease prevention, diagnosis, and treatment—through the development of more precise, individualized care [3]. Because of the chaotic genetic background of OS and its lack of treatment options, which still mainly involve radical surgery and non-specific combination chemotherapy, the concept of precision medicine could be the most highly desired platform for patients with OS. This chaos of OS biology probably started 1.7 million or even more years ago.

The complicated genetic background of OS is characterized by an extremely heterogeneous genetic alteration spectrum. The most historical and thoroughly described genetic alterations in patients with OS are aberrations of the tumor suppressors p53 and Rb, which cause hereditary dispositions to Li-Fraumeni syndrome and retinoblastoma, respectively [4]. Because both the p53 and Rb pathways are involved in cell cycle regulation, other cell cycle regulators such as p16INK4a/p19ARF and MDM2 have also been investigated [5]. These tumor suppressors and their associated pathways are still a staple of research for potential therapeutic targets in patients with OS. However, treatments targeting these pathways thus far have failed to show substantial impact.

Recent advances in next-generation sequencing, including whole-genome sequencing, whole-exome sequencing, and RNA sequencing, have revealed several possible candidate pathways involved in OS development. In a study performed at St. Jude Children's Research Hospital, Chen et al. [6] reported that next-generation sequencing of pediatric OS specimens revealed recurrent somatic alterations: structural variations and/or single-nucleotide variation in the ATRX and DLG2 genes. Among those, the PI3K/mTOR signaling pathways, including the PTEN, PI3K/Akt, and IGF1/mTOR pathways, have emerged as possible therapeutic targets in patients with OS [7]. A genome-wide siRNA screening with a screen of therapeutically relevant small molecules have identified the dual inhibition of the PI3K-mTOR pathway as a sensitive druggable target in OS [8]. A Sleeping Beauty transposon-based forward genetic screen also highlighted that OS driver genes are enriched in the ERBB, PI3K–AKT–mTOR, MAPK, PTEN, and NF2 signaling pathways [9]. Several specific inhibitors of the PI3K–AKT–mTOR pathway have been developed, and their efficacy against OS has been investigated; some of these inhibitors have already been applied in clinical trials [10].

High-throughput screening technologies, including those that involve microRNA (miRNA), have also had a huge impact on the cancer research field. miRNAs are small non-coding RNAs that play critical roles in the regulation of gene expression at the post-transcriptional level and in the control of cellular processes such as proliferation, differentiation, initiation, and progression of various diseases including cancer. More than 2500 miRNAs have been identified, and many of them function as oncogenes or tumor suppressors that regulate gene and protein expression. Some miRNAs like miR-34a and miR-21, target genes involved in OS development such as the p53 and Rb genes as well as the PI3K/Akt/mTOR, IGF-R1, and MAPK pathways. Some miRNAs could be proposed as potential biomarkers of disease progression and metastasis, and may serve as therapeutic targets for OS [11].

For precise, personalized therapeutic approaches, especially in the prediction of the response to chemotherapy, the establishment of predictive biomarkers is a long-standing goal in OS research. The "-omics" approach at the genome, transcriptome, and proteome levels has been applied to identify the predictive biomarkers of OS, and several potential candidates have been identified [12]. Hagleitner et al. [13] recently identified the association between five-year progression-free survival and five genetic variants [the Fas Ligand (FasL), MutS homologue 2 (MSH2), ATP-binding cassette sub-family C (ABCC5), caspase 3 (CASP3), and cytochrome P450 3A4 (CYP3A4)] using a linkage disequilibrium-based tag single-nucleotide polymorphism strategy. They found that patients with fewer risk alleles showed a more favorable prognosis. They concluded that these pharmacogenetic risk factors might be useful to predict treatment outcomes and to stratify patients, thus allowing for more personalized treatment [13]. Recent studies have also uncovered the important roles of the tumor microenvironment, including tumor stromal cells and extracellular matrices, in the development of OS. Mesenchymal stromal/stem cells (MSCs) or MSC-derived lineage-specific progenitors have long been considered as the cells of origin for certain types of sarcomas, including OS [14]. Additionally, OS development is closely linked to certain oncogenic lesions, such as p53 and Rb deficiency in MSCs, and to bone microenvironment signals such as calcified substrates and bone morphogenetic protein-2 [15]. MSCs are not only the putative cells of origin for sarcomas, but are also thought to be the source of cancer-associated fibroblasts, one of the key players in the tumor microenvironment for cancer progression [16]. Several studies have proposed that the mechanism of the interaction between MSCs and tumor cells could be a potential therapeutic target against OS. A recent study by an Italian group demonstrated that MSCs in the tumor stroma driven by oxidative stress induced by OS cells could be potential modulators of the metabolism of OS cells that underwent mitochondrial biogenesis to increase the mitochondrial activity [17]. The authors suggested that this mutual metabolic reprogramming of OS cells and their stroma could also represent a possible target for OS therapies.

Despite remarkable progress in these fields, the results of studies of specific inhibitors of possible targetable pathways and specific biomarkers have not yet been applicable to the clinical setting. However, continued progress in -omics technology, next-generation sequencing, and high-throughput screening will provide new insights into the pathogenesis of OS and will help to identify novel biomarkers that will contribute to improved therapeutic strategies, prognoses, and quality of life.

The role of immunotherapy has been investigated in both the preclinical and clinical settings in OS. Immunotherapeutic techniques include the use of nonspecific immunomodulators such as muramyl tripeptide phosphatidylethanolamine [18], interferons [19], interleukin-2 [20], adoptive T-cell immunotherapy, vaccines, immunologic checkpoint blockades such as CTLA-4/PD-1 blockade, and oncolytic viral therapy. It is very important to continue the development of immunotherapeutic strategies, especially for patients with metastatic disease in whom effective systemic therapy is not a treatment option.

Advances in imaging modalities, surgical procedures, and neoadjuvant chemotherapy have allowed more limb salvaged and less amputation to be performed. Megaprosthetic replacement has become more popular for limb salvage than any other technique, including the use of allografts and vascularized autografts. However, when preoperative chemotherapy is effective and tumor locates far enough from the joint surface, joint preservation rather than megaprosthetic replacement has been utilized. Joint preservation can be achieved using so-called biological reconstruction methods including allografts, vascularized autografts, and processed autologous bone grafts. Processed autologous bone grafts have been developed to utilize the patient's own diseased bone sterilized by irradiation, pasteurization, and liquid nitrogen freezing. However, precise evaluation and surgical planning are required for joint-preserving reconstruction.

Recent advances in three-dimensional (3D) imaging and printing techniques have already had a significant impact on orthopedic surgery. Especially for musculoskeletal tumor resection and reconstruction, 3D visualization of computed tomographic and magnetic resonance images has become an effective supportive tool for surgical planning and determination of surgical margins. In addition, a precise personalized anatomical model of the surgical site by 3D printing can be created for each patient, and personalized guiding templates fabricated by 3D printing with computer-assisted designs have been utilized for many orthopedic surgeries, including resection of OS [21]. The jaw, including the mandible and maxilla, is a region where OS is occasionally involved, representing 7% of all cases of OS and 1% of all head and neck malignancies [22]. Although definitive surgery is still the mainstay of jaw OS treatment, precise tumor resection is sometimes difficult to achieve because of the anatomical complexity of the maxillofacial region. In this clinical setting of OS of the jaw, as well as in joint-preserving surgery, 3D imaging and printing techniques will be of great help for precise surgical treatment of OS.

A multi-disciplinary approach is essential for the management of OS. Among many clinical symptoms of OS, pain is the most prominent symptom and sometimes requires multimodal treatments. Recent studies have demonstrated that molecular pathways such as the MAPK and PI3K pathways, which are closely involved in OS development as described earlier, play critical roles in regulating the cell signaling of transient receptor potential vannilloid subfamily member 1 (TRPV1), a nocioceptive receptor among peripheral nerve fibers that is closely linked in cancer pain [23, 24]. Therefore, these pathways could be possible targets for both cancer-induced pain as well as OS development.

Comparative oncology approaches through translational research involving rodent, canine, and human, models could provide new insights for OS treatment strategies. Genetically engineered mouse models of OS have been created, such as those exhibiting Cre/LoxP–mediated deletion of p53 and/or Rb [25]. A novel model of OS developed using the Sleeping Beauty transposon mutagenesis system was recently established [9]. These mouse models will be useful to identify new candidate driver genes of OS development. While the incidence of OS in humans is roughly 25 per 10 million cases per year in the US, it is about 15 times more common in dogs. The natural history of OS and the genome-wide expression profiles are very similar between humans and canines OS [26]. Comparative studies using a multi-species approach will be indispensable for OS research and will allow us to identify true driver genes and pathways that will provide novel therapeutic targets and new therapeutic strategies encompassing the fields of chemotherapy, immunotherapy, and surgery.

Precision medicine in the management of OS should be a multidisciplinary effort involving the collaboration of both medical and non-medical professions. Involved individuals should include family members, friends, teachers, and colleagues in the patients' schools and work places. We hope that the findings provided herein will be helpful for all individuals dealing with OS, including physicians, researchers, and patients and their family members.

Acknowledgments

We thank our families, colleagues, patients, and their family members. We also express our gratitude to all participants in this book, especially Ms. Martina Usljebrka for her tremendous efforts during book editing process.

Author details

Kanya Honoki[1]* and Kurt Richard Weiss[2]

*Address all correspondence to: kahonoki@naramed-u.ac.jp

1 Department of Orthopedic Surgery, Nara Medical University, Kashihara, Japan

2 Division of Musculoskeletal Oncology, Department of Orthopedic Surgery, Cancer Stem Cell Laboratory, School of Medicine, University of Pittsburgh, Pittsburgh, USA

References

[1] Odes EJ, Randolph-Quinney PS, Steyn M, Throckmorton Z, Smilg JS, Zipfel B, Augustine T, De Beer F, Hoffman JW, Franklin RD, Berger LR. Earliest Hominin Cancer: 1.7-Million-Year-Old Osteosarcoma from Swartkrans Cave, South Africa. South African Journal of Science. 2016;1-5, 112. DOI: 17159/sajs.2016/20150471

[2] Egas-Bejar D, Anderson PM, Agarwal R, Corrales-Medina F, Devarajan E, Huh WW, Brown RE, Subbiah V. Theranostic Profiling for Actionable Aberrations in Advanced High Risk Osteosarcoma with Aggressive Biology Reveals High Molecular Diversity: The Human Fingerprint Hypothesis. Oncoscience. 2014;12:167–179. PMID:25126591; PMCID:PMC4128257. DOI: 10.18632/oncoscience.21

[3] Collins FS, Varmus H. A New Initiative on Precision Medicine. The New England Journal of Medicine. 2015;372(9):793–795. PMID:25635347. DOI: 10.1056/NEJMp1500523

[4] Miller CW, Aslo A, Won A, Tan M, Lampkin B, Koeffler HP. Alterations of the p53, Rb and MDM2 Genes in Osteosarcoma. Journal of Cancer Research and Clinical Oncology. 1996;122(9):559–565. PMID:8781571

[5] Miller CW, Aslo A, Campbell MJ, Kawamata N, Lampkin BC, Koeffler HP. Alterations of the p15, p16, and p18 Genes in Osteosarcoma. Cancer Genetics and Cytogenetics. 1996;86 (2):136–142. PMID:8603340

[6] Chen X, Bahrami A, Pappo A, Easton J, Dalton J, Hedlund E, Ellison D, Shurtleff S, Wu G, Wei L, Parker M, Rusch M, Nagahawatte P, Wu J, Mao S, Boggs K, Mulder H, Yergeau D, Lu C, Ding L, Edmonson M, Qu C, Wang J, Li Y, Navid F, Daw NC, Mardis ER, Wilson RK, Downing JR, Zhang J, Dyer MA. St. Jude Children's Research Hospital–Washington University Pediatric Cancer Genome Project. Recurrent Somatic Structural Variations Contribute to Tumorigenesis in Pediatric Osteosarcoma. Cell Rep. 2014;7(1):104–112. PMID:24703847; PMCID:PMC4096827. DOI: 10.1016/j.celrep.2014.03.003

[7] Perry JA, Kiezun A, Tonzi P, Van Allen EM, Carter SL, Baca SC, Cowley GS, Bhatt AS, Rheinbay E, Pedamallu CS, Helman E, Taylor-Weiner A, McKenna A, DeLuca DS,

Lawrence MS, Ambrogio L, Sougnez C, Sivachenko A, Walensky LD, Wagle N, Mora J, de Torres C, Lavarino C, Dos Santos Aguiar S, Yunes JA, Brandalise SR, Mercado-Celis GE, Melendez-Zajgla J, Cárdenas-Cardós R, Velasco-Hidalgo L, Roberts CW, Garraway LA, Rodriguez-Galindo C, Gabriel SB, Lander ES, Golub TR, Orkin SH, Getz G, Janeway KA. Complementary Genomic Approaches Highlight the PI3K/mTOR Pathway as a Common Vulnerability in Osteosarcoma. Proc Natl Acad Sci U S A. 2014;111(51):E5564–E5573. PMID:25512523; PMCID:PMC4280630. DOI: 10.1073/pnas.1419260111

[8] Gupte A, Baker EK, Wan SS, Stewart E, Loh A, Shelat AA, Gould CM, Chalk AM, Taylor S, Lackovic K, Karlström Å, Mutsaers AJ, Desai J, Madhamshettiwar PB, Zannettino AC, Burns C, Huang DC, Dyer MA, Simpson KJ, Walkley CR. Systematic Screening Identifies Dual PI3K and mTOR Inhibition as a Conserved Therapeutic Vulnerability in Osteosarcoma. Clin Cancer Res. 2015;21(14):3216–3229. PMID:25862761; PMCID:PMC4506243. DOI: 10.1158/1078-0432.CCR-14-3026

[9] Moriarity BS, Otto GM, Rahrmann EP, Rathe SK, Wolf NK, Weg MT, Manlove LA, LaRue RS, Temiz NA, Molyneux SD, Choi K, Holly KJ, Sarver AL, Scott MC, Forster CL, Modiano JF, Khanna C, Hewitt SM, Khokha R, Yang Y, Gorlick R, Dyer MA, Largaespada DA. A Sleeping Beauty Forward Genetic Screen Identifies New Genes and Pathways Driving Osteosarcoma Development and Metastasis. Nat Genet. 2015;47(6):615–624. PMID:25961939; PMCID:PMC4767150. DOI: 10.1038/ng.3293

[10] Demetri GD, Chawla SP, Ray-Coquard I, Le Cesne A, Staddon AP, Milhem MM, Penel N, Riedel RF, Bui-Nguyen B, Cranmer LD, Reichardt P, Bompas E, Alcindor T, Rushing D, Song Y, Lee RM, Ebbinghaus S, Eid JE, Loewy JW, Haluska FG, Dodion PF, Blay JY. Results of an International Randomized Phase III Trial of the Mammalian Target of Rapamycin Inhibitor Ridaforolimus Versus Placebo to Control Metastatic Sarcomas in Patients after Benefit from Prior Chemotherapy. J Clin Oncol. 2013;31(19):2485–2492. PMID:23715582. DOI: 10.1200/JCO.2012.45.5766

[11] Sampson VP, Yoo S, Kumar A, Vetter NS, Kolb EA. MicroRNAs and Potential Targets in Osteosarcoma: Review. Front Pediatr. 2015;3:69. PMID:26380245; PMCID:PMC4547013 DOI: 10.3389/fped.2015.00069

[12] Wan-Ibrahim WI, Singh VA, Hashim OH, Abdul-Rahman PS. Biomarkers for Bone Tumours: Discovery from Genomics and Proteomics Studies and Their Challenges. Mol Med. 2015. PMID:26581086; PMCID:PMC4818258. DOI: 10.2119/molmed.2015.00183

[13] Hagleitner MM, Coenen MJ, Gelderblom H, Makkinje RR, Vos HI, de Bont ES, van der Graaf WT, Schreuder HW, Flucke U, van Leeuwen FN, Hoogerbrugge PM, Guchelaar HJ, te Loo DM. A First Step Toward Personalized Medicine in Osteosarcoma: Pharmacogenetics as Predictive Marker of Outcome after Chemotherapy-Based Treatment. Clinical Cancer Research. 2015;21(15):3436–3441. PMID:25829401. DOI: 10.1158/1078-0432.CCR-14-2638

[14] Rodriguez R, Rubio R, Menendez P. Modeling Sarcomagenesis Using Multipotent Mesenchymal Stem Cells. Cell Res. 2012;22(1):62–77. PMID: 21931359; PMCID:PMC3351912. DOI: 10.1038/cr.2011.157

[15] Rubio R, Abarrategi A, Garcia-Castro J, Martinez-Cruzado L, Suarez C, Tornin J, Santos L, Astudillo A, Colmenero I, Mulero F, Rosu-Myles M, Menendez P, Rodriguez R. Bone Environment is Essential for Osteosarcoma Development from Transformed Mesenchymal Stem Cells. Stem Cells. 2014;32(5):1136–1148. PMID:24446210. DOI: 10.1002/stem.1647

[16] Bergfeld SA, DeClerck YA. Bone Marrow-Derived Mesenchymal Stem Cells and the Tumor Microenvironment. Cancer and Metastasis Reviews. 2010;29(2):249–261. PMID:20411303. DOI: 10.1007/s10555-010-9222-7

[17] Bonuccelli G, Avnet S, Grisendi G, Salerno M, Granchi D, Dominici M, Kusuzaki K, Baldini N. Role of Mesenchymal Stem Cells in Osteosarcoma and Metabolic Reprogramming of Tumor Cells. Oncotarget. 2014;5(17):7575–7588. PMID:25277190; PMCID:PMC4202145. DOI: 10.18632/oncotarget.2243

[18] Anderson PM, Meyers P, Kleinerman E, Venkatakrishnan K, Hughes DP, Herzog C, Huh W, Sutphin R, Vyas YM, Shen V, Warwick A, Yeager N, Oliva C, Wang B, Liu Y, Chou A. Mifamurtide in Metastatic and Recurrent Osteosarcoma: A Patient Access Study with Pharmacokinetic, Pharmacodynamic, and Safety Assessments. Pediatr Blood Cancer. 2014;61(2):238–244. PMID:23997016; PMCID:PMC4533988. DOI: 10.1002/pbc.24686

[19] Guma SR, Lee DA, Yu L, Gordon N, Hughes D, Stewart J, Wang WL, Kleinerman ES. Natural Killer Cell Therapy and Aerosol Interleukin-2 for the Treatment of Osteosarcoma Lung Metastasis. Pediatr Blood Cancer. 2014;61(4):618–626. PMID:24136885; PMCID: PMC4154381. DOI: 10.1002/pbc.24801

[20] DeRenzo C, Gottschalk S. Genetically modified T-cell therapy for osteosarcoma. Adv ExpMed Biol. 2014;804:323–340. PMID:24924183; PMCID: PMC4617538. DOI: 10.1007/978-3-319-04843

[21] Ma L, Zhou Y, Zhu Y, Lin Z, Wang Y, Zhang Y, Xia H, Mao C. 3D-Printed Guiding Templates for Improved Osteosarcoma Resection. Sci Rep. 2016;6:23335. PMID:26997197; PMCID:PMC4800413. DOI: 10.1038/srep23335

[22] Clark JL, Unni KK, Dahlin DC, Devine KD. Osteosarcoma of the Jaw. Cancer. 1983;51 (12):2311–2316. PMID:6573939.

[23] Chen Y, Geis C, Sommer C. Activation of TRPV1 Contributes to Morphine Tolerance: Involvement of the Mitogen-Activated Protein Kinase Signaling Pathway. Journal of Neuroscience. 2008;28(22):5836–5845. PMID:18509045. DOI: 10.1523/JNEUROSCI.4170-07.2008

[24] Pezet S, Marchand F, D'Mello R, Grist J, Clark AK, Malcangio M, Dickenson AH, Williams RJ, McMahon SB. Phosphatidylinositol 3-Kinase is a Key Mediator of Central Sensitization in Painful Inflammatory Conditions. J Neurosci. 2008;28(16):4261–4270. PMID:18417706; PMCID:PMC2935680. DOI: 10.1523/JNEUROSCI.5392-07.2008

[25] Guijarro MV, Ghivizzani SC, Gibbs CP. Animal Models in Osteosarcoma. Front Oncol. 2014;4:189. PMID:25101245; PMCID:PMC4102850. DOI: 10.3389/fonc.2014.00189

[26] Scott MC, Sarver AL, Gavin KJ, Thayanithy V, Getzy DM, Newman RA, Cutter GR, Lindblad-Toh K, Kisseberth WC, Hunter LE, Subramanian S, Breen M, Modiano JF. Molecular Subtypes of Osteosarcoma Identified by Reducing Tumor Heterogeneity Through an Interspecies Comparative Approach. Bone. 2011;49(3):356–367. PMID:21621658; PMCID: PMC3143255. DOI: 10.1016/j.bone.2011.05.008

Section 2

Basic Sciences

Chapter 2

Characterizing Osteosarcoma Through PTEN and PI3K: What p53 and Rb1 Can't Tell Us

Matthew G. Cable and R. Lor Randall

Additional information is available at the end of the chapter

http://dx.doi.org/10.5772/67071

Abstract

Attention has been given to the fact that overall survival of osteosarcoma has plateaued over the last 30 years despite the addition of chemotherapy regimens. Elucidating the involvement of p53 and Rb1 in osteosarcoma has not yielded many novel treatments, but recent studies have started to characterize how the PTEN and the PI3K pathway can contribute to osteosarcoma. PTEN is a tumor suppressor that regulates a variety of signal transduction pathways and cellular processes, mainly by antagonizing PI3K activity and shutting down the PI3K/Akt pathway. Loss of PTEN function with concurrent PI3K activation has been detected frequently in a multitude of cancers, including osteosarcoma. This chapter aims to characterize PTEN and the PI3K/Akt pathway in osteosarcoma, their effects on primary bone tumor behavior, and potential therapeutic targets.

Keywords: osteosarcoma, phosphatase and tensin homolog, phosphatidylinositol 3-kinase, therapeutic applications

1. Introduction

Osteosarcoma (OS) is a malicious cancer that affects predominantly children and adolescents, and is the most common primary sarcoma of bone. After the advents of adjuvant multi-agent chemotherapy, in combination with surgery, the 5-year survival rate for OS has increased from 40 to 76% in children under 15 and from 56 to 66% in adolescents 15–19 years old [1]. Despite these advances, the prognosis for the 20% of patients that present with stage IV disease remains poor, and survival rates have plateaued [2]. In addition, with roughly 60% of cases occurring in just the second decade of life, the societal cost of OS exceeds that of many other cancers.

OS also represents a unique entity among pediatric cancers, with cases arising de novo and already exhibiting high-grade pathology, heterogeneous karyotypes, and frequent genomic mutations. This genomic instability is further characterized by unusually high numbers of chromosomal structural variants and not single nucleotide mutations [3]. An OS genome can often contain over 200 of these structural variants, making it the most disordered among childhood cancers [4] (**Figure 1**).

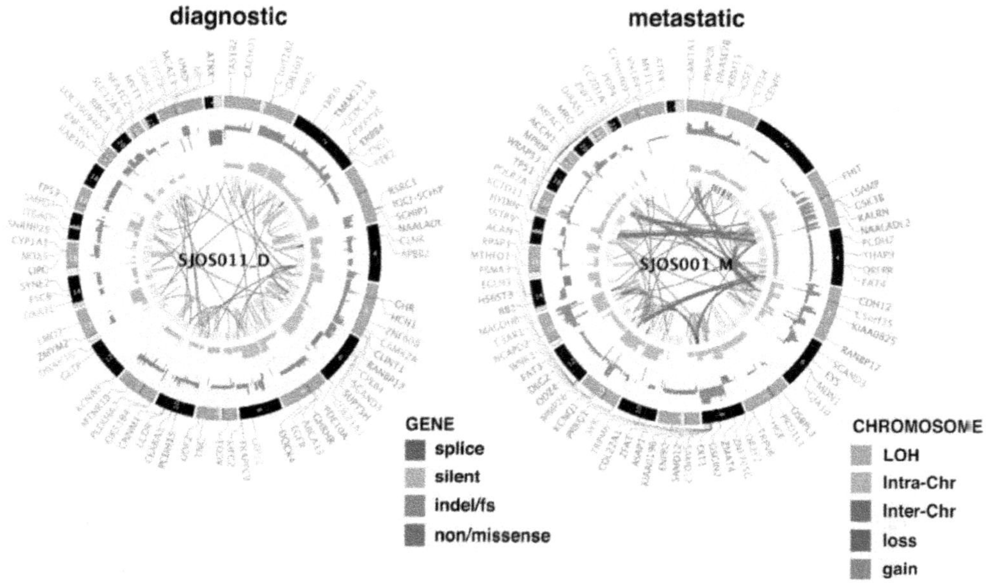

Figure 1. CIRCOS plots of osteosarcoma tumors. Representative CIRCOS plots of validated mutations and chromosomal lesions in diagnostic and metastatic osteosarcoma tumors from different patients. Loss of heterozygosity (orange), gain (red), and loss (blue) is shown. Intra-chromosomal (green lines) and inter-chromosomal (purple lines) translocations are indicated. Sequence mutations in RefSeq genes included silent single nucleotide variations (green), nonsense and missense single nucleotide variations (brown), splice-site mutations (dark blue), and insertion/deletion mutations (red). An additional track was added to the innermost ring of the plot showing the density of single nucleotide variations to highlight regions adjacent to structural variations characteristic of kataegis. Adapted from **Figure 1A**, Chen et al. [3].

To overcome the stagnation in survival rates, the cellular etiology and biology of OS need to be more completely understood. Toward this end, molecular targets that actively modulate essential cell processes such as cell cycle regulation, migration, mitosis, metabolism, and apoptosis have been studied to develop potential therapies. The most well-known and frustrating examples are the frequent inactivation mutations of cell cycle regulator gene tumor protein 53 (TP53) or tumor suppressor gene retinoblastoma protein 1 (Rb1), and attempts in translating these targets into applicable therapies have been met with much difficulty. Recent advances in cell signaling have broadly identified tyrosine kinase receptors (TKRs) as prominent targets for cancer therapies, with many receptors confluencing on the second messenger phosphatidylinositol (3,4,5)-triphosphate (PIP3), and it is activation by phosphatidylinositol-4,5-bisphosphonate 3-kinase (PI3K). More importantly, PI3K and its inhibitor, phosphatase and tensin homolog (PTEN), may play significant roles in

OS and represent therapeutic targets [4]. Investigations have also been centered on the effects of PTEN on osteoclastogenesis, and how the bone microenvironment may facilitate tumor expansion with PTEN loss. Therapeutic targets are expanding as strategies focus on restoring normal PTEN function and inhibiting PI3K pathway activation.

2. The PI3K pathway and PTEN

Class I PI3K is a family of heterodimeric signal transduction enzymes that phosphorylates the 3′ hydroxyl group of the inositol ring on phosphatidylinositol-4,5-bisphosphate (PIP2) to PIP3. The implications of that biochemical mouthful are that PI3K activates one of the most influential pathways in cell cycle regulation and cell proliferation, the PI3K/Akt pathway (**Figure 2**).

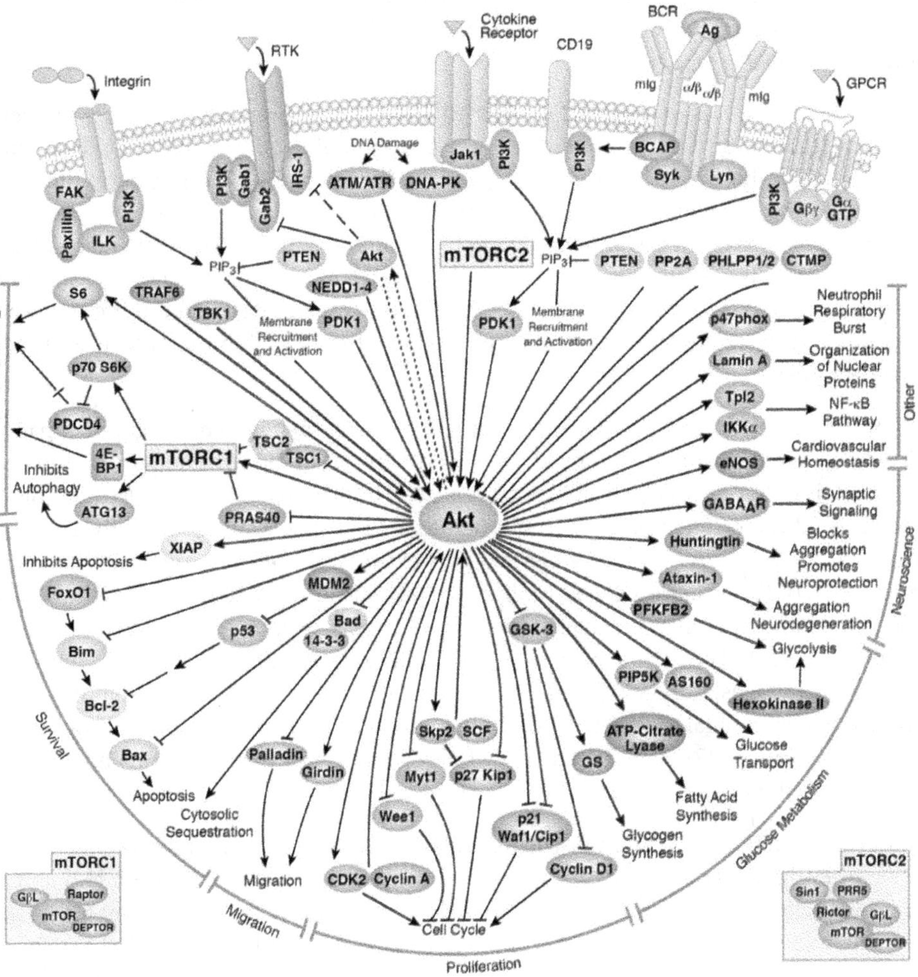

Figure 2. PI3K/Akt signaling pathway. Illustration reproduced courtesy of Cell Signaling Technology, Inc. (www.cellsignal.com).

The PI3K/Akt pathway was first identified when attempting to characterize insulin signaling and discovering the tyrosine kinase receptor type-1 insulin-like growth factor receptor (IGF1R) [5]. IGFR1 is one of the many tyrosine kinase receptors (TKRs) in the cell membrane, in addition to G protein-coupled receptors, that can instigate signaling through the canonical PI3K pathway. Although there are three classes of PI3Ks, class I is the most involved in oncogenesis and divided into class IA (PI3K alpha, PI3K beta, and PI3K delta) and class IB (PI3K gamma) [6]. All class I PI3Ks form a heterodimer consisting of a catalytic and regulatory subunit. The catalytic subunits forming class IA PI3Ks are p110 alpha, beta, and delta, and encodedby the genes PIK3CA, PIK3CB, and PIK3CD, respectively. The regulatory subunits for class IA PI3Ks are p85 alpha, p85 beta, and p55 gamma encoded by PIK3R1, PIK3R2, and PIK3R3, respectively [7]. Class IB PI3K is formed exclusively from the catalytic subunit p110 gamma (encoded by PIK3CG) and and the regulatory subunit p101 (encoded by PIK3R5). Class IA PI3Ks can be activated by TKRs including IGFR1, platelet-derived growth factor (PDGF), and epidermal growth factor receptor (EGFR). Class IB PI3Ks are activated only by G protein-coupled receptors.

Once activated, PI3K converts PIP2 to PIP3 [8]. PIP3 acts as a second messenger by recruiting and activating proteins containing a pleckstrin homology domain to the plasma membrane, notably the phosphoinositide-dependent kinase 1 (PDK1) and serine-threonine kinase Akt (also known as protein kinase B) [9]. Akt is activated via two phosphorylation sites, and the first occurs at threonine 308 by none other than PDK1. The second phosphorylation required for Akt activation occurs at serine 473 by a number of kinases including PDK1 or even Akt itself [7]. Once activated, Akt translocates to the cell cytoplasm or nucleus to set in motion a number of downstream effects to inhibit apoptosis and induce protein synthesis.

One of the most important downstream targets of Akt is mammalian target of rapamycin (mTOR), a 289 kDa serine/threonine kinase that drives one of the two complexes in mammalian cells, mTORC1 or mTORC2. mTORC1 has been implicated as a driver of many cancers, and mTORC2 can create a positive feedback loop by phosphorylating and activating Akt at serine 473 [10]. mTOR is activated when Akt phosphorylates and inactivates a regulatory protein in the mTORC1 complex called proline-rich Akt substrate of 40 kDa (PRAS40). Akt also inhibits the tumor suppressor protein tuberous sclerosis protein 2 (TSC2) which can result in activation of mTOR [11]. The activation of mTORC1 promotes protein synthesis and cellular proliferation by phosphorylation of eukaryotic translation initiation factor 4E-binding protein 1 (4EBP1) and ribosomal protein S6 kinase polypeptide 1 (S6K1) which in turn phosphorylates ribosomal protein S6 (RPS6). The majority of mTOR inhibitors (including rapamycin derivatives) function by inhibiting mTORC1.

In addition to mTOR, important downstream targets of the PI3K/Akt pathway include promotion of cyclin-dependent kinase 4 (CDK4) to support cell cycle progression [12] and activation of nuclear factor-kappa B (NF-κB) which initiates transcription of many target genes including those seen in drug-resistant malignancies [13]. Akt also inhibits Bcl-2-associated death promoter (BAD), caspase-9, and forkhead box O3 (FOXO3), while activating cyclic AMP response element-binding protein (CREB), all of which serve to prevent apoptosis [14–16].

The grandiosity and arborous nature of the of the PI3K/Akt pathway emphasize the current attention being given to phosphatase and tensin homolog (PTEN) (**Figure 3**), a lipid phosphatase that directly antagonizes PI3K during the initiation steps of the PI3K/Akt pathway [17]. PTEN is a 200 kb gene located on chromosome 10q23.3 [18], which encodes a 60-kDa dual-specificity phosphatase that cleaves phosphate groups from phospholipids (including phosphatidylinositols) as well as proteins (serine, threonine, and tyrosine residues including those on TKRs) [19]. PTEN functions as a tumor suppressor by dephosphorylating and inactivating the second messenger PIP3 to PIP2, cogently shutting down the PI3K/Akt pathway and promoting cell cycle regulation and apoptosis [20]. The function of PTEN is further supported by phosphorylation at tyrosine 336 by RAK, which prevents ubiquitin-mediated proteosomal degradation [21]. PTEN also has tumor suppressor functions outside of the canonical PI3K pathway and regulates a variety of cellular processes and signal transduction pathways, such as controlling cell proliferation through cyclin D1 levels [22, 23]. A 576 amino acid translational variant of PTEN has been discovered, termed PTEN long, that can be secreted and enter other cells, enabling tumor suppressor effects in a paracrine-like manner [24]. The C-terminus of PTEN is thought to be essential in maintaining heterochromatin structure and genomic stability [25].

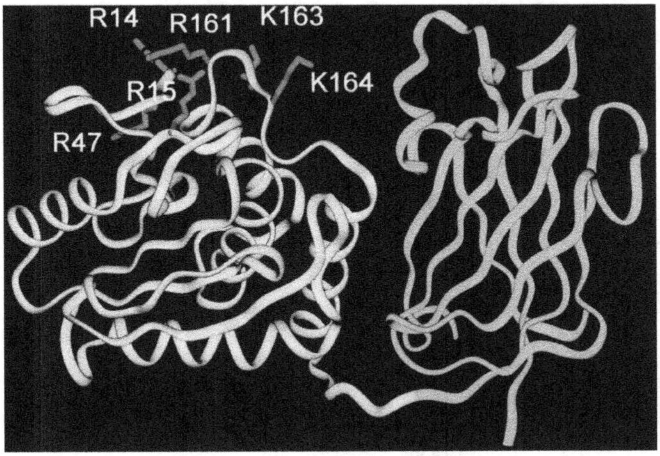

Figure 3. A ribbon diagram of the PTEN tumor suppressor. The phosphatase domain and the C2 domains are shown in yellow and green ribbons, respectively. Reproduced from Das et al. [98].

3. Relevance of PTEN and PI3K to cancer processes

OS is already prone for structural genomic variations and chromothripsis, and whether this is due to selective loss of the TP53 gene or an intrinsic feature of OS itself is beyond the scope of this paper. What this intrinsic genomic instability does allow for is the selection of cancer cells that consistently develop predictable mutations that are beneficial for tumor survival [3]. This phenomenon of localized hypermutation in a cancer genome is called kataegis. Two of these predictable mutations in OS are the frequent loss of PTEN and activation of the PI3K/Akt pathway [26, 27]. The PI3K/Akt pathway is activated in a multitude of cancers, as its overall effects are to promote cellular proliferation and survival while reducing apoptosis. Akt upregulates expression of murine double minute 2 (MDM2) which further inhibits release of tumor protein 53 (p53) [28] and can result in very aggressive phenotypes since p53 is already stunted in many OS cancers. p53 itself has been shown to be a potent dual inhibitor of mTORC1 and mTORC2 in OS cells, further supporting a highly active PI3K/Akt pathway in OS tumors [29].

Loss of PTEN function has been detected frequently in many different forms of cancer including breast, prostate, lung, gastric, colon, and skin cancer, as well as endometrial carcinoma. The frequency of mono-allelic mutations of the PTEN locus is estimated to be 50–80% in sporadic tumors, with complete loss generally associated with advanced malignancies and metastases [30]. In fact, the PTEN protein was initially referred to as MMAC1 for "mutated in multiple advanced cancers" [18]. PTEN deletion mutations were first identified in canine OS cell lines [31], and retrospectively, it is interesting to note that chromosomal loss of 10q has been a frequent occurrence in over 50% of human OS tumor samples analyzed in some studies [32]. Specific mutations in PTEN have been identified in 44% of pediatric OS [3].

The genetic disruption of PTEN often leads to unchecked PI3K/Akt signaling [33]. In breast cancer cell lines, a functional PTEN can directly inhibit cell growth [21]. More recently, the PI3K/Akt pathway and PTEN have risen to the forefront of OS research since the surprise finding by Perry et al. that identified biologically and clinically relevant alterations in the PI3K/Akt pathway in 24% of OS samples [4]. Furthermore, when comparing the same OS tumors to a murine model of OS (with conditional deletions of TP53 and Rb1 in the preosteoblast), both contained somatic mutations in PTEN and PIK3R1.

4. How is PTEN lost in cancer?

There are numerous methods by which the PI3K/Akt pathway is activated in malignancies, often the consequence of upregulation via a multitude of TKRs and G-protein-coupled receptors. With PTEN having a pronounced effect on the PI3K/Akt pathway, PTEN function is accordingly inhibited in many ways. Recurrent PTEN germline mutations often involve exon 5, which codes for its phosphatase domain, and missense and nonsense somatic mutations also can occur in exons 5–8 [34]. Cowden's disease (also known as multiple hamartoma syndrome) is an autosomal dominant condition with increased risk of thyroid, breast, uterine, and kidney cancers that results from similar somatic inactivating mutations of PTEN [35]. The end result is a functional loss of heterozygosity, which is sufficient to produce oncogenesis, as PTEN is essential for embryonic development, and homozygous loss results in embryonic lethal phenotype in mice [36].

At the epigenetic level, PTEN is inhibited by aberrant promoter hypermethylation of CpG islands, which is a poor prognostic indicator in numerous cancer types including breast, colorectal, uterine, and malignant melanoma [37–40]. While hypermethylation has been identified in several soft tissue sarcomas and in murine models of OS, it has only been studied in human OS tumors in vitro [41]. PTEN protein translation can be negatively regulated by many microRNAs including miR-92a, miR-17, miR-128, and miR-130/131 [42–44]. Theoretically, structural features of PTEN itself could prove to be potential sites for compromising protein stability. Post-translational modification such as phosphorylation at tyrosine 336 could be abrogated, thus promoting protein degradation. Protein localization to the cell membrane or nucleus could be affected if the C2 or PDZ-binding domains of PTEN were impaired. Although the majority of inactivating mutations affect the phosphatase domain of PTEN, preventing it from cleaving PIP3 to PIP2, there are several ways that PTEN expression and dysregulation can be imparted in malignancies.

5. PTEN in bone and osteosarcoma

PTEN is frequently deactivated through deletions in human OS tumor samples [26]. A sleeping beauty forward genetic screen by Moriarity et al. supports the role of PTEN loss as a key driver in osteosarcomagenesis in mice, with a concordant enrichment of genes involved in the PI3K/Akt pathway [45]. The PI3K/Akt pathway is already recognized as a common effector for RTK-activating mutations in cancer [46]. The loss of PTEN only further promotes this, but what factors in the bone microenvironment that facilitate tumor expansion in the absence of PTEN is unknown. It would be very un-Darwinian for OS, multiple myeloma, and bone metastases to all have PTEN derangements for unrelated reasons. The effects of PTEN on osteoclastogenesis and receptor activator of nuclear factor-kappa-B ligand (RANKL) may be the commonality among these cancers.

There is a vicious cycle that begins when a malignancy metastasizes or originates in bone that allows it to propagate and induce osteolysis. Metastatic tumor cells can secrete interleukin-1 (IL-1) and parathyroid hormone-related protein (PTHrP), which stimulate RANKL production and secretion from osteoblasts. IL-1 also stimulates osteoblasts to secrete IL-6 via the PI3K/Akt pathway, and IL-6 is a potent stimulator of osteoclastogenesis [47]. OS cells also directly produce RANKL. RANKL binding to the RANK receptor on osteoclast precursors activates osteoclast differentiation and osteolysis. The increased bone resorption results in the release of bone morphogenetic proteins (BMPs) and insulin-like growth factor 1 (IGF-1) that further attract and stimulate the growth of cancer cells in bone, thus initiating a vicious cycle of tumor expansion and osteolysis [48, 49].

PI3K/Akt acts as a cog in the wheel of this vicious cycle, being activated by RANKL and resulting in downstream expression of NFATc1, a key transcription factor of osteoclastogenesis [50]. This gives PTEN the opportunity to prevent bone resorption by inhibiting the PI3K/Akt pathway, thus suppressing RANKL-induced osteoclast differentiation and stopping the vicious cycle [51]. This would support the loss of PTEN in aggressive bony malignancies, preventing stimulation of osteoblasts by IL-1 and osteoclasts by RANKL. Murine models with PTEN deletions have shown increased osteoblast proliferation and bone mass [52], in addition to increased osteoclast differentiation [53]. Fibroblast growth factor 18 (FGF18) is another stimulator of bone growth, and with all FGF receptors being RTK's, its effects are mediated via the PI3K/Akt pathway and can be inhibited by PTEN [54]. Vascular endothelial growth factor (VEGF) and EGFR are both upregulated in OS and are key activators of the PI3K/Akt pathway [26, 55].

The finding that WNT5A may phosphorylate Akt is further support for the bone microenvironment being conducive to tumor growth [56]. WNT5A is expressed on osteoblast-precursor cells and activates RTK-like orphan receptors (Ror) on osteoclast precursors, culminating in increased expression of RANK on osteoclasts and enhancing RANKL osteoclastogenesis [57]. The result of PTEN loss in OS would be twofold in promoting the effects of WNT5A: (1) further increasing RANKL production by osteoblasts and (2) enabling WNT5A-related Akt activation, both increasing osteoclastogenesis and osteolysis.

6. PTEN in osteosarcoma and metastasis

WNT5A also provides segue into the realm of OS metastases. Metastatic melanoma cell motility and invasiveness are increased through WNT5A and Akt. Akt is increased in metastatic OS specimens, and inhibiting Akt in mice decreases pulmonary metastases [7]. WNT5A is even implicated in helping to initiate the epithelial to mesenchymal transition (EMT), a key event in malignant cancers developing metastatic potential [58, 59]. The effect of PTEN loss in promoting EMT has been shown in prostate, colorectal, and OS cancer cells [60–62]; however, the role of EMT in mesenchymal tumors including OS is still a topic of debate and a focus of current research.

IL-6 is also increased in OS tissues and can promote ICAM-1 expression and cell motility in OS in vitro, possibly correlating to metastatic potential. These effects of IL-6 in OS can be negated by Akt inhibition [63], suggesting that PTEN could also negate this effect in bone by preventing IL-1 from stimulating IL-6 through PI3K/Akt. Another promoter of metastasis is the chemokine CXCL12 and its receptor CXCR4, both induced by IL-1 and strongly linked to bone metastasis [64]. PTEN is involved in the negative regulation of CXCR4, and in prostate cancer, PTEN loss induces CXCL12/CXCR4 expression [65].

Focal adhesion kinase (FAK) deserves special recognition as a direct target of PTEN outside of the canonical PI3K pathway, as it is a target of the protein phosphatase (not lipophosphatase) domain of PTEN [66]. Activation of FAK by phosphorylation (pFAK) promotes proliferation and invasion of tumor cells and increases matrix metalloproteinases that can degrade the extracellular matrix. FAK and pFAK are overexpressed in human OS samples and independently predict overall and metastasis-free survival [67]. This effect may be reversed in OS cells with PTEN transfections, which exhibit decreased migration and adhesion capabilities and concomitant downregulation of pFAK and MMP-9, further supporting the loss of PTEN in OS [68]. Just as FAK can be prognostic in human OS, the presence of PTEN in tumor resections is significantly associated with improved survival prognosis [69]. Unfortunately neither can be correlated with response to current chemotherapy regimens.

7. Therapeutic applications targeting PI3K/Akt pathway and PTEN in osteosarcoma

There is an abundance of convincing evidence supporting a key role for PTEN in OS, but from a therapeutic standpoint, this assumes that there is causality and not just correlation between PTEN loss and poor patient prognosis. Two major therapeutic strategies are restoring normal PTEN function and inhibiting the PI3K pathway. Comparing these two strategies could also aid in distinguishing how PTEN serves as a tumor suppressor beyond the canonical PI3K pathway.

Many chemotherapy agents already target various levels of the PI3K/Akt pathway, and several are in various phases of clinical trials involving OS. These include small molecule inhibitors of PI3K, Akt, and numerous mTOR inhibitors (**Table 1**). Countless PI3K small molecule inhibitors have been developed, but several have specifically been effective in OS including GSK458, LY294002, BYL719, and BKM120 (Buparlisib) [4, 70–72]. Pictilisib (GDC-0941) is a pan PI3K inhibitor that has entered phase I clinical trials for advanced solid tumors [73]. Aminopeptidase N (also known as CD13) is a surface receptor activated by IL-6 that can stimulate PI3K and is involved in tumor invasion. An aminopeptidase N inhibitor, ubenimex, is currently used for acute myeloid leukemia treatments and may help prevent OS metastases [74]. The Akt inhibitors perifosine and MK-2206 both exert anti-OS activity in vitro [75, 76]. Inhibitors of the mTOR complex are the most numerous of this pathway, being extensively studied and developed since the discovery of the mTORC1 inhibitor rapamycin in 1975. Many new inhibitors of the mTORC1/2 complex are currently being developed, but several in particular have been tested on OS either in vivo or are in various phases of clinical trials: temsirolimus [77], ridaforolimus [78], everolimus [79], XL388 [80], and NVP-BEZ235 [81]. Apitolisib (GDC-0980) has entered phase I clinical trials for patients with advanced solid tumors and could precede future studies involving OS patients [82].

With current chemotherapy regimens for OS having reached seemingly maximum efficacy, attention has been generous in identifying new agents to increase PTEN function in OS. MicroRNA-21 (miR-21) is one of the first mammalian microRNA's discovered that happens to be highly expressed in bone marrow and post-transcriptionally regulates a number of tumor suppressors including PTEN. miR-21 is overexpressed, suppresses PTEN in OS, and has been identified as a potential therapeutic target [83]. MicroRNAs are small non-coding pieces of RNA, similar to small interfering RNA (siRNAs) that bind to complimentary pieces of messenger RNA, effectively preventing translation of the mRNA into proteins. In multiple myeloma, miR-21 inhibitors have been used in vivo using murine models to cause tumor suppression, with tumors exhibiting increased PTEN and decreased p-Akt levels [84]. Targeting microRNAs could show promise, as numerous microRNAs are specifically upregulated in OS cell lines [44]. In addition to miR-21, miR-17 and miR-221 are also increased and can inhibit PTEN in OS cells and tissues, potentially being therapeutic targets [42, 85]. Further incentive for therapeutic inhibition of miR-221 is its association with cisplatin resistance, an agent frequently included in chemotherapy regimens for OS.

Agent	Target	Therapies
GSK458	PI3K	Phase I trial for advanced solid tumors
LY294002	PI3K	Efficacy against OS cells in vitro
BYL719 (Alpelisib)	PI3K alpha	Phase I for advanced solid tumors
BKM120 (Buparlisib)	PI3K	Phase Ib for advanced solid tumors
GDC0941 (Pictilisib)	PI3K	Phase I for advanced solid tumors
Bestatin (Ubenimex)	Aminopeptidase N	Efficacy against OS cells in vitro
KRX0401 (Perifosine)	PI3K, Akt	Efficacy against OS cells in vitro
MK-2206	Akt	Phase I for advanced solid tumors and metastatic breast cancer
Rapamycin (Sirolimus)	mTORC1	Phase II for soft tissue sarcoma and osteosarcoma
CCI779 (Temsirolimus)	mTORC1	Phase II for soft tissue sarcoma and recurrent, refractory sarcoma
MK8669 (Ridaforolimus)	mTORC1	Phase II and III for advanced soft tissue sarcoma and osteosarcoma
RAD001 (Everolimus)	mTORC1	Phase II for advanced osteosarcoma
XL388	mTORC1/2	Efficacy against OS cells in vitro
NVP-BEZ235 (Dactolisib)	PI3K, mTORC1/2	Phase I for advanced solid tumors Efficacy in vivo against OS in mice
GDC0980 (Apitolisib)	PI3K, mTORC1/2	Phase I for advanced solid tumors
Sorafenib	RTK	Phase II for advanced osteosarcoma

"Advanced" denotes tumors that have metastasized, recurred, failed prior chemotherapies, or are not surgically resectable.

Table 1. Current agents targeting PI3K/Akt pathway with potential against osteosarcoma.

Targeted molecular therapy using RTK inhibitors has been fruitful in many cancers. EGFR causes activation of Akt in OS, and resistance to EGFR inhibitors can be seen in tumors with PTEN deletions leading to unchecked Akt activity. This is encouraging for possible combination therapies that restore PTEN function and inhibit either the PI3K pathway or RTKs. One RTK inhibitor in particular, sorafenib, may have interactions with PTEN. Sorafenib is a small molecule inhibitor of many RTKs including platelet-derived growth factor receptors (PDGFR), VEGF, EGFR, and Raf family kinases and is currently used in advanced renal cell carcinoma, thyroid cancer, and hepatocellular carcinoma. In thyroid cancers in vivo, sorafenib reversed tumor growth that had been attributed to PTEN loss [86]. Interactions between sorafenib and PTEN can also explain why acquired resistance to sorafenib in hepatocellular carcinomas is partly due to miR-21-mediated inhibition of PTEN [87]. Notably, sorafenib is the first targeted chemotherapy agent used for treatment of OS. Sorafenib did demonstrate some activity as a single agent in patients with unresectable OS, with median progression free and overall survival of 4 and 7 months, respectively [88]. Additional effect was seen with combination of sorafenib and the mTOR inhibitor everolimus [78], and further improvement could be achieved with combination therapy specifically targeting PTEN or miR-21.

Demethylating agents may be able to restore PTEN function by removing hypermethylated promoter regions in cancer cells. In many cancerous processes, methyl groups are added throughout the genome preferentially in the promoter regions of tumor suppressor genes, to the five position of cytosine of a CpG dinucleotide (i.e., where a guanine is preceded by a cytosine). These 5-methylcytosines act as roadblocks on a cell's DNA, preventing transcription of tumor suppressor genes. Although hypermethylation occurs in many cancers, it is difficult to show that this occurs in OS in vivo. 5-Azacytidine is a commonly used demethylating agent approved for treatment of myelodysplastic syndrome. It has been shown in human OS in vitro that the PTEN gene promoter is hypermethylated and that 5-azacytidine treatments activate PTEN expression [89]. Initial uses of 5-azacytidine as an isolated agent in OS were disappointing [90]; however, recent investigations show a role for combination therapies targeting PTEN through epigenetic regulation [91].

Many other specific activators of PTEN have been recently identified, but at this time, they remain tested only in vitro. Tepoxalin, a 5-lipogenase inhibitor, appears to increase PTEN activity by preventing its alkylation or oxidation in canine OS cell lines [92]. Evodiamine, derived from the fruit of the *Evodia rutaecarpa* plant, inhibits human OS cell proliferation by increasing both protein and gene levels of PTEN [93]. Celecoxib, a cyclooxygenase-2 inhibitor, inhibits hepatocarcinoma tumor growth and angiogenesis in mice by concurrently increasing PTEN and decreasing PI3K levels [94]. Similarly, using a VEGF inhibitor in combination with celecoxib may prove beneficial in human OS [95]. Even caffeine has been shown to induce PTEN activation and many other tumor suppressor genes, while decreasing expression of IL-6 and matrix metallopeptidase 2 [96, 97]. Overall there is much promise for improving OS treatments by honing our understanding of PTEN and the PI3K pathway (**Table 2**).

Agent	Target	Effect on PTEN
None yet available	miR17, miR21, miR221	Reduced inhibition of PTEN by miR
5-Azacytidine	Demethylating agent	Increases PTEN in human OS cells
Tepoxalin	5-Lipogenase inhibitor	Increases PTEN in canine OS cells
Evodiamine	Unknown	Increases PTEN in human OS cells
Celecoxib	Cyclooxygenase-2 inhibitor	Increases PTEN and decreases PI3K in vitro
Caffeine	Unknown	Activates PTEN, decreases expression of IL-6 and MMP2

Table 2. Potential future agents for targeting PTEN in osteosarcoma.

8. Conclusion

The stagnation of current chemotherapy regimens has forced us to look beyond the usual players in oncogenesis. The mentality behind the recent targeted developments against OS involving PI3K and PTEN could be expanded to benefit many tumor types. We have been able to see through the genetic chaos of OS, finding predictability in the form of kataegis and the seemingly random mutations that converge on the PI3K/Akt pathway. Significant inroads still need to be made to clinically validate what has been proven on the bench and in animal models, but sarcomatologists are optimistic that potential therapies and improved patient survival lie within the PI3K and PTEN axis.

Author details

Matthew G. Cable and R. Lor Randall*

*Address all correspondence to: Lor.Randall@hci.utah.edu

Huntsman Cancer Institute, The University of Utah, Salt Lake City, Utah, USA

References

[1] Smith MA, Altekruse SF, Adamson PC, Reaman GH, Seibel NL. Declining childhood and adolescent cancer mortality. Cancer. 2014 Aug 15;120(16):2497–2506. doi:10.1002/cncr.28748

[2] Meyers PA, Schwartz CL, Krailo M, Kleinerman ES, Betcher D, Bernstein ML, et al. Osteosarcoma: a randomized, prospective trial of the addition of ifosfamide and/or muramyl tripeptide to cisplatin, doxorubicin, and high-dose methotrexate. J Clin Oncol. 2005 Mar 20;23(9):2004–2011.

[3] Chen X, Bahrami A, Pappo A, Easton J, Dalton J, Hedlund E, et al. Recurrent somatic structural variations contribute to tumorigenesis in pediatric osteosarcoma. Cell Rep. 2014 Apr 10;7(1):104–112. doi:10.1016/j.celrep.2014.03.003

[4] Perry JA, Kiezun A, Tonzi P, Van Allen EM, Carter SL, Baca SC, et al. Complementary genomic approaches highlight the PI3K/mTOR pathway as a common vulnerability in osteosarcoma. Proc Natl Acad Sci USA. 2014 Dec 23;111(51):E5564–E5573. doi:10.1073/pnas.1419260111

[5] Baserga R. The IGF-I receptor in cancer research. Exp Cell Res. 1999 Nov 25;253(1):1–6.

[6] Vadas O, Burke JE, Zhang X, Berndt A, Williams RL. Structural basis for activation and inhibition of class I phosphoinositide 3-kinases. Sci Signal. 2011 Oct 18(4):195:re2. doi:10.1126/scisignal.2002165

[7] Zhang J, Yu XH, Yan YG, Wang C, Wang WJ. PI3K/Akt signaling in osteosarcoma. Clin Chem Acta. 2015 Apr 15;444:182–192. doi:10.1016/j.cca.2014.12.041

[8] Cantley LC. The phosphoinositide 3-kinase pathway. Science. 2002 May 31;296(5573): 1655–1657.

[9] Georgescu MM. PTEN tumor suppressor network in PI3K-Akt pathway control. Genes Cancer. 2010 Dec;1(12):1170–1177. doi:10.1177/1947601911407325

[10] Chang W, Wei K, Ho L, Berry GJ, Jacobs SS, Chang CH, et al. A critical role for the mTORC2 pathway in lung fibrosis. PLoS One. 2014 Aug 27;9(8):e106155. doi:10.1371/journal.pone.0106155

[11] Vander Haar E, Lee SI, Bandhakavi S, Griffin TJ, Kim DH. Insulin signalling to mTOR mediated by the Akt/PKB substrate PRAS40. Nat Cell Biol. 2007 Mar;9(3):316–323.

[12] Shin I, Yakes FM, Rojo F, Shin NY, Bakin AV, Baselga J, et al. PKB/Akt mediates cell-cycle progression by phosphorylation of p27Kip1 at threonine 157 and modulation of its cellular localization. Nat Med. 2002 Oct;8(10):1145–1152.

[13] Grandage VL, Gale RE, Linch DC, Khwaja A. PI3-kinase/Akt is constitutively active in primary acute myeloid leukaemia cells and regulates survival and chemoresistance via NF-kB, MAPkinase and p53 pathways. Leukemia. 2005 Apr;19(4):586–594.

[14] Datta SR, Dudek H, Tao X, Masters S, Fu H, Gotoh Y, et al. Akt phosphorylation of BAD couples survival signals to the cell-intrinsic death machinery. Cell. 1997 Oct 17; 91(2):231–241.

[15] Pugazhenthi S, Nesterova A, Sable C, Heidenreich KA, Boxer LM, Heasley LE, et al. Akt/protein kinase B up-regulates Bcl-2 expression through cAMP-response element-binding protein. J Biol Chem. 2000 Apr 14;275(15):10761–10766.

[16] Brunet A, Bonni A, Zigmond MJ, Lin MZ, Juo P, Hu LS, et al. Akt promotes cell survival by phosphorylating and inhibiting a Forkhead transcription factor. Cell. 1999 Mar 14; 96(6):857–868.

[17] Stambolic V, Suzuki A, de la Pompa JL, Brothers GM, Mirtsos C, Sasaki T, et al. Negative regulation of PKB/Akt-dependent cell survival by the tumor suppressor PTEN. Cell. 1998 Oct 2;95(1):29–39.

[18] Steck PA, Pershouse MA, Jasser SA, Yung WA, Lin H, Ligon AH, et al. Identification of a candidate tumour suppressor gene, MMAC1, at chromosome 10q23. 3 that is mutated in multiple advanced cancers. Nat Genet. 1997 Apr;15(4):356–362.

[19] Maehama T, Dixon JE. The tumor suppressor, PTEN/MMAC1, dephosphorylates the lipid second messenger, phosphatidylinositol 3,4,5-trisphosphate. J Biol Chem. 1998 Mar 29; 273(22):13375–13378.

[20] Myers MP, Pass I, Batty IH, Van der Kaay J, Stolarov JP, Hemmings BA, et al. The lipid phosphatase activity of PTEN is critical for its tumor supressor function. Proc Natl Acad Sci USA. 1998 Nov 10;95(23):13513–13518.

[21] Yim EK, Peng G, Dai H, Hu R, Li K, Lu Y, et al. Rak functions as a tumor suppressor by regulating PTEN protein stability and function. Cancer Cell. 2009 Apr 7;15(4):304–314. doi:10.1016/j.ccr.2009.02.012

[22] Di Cristofano A, Pandolfi PP. The multiple roles of PTEN in tumor suppression. Cell. 2000 Feb 18;100(4):387–390.

[23] Weng LP, Brown JL, Eng C. PTEN coordinates G1 arrest by down-regulating cyclin D1 via its protein phosphatase activity and up-regulating p27 via its lipid phosphatase activity in a breast cancer model. Hum Mol Genet. 2001 Mar 15;10(6):599–604.

[24] Hopkins BD, Fine B, Steinbach N, Dendy M, Rapp Z, Shaw J, et al. A secreted PTEN phosphatase that enters cells to alter signaling and survival. Science. 2013 Jul 26; 341(6144):399–402. doi:10.1126/science.1234907

[25] Gong L, Govan JM, Evans EB, Dai H, Wang E, Lee SW, et al. Nuclear PTEN tumor-suppressor functions through maintaining heterochromatin structure. Cell Cycle. 2015;14(14):2323–2332. doi:10.1080/15384101.2015.1044174

[26] Freeman SS, Allen SW, Ganti R, Wu J, Ma J, Su X, et al. Copy number gains in EGFR and copy number losses in PTEN are common events in osteosarcoma tumors. Cancer. 2008 Sept 15;113(6):1453–1461. doi:10.1002/cncr.23782

[27] Choy E, Hornicek F, MacConaill L, Harmon D, Tariq Z, Garraway L, et al. High-throughput genotyping in osteosarcoma identifies multiple mutations in phosphoinositide-3-kinase and other oncogenes. Cancer. 2012 Jun 1;118(11):2905–2914. doi:10.1002/cncr.26617

[28] Ji H, Ding Z, Hawke D, Xing D, Jiang BH, Mills GB, et al. AKT-dependent phosphorylation of Niban regulates nucleophosmin-and MDM2-mediated p53 stability and cell apoptosis. EMBO Rep. 2012 Jun1;13(6):554–560. doi:10.1038/embor.2012.53

[29] Song R, Tian K, Wang W, Wang L. P53 suppresses cell proliferation, metastasis, and angiogenesis of osteosarcoma through inhibition of the PI3K/AKT/mTOR pathway. Int J Surg. 2015 Aug;20:80–87. doi:10.1016/j.ijsu.2015.04.050

[30] Salmena L, Carracedo A, Pandolfi PP. Tenets of PTEN tumor suppression. Cell. 2008 May 2; 133(3):403–414. doi:10.1016/j.cell.2008.04.013

[31] Levine RA, Forest T, Smith C. Tumor suppressor PTEN is mutated in canine osteosarcoma cell lines and tumors. Vet Pathol. 2002 May;39(3):372–378.

[32] Yamaguchi T, Toguchida J, Yamamuro T, Kotoura Y, Takada N, Kawaguchi N, et al. Allelotype analysis in osteosarcomas: frequent allele loss on 3q, 13q, 17p, and 18q. Cancer Res. 1992 May 1;52(9):2419–2423.

[33] Sun H, Lesche R, Li DM, Liliental J, Zhang H, Gao J, et al. PTEN modulates cell cycle progression and cell survival by regulating phosphatidylinositol 3,4,5,-trisphosphate and Akt/protein kinase B signaling pathway. Proc Natl Acad Sci USA. 1999 May 25;96(11):6199–6204.

[34] Wang SI, Puc J, Li J, Bruce JN, Cairns P, Sidransky D, et al. Somatic mutations of PTEN in glioblastoma multiforme. Cancer Res. 1997 Oct 1;57(19):4183–4186.

[35] Liaw D, Marsh DJ, Li J, Dahia PL, Wang SI, Zheng Z, et al. Germline mutations of the PTEN gene in Cowden disease, an inherited breast and thyroid cancer syndrome. Nat Genet. 1997 May;16(1):64–67.

[36] Cristofano AD, Pesce B, Cordon-Cardo C, Pandolfi PP. Pten is essential for embryonic development and tumour suppression. Nat Genet. 1998 Aug;19(4):348–355.

[37] Lahtz C, Stranzenbach R, Fiedler E, Helmbold P, Dammann RH. Methylation of PTEN as a prognostic factor in malignant melanoma of the skin. J Invest Dermatol. 2010 Feb;130(2):620–622. doi:10.1038/jid.2009.226

[38] Kang YH, Lee HS, Kim WH. Promoter methylation and silencing of PTEN in gastric carcinoma. Lab Invest. 2002 Mar;82(3):285–291.

[39] García JM, Silva J, Peña C, Garcia V, Rodríguez R, Cruz MA, et al. Promoter methylation of the PTEN gene is a common molecular change in breast cancer. Genes Chromosomes Cancer. 2004 Oct;41(2):117–124.

[40] Salvesen HB, MacDonald N, Ryan A, Jacobs IJ, Lynch ED, Akslen LA, et al. PTEN methylation is associated with advanced stage and microsatellite instability in endometrial carcinoma. Int J Cancer. 2001 Jan;91(1):22–26.

[41] Kawaguchi KI, Oda Y, Saito T, Yamamoto H, Takahira T, Kobayashi C, et al. DNA hypermethylation status of multiple genes in soft tissue sarcomas. Mod Pathol. 2006 Jan; 19(1):106–114.

[42] Gao Y, Luo LH, Li S, Yang C. miR-17 inhibitor suppressed osteosarcoma tumor growth and metastasis via increasing PTEN expression. Biochem Biophys Res Commun. 2014 Feb 7;444(2):230–234. doi:10.1016/j.bbrc.2014.01.061

[43] Shen L, Chen XD, Zhang YH. MicroRNA-128 promotes proliferation in osteosarcoma cells by downregulating PTEN. Tumour Biol. 2014 Mar;35(3):2069–2074. doi:10.1007/s13277-013-1274-1

[44] Namløs HM, Meza-Zepeda LA, Barøy T, Østensen IH, Kresse SH, Kuijjer ML, et al. Modulation of the osteosarcoma expression phenotype by microRNAs. PLoS One. 2012;7(10):e48086. doi:10.1371/journal.pone.0048086

[45] Moriarity BS, Otto GM, Rahrmann EP, Rathe SK, Wolf NK, Weg MT, et al. A Sleeping Beauty forward genetic screen identifies new genes and pathways driving osteosarcoma development and metastasis. Nat Genet. 2015 Jun;47(6):615–624. doi:10.1038/ng.3293

[46] Engelman JA. Targeting PI3K signalling in cancer: opportunities, challenges and limitations. Nat Rev Cancer. 2009 Aug;9(8):550–562. doi:10.1038/nrc2664

[47] Cahill CM, Rogers JT. Interleukin (IL) 1β induction of IL-6 is mediated by a novel phosphatidylinositol 3-kinase-dependent AKT/IκB kinase α pathway targeting activator protein-1. J Biol Chem. 2008 Sep 19;283(38):25900–25912. doi:10.1074/jbc.M707692200

[48] Weiss KR, Cooper GM, Jadlowiec JA, McGough RL 3rd, Huard J. VEGF and BMP expression in mouse osteosarcoma cells. Clin Orthop Relat Res. 2006 Sep;450:111–117. doi:10.1097/01.blo.0000229333.98781.56

[49] Xi Y, Chen Y. Oncogenic and therapeutic targeting of PTEN loss in bone malignancies. J Cell Biochem. 2015 Sep;116(9):1837–1847. doi:10.1002/jcb.25159

[50] Moon JB, Kim JH, Kim K, Youn BU, Ko A, Lee SY, et al. Akt induces osteoclast differentiation through regulating the GSK3β/NFATc1 signaling cascade. J Immunol. 2012 Jan 1;188(1):163–169. doi:10.4049/jimmunol.1101254

[51] Sugatani T, Alvarez U, Hruska KA. PTEN regulates RANKL-and osteopontin-stimulated signal transduction during osteoclast differentiation and cell motility. J Biol Chem. 2003 Feb 14;278(7):5001–5008.

[52] Filtz EA, Emery A, Lu H, Forster CL, Karasch C, Hallstrom TC. Rb1 and Pten co-deletion in osteoblast precursor cells causes rapid lipoma formation in mice. PLoS One. 2015 Aug 28;10(8):e0136729. doi:10.1371/journal.pone.0136729

[53] Blüml S, Friedrich M, Lohmeyer T, Sahin E, Saferding V, Brunner J, et al. Loss of phosphatase and tensin homolog (PTEN) in myeloid cells controls inflammatory bone destruction by regulating the osteoclastogenic potential of myeloid cells. Ann Rheum Dis. 2015 Jan;74(1):227–233. doi:10.1136/annrheumdis-2013-203486

[54] Guntur AR, Reinhold MI, Cuellar J, Naski MC. Conditional ablation of Pten in osteoprogenitors stimulates FGF signaling. Development. 2011 Apr;138(7):1433–1444. doi:10.1242/dev.058016

[55] Zhao J, Zhang ZR, Zhao N, Ma BA, Fan QY. VEGF silencing inhibits human osteosarcoma angiogenesis and promotes cell apoptosis via PI3K/AKT signaling pathway. Cell Biochem Biophys. 2015 Nov;73(2):519–525. doi:10.1007/s12013-015-0692-7

[56] Zhang A, He S, Sun X, Ding L, Bao X, Wang N. Wnt5a promotes migration of human osteosarcoma cells by triggering a phosphatidylinositol-3 kinase/Akt signals. Cancer Cell Int. 2014 Feb 14;14(1):15. doi:10.1186/1475-2867-14-15

[57] Maeda K, Kobayashi Y, Udagawa N, Uehara S, Ishihara A, Mizoguchi T, et al. Wnt5a-Ror2 signaling between osteoblast-lineage cells and osteoclast precursors enhances osteoclastogenesis. Nat Med. 2012 Feb 19;18(3):405–412. doi:10.1038/nm.2653

[58] Dissanayake SK, Wade M, Johnson CE, O'Connell MP, Leotlela PD, French AD, et al. The Wnt5A/protein kinase C pathway mediates motility in melanoma cells via the inhibition

of metastasis suppressors and initiation of an epithelial to mesenchymal transition. J Biol Chem. 2007 Jun 8;282(23):17259–17271.

[59] Weeraratna AT, Jiang Y, Hostetter G, Rosenblatt K, Duray P, Bittner M, et al. Wnt5a signaling directly affects cell motility and invasion of metastatic melanoma. Cancer Cell. 2002 Apr;1(3):279–288.

[60] Mulholland DJ, Kobayashi N, Ruscetti M, Zhi A, Tran LM, Huang J, et al. Pten loss and RAS/MAPK activation cooperate to promote EMT and metastasis initiated from prostate cancer stem/progenitor cells. Cancer Res. 2012 Apr 1;72(7):1878–1889. doi:10.1158/0008-5472.CAN-11-3132

[61] Wang H, Quah SY, Dong JM, Manser E, Tang JP, Zeng Q. PRL-3 down-regulates PTEN expression and signals through PI3K to promote epithelial-mesenchymal transition. Cancer Res. 2007 Apr 1;67(7):2922–2926.

[62] Chen J, Yan D, Wu W, Zhu J, Ye W, Shu Q. MicroRNA-130a promotes the metastasis and epithelial-mesenchymal transition of osteosarcoma by targeting PTEN. Oncol Rep. 2016 Jun; 35(6):3285–3292. doi:10.3892/or.2016.4719

[63] Lin YM, Chang ZL, Liao YY, Chou MC, Tang CH. IL-6 promotes ICAM-1 expression and cell motility in human osteosarcoma. Cancer Lett. 2013 Jan 1;328(1):135–143. doi:10.1016/j.canlet.2012.08.029

[64] Wang J, Loberg R, Taichman RS. The pivotal role of CXCL12 (SDF-1)/CXCR4 axis in bone metastasis. Cancer Metastasis Rev. 2006 Dec;25(4):573–587.

[65] Conley-LaComb MK, Saliganan A, Kandagatla P, Chen YQ, Cher ML, Chinni SR. PTEN loss mediated Akt activation promotes prostate tumor growth and metastasis via CXCL12/CXCR4 signaling. Mol Cancer. 2013 Jul 31;12(1):85. doi:10.1186/1476-4598-12-85

[66] Tamura M, Gu J, Matsumoto K, Aota SI, Parsons R, Yamada KM. Inhibition of cell migration, spreading, and focal adhesions by tumor suppressor PTEN. Science. 1998 Jun 5; 280(5369):1614–1617.

[67] Ren K, Lu X, Yao N, Chen Y, Yang A, Chen H, et al. Focal adhesion kinase overexpression and its impact on human osteosarcoma. Oncotarget. 2015 Oct 13;6(31):31085–31103. doi:10.18632/oncotarget.5044

[68] Hu Y, Xu S, Jin W, Yi Q, Wei W. Effect of the PTEN gene on adhesion, invasion and metastasis of osteosarcoma cells. Oncol Rep. 2014 Oct;32(4):1741–1747. doi:10.3892/or.2014.3362

[69] Robl B, Pauli C, Botter SM, Bode-Lesniewska B, Fuchs B. Prognostic value of tumor suppressors in osteosarcoma before and after neoadjuvant chemotherapy. BMC Cancer. 2015 May 9;15:379. doi:10.1186/s12885-015-1397-4

[70] Zhou Y, Zhu LB, Peng AF, Wang TF, Long XH, Gao S, et al. LY294002 inhibits the malignant phenotype of osteosarcoma cells by modulating the phosphatidylinositol 3-kinase/

Akt/fatty acid synthase signaling pathway in vitro. Mol Med Rep. 2015 Feb;11(2):1352–1357. doi:10.3892/mmr.2014.2787

[71] Gobin B, Huin MB, Lamoureux F, Ory B, Charrier C, Lanel R, et al. BYL719, a new α-specific PI3K inhibitor: single administration and in combination with conventional chemotherapy for the treatment of osteosarcoma. Int J Cancer. 2015 Feb 15;136(4):784–796. doi:10.1002/ijc.29040

[72] Anderson JL, Park A, Akiyama R, Tap WD, Denny CT, Federman N. Evaluation of in vitro activity of the class I PI3K inhibitor buparlisib (BKM120) in pediatric bone and soft tissue sarcomas. PLoS One. 2015 Sep 24;10(9):e0133610. doi:10.1371/journal.pone.0133610

[73] Sarker D, Ang JE, Baird R, Kristeleit R, Shah K, Moreno V, et al. First-in-human phase I study of pictilisib (GDC-0941), a potent pan–class I phosphatidylinositol-3-kinase (PI3K) inhibitor, in patients with advanced solid tumors. Clin Cancer Res. 2015 Jan 1;21(1):77–86. doi:10.1158/1078-0432.CCR-14-0947

[74] Liang W, Gao B, Xu G, Weng D, Xie M, Qian Y. Possible contribution of aminopeptidase N (APN/CD13) to migration and invasion of human osteosarcoma cell lines. Int J Oncol. 2014 Dec;45(6):2475–2485. doi:10.3892/ijo.2014.2664

[75] Yao C, Wei JJ, Wang ZY, Li D, Yan SC, Yang YJ, et al. Perifosine induces cell apoptosis in human osteosarcoma cells: new implication for osteosarcoma therapy? Cell Biochem Biophys. 2013 Mar;65(2):217–227. doi:10.1007/s12013-012-9423-5

[76] Jiang H, Zeng Z. Dual mTORC1/2 inhibition by INK-128 results in antitumor activity in preclinical models of osteosarcoma. Biochem Biophys Res Commun. 2015 Dec 4–11;468(1):255–261. doi:10.1016/j.bbrc.2015.10.119

[77] Bagatell R, Norris R, Ingle AM, Ahern C, Voss S, Fox E, et al. Phase 1 trial of temsirolimus in combination with irinotecan and temozolomide in children, adolescents and young adults with relapsed or refractory solid tumors: a Children's Oncology Group Study. Pediatr Blood Cancer. 2014 May;61(5):833–839. doi:10.1002/pbc.24874

[78] Chawla SP, Staddon AP, Baker LH, Schuetze SM, Tolcher AW, D'Amato GZ, et al. Phase II study of the mammalian target of rapamycin inhibitor ridaforolimus in patients with advanced bone and soft tissue sarcomas. J Clin Oncol. 2012 Jan 1;30(1):78–84. doi:10.1200/JCO.2011.35.6329

[79] Grignani G, Palmerini E, Ferraresi V, D'Ambrosio L, Bertulli R, Asaftei SD, et al. Sorafenib and everolimus for patients with unresectable high-grade osteosarcoma progressing after standard treatment: a non-randomised phase 2 clinical trial. Lancet Oncol. 2015 Jan;16(1):98–107. doi:10.1016/S1470-2045(14)71136-2

[80] Zhu YR, Zhou XZ, Zhu LQ, Yao C, Fang JF, Zhou F, et al. The anti-cancer activity of the mTORC1/2 dual inhibitor XL388 in preclinical osteosarcoma models. Oncotarget. 2016;Jul 2. doi:10.18632/oncotarget.10389 [Epub ahead of print].

[81] Zhu YR, Min H, Fang JF, Zhou F, Deng XW, Zhang YQ. Activity of the novel dual phosphatidylinositol 3-kinase/mammalian target of rapamycin inhibitor NVP-BEZ235 against osteosarcoma. Cancer Biol Ther. 2015;16(4):602–609. doi:10.1080/15384047.2015.1017155

[82] Dolly SO, Wagner AJ, Bendell JC, Kindler HL, Krug LM, Seiwert TY, et al. Phase I study of Apitolisib (GDC-0980), dual phosphatidylinositol-3-kinase and mammalian target of rapamycin kinase inhibitor, in patients with advanced solid tumors. Clin Cancer Res. 2016 Jun 15;22(12):2874–2884. doi:10.1158/1078-0432.CCR-15-2225

[83] Lv C, Hao Y, Tu G. MicroRNA-21 promotes proliferation, invasion and suppresses apoptosis in human osteosarcoma line MG63 through PTEN/Akt pathway. Tumour Biol. 2016 Jul;37(7):9333–9342. doi:10.1007/s13277-016-4807-6

[84] Leone E, Morelli E, Di Martino MT, Amodio N, Foresta U, Gullà A, et al. Targeting miR-21 inhibits in vitro and in vivo multiple myeloma cell growth. Clin Cancer Res. 2013 Apr 15; 19(8):2096–2106. doi:10.1158/1078-0432.CCR-12-3325

[85] Zhao G, Cai C, Yang T, Qiu X, Liao B, Li W, et al. MicroRNA-221 induces cell survival and cisplatin resistance through PI3K/Akt pathway in human osteosarcoma. PLoS One. 2013;8(1):e53906. doi:10.1371/journal.pone.0053906

[86] Mirantes C, Dosil MA, Eritja N, Felip I, Gatius S, Santacana M, et al. Effects of the multikinase inhibitors Sorafenib and Regorafenib in PTEN deficient neoplasias. Eur J Cancer. 2016 Aug;63:74–87. doi:10.1016/j.ejca.2016.04.019

[87] He C, Dong X, Zhai B, Jiang X, Dong D, Li B, et al. MiR-21 mediates sorafenib resistance of hepatocellular carcinoma cells by inhibiting autophagy via the PTEN/Akt pathway. Oncotarget. 2015 Oct 6;6(30):28867–28881. doi:10.18632/oncotarget.4814

[88] Grignani G, Palmerini E, Dileo P, Asaftei SD, D'Ambrosio L, Pignochino Y, et al. A phase II trial of sorafenib in relapsed and unresectable high-grade osteosarcoma after failure of standard multimodal therapy: an Italian Sarcoma Group study. Ann Oncol. 2012 Feb;23(2):508–516. doi:10.1093/annonc/mdr151

[89] Song D, Ni J, Xie H, Ding M, Wang J. DNA demethylation in the PTEN gene promoter induced by 5-azacytidine activates PTEN expression in the MG-63 human osteosarcoma cell line. Exp Ther Med. 2014 May;7(5):1071–1076.

[90] Srinivasan U, Reaman GH, Poplack DG, Glaubiger DL, Levine AS. Phase II study of 5-azacytidine in sarcomas of bone. Am J Clin Oncol. 1982 Aug;5(4):411–416.

[91] Thayanithy V, Park C, Sarver AL, Kartha RV, Korpela DM, Graef AJ, et al. Combinatorial treatment of DNA and chromatin-modifying drugs cause cell death in human and canine osteosarcoma cell lines. PLoS One. 2012;7(9):e43720. doi:10.1371/journal.pone.0043720

[92] Loftus JP, Cavatorta D, Bushey JJ, Levine CB, Sevier CS, Wakshlag JJ. The 5-lipoxygenase inhibitor tepoxalin induces oxidative damage and altered PTEN status prior to apoptosis in canine osteosarcoma cell lines. Vet Comp Oncol. 2016 Jun;14(2):e17–30. doi:10.1111/vco.12094

[93] Meng ZJ, Wu N, Liu Y, Shu KJ, Zou X, Zhang RX, et al. Evodiamine inhibits the proliferation of human osteosarcoma cells by blocking PI3K/Akt signaling. Oncol Rep. 2015 Sep;34(3):1388–1396. doi:10.3892/or.2015.4084

[94] Sui W, Zhang Y, Wang Z, Wang Z, Jia Q, Wu L, et al. Antitumor effect of a selective COX-2 inhibitor, celecoxib, may be attributed to angiogenesis inhibition through modulating the PTEN/PI3K/Akt/HIF-1 pathway in an H22 murine hepatocarcinoma model. Oncol Rep. 2014 May;31(5):2252–2260. doi:10.3892/or.2014.3093

[95] Liu J, Wu J, Zhou L, Pan C, Zhou Y, Du W, et al. ZD6474, a new treatment strategy for human osteosarcoma, and its potential synergistic effect with celecoxib. Oncotarget. 2015 Aug 28;6(25):21341–21352.

[96] Miwa S, Sugimoto N, Shirai T, Hayashi K, Nishida H, Ohnari I, et al. Caffeine activates tumor suppressor PTEN in sarcoma cells. Int J Oncol. 2011 Aug;39(2):465–472. doi:10.3892/ijo.2011.1051

[97] Al-Ansari MM, Aboussekhra A. Caffeine mediates sustained inactivation of breast cancer-associated myofibroblasts via up-regulation of tumor suppressor genes. PLoS One. 2014 Mar 3;9(3):e90907. doi:10.1371/journal.pone.0090907

[98] Das S, Dixon JE, Cho W. Membrane-binding and activation mechanism of PTEN. PNAS. 2003 Jun;100(13):7491–7496. doi:10.1073/pnas.0932835100

Chapter 3

The Use of Molecular Pathway Inhibitors in the Treatment of Osteosarcoma

Adel Mahjoub, Jared A. Crasto, Jonathan Mandell,
Mitchell S. Fourman, Rashmi Agarwal and
Kurt R. Weiss

Additional information is available at the end of the chapter

http://dx.doi.org/10.5772/67627

Abstract

Presently, the 5-year survival rate for metastatic osteosarcoma remains low despite advances in chemotherapeutics and neoadjuvant therapy. A majority of the morbidity and nearly all of the mortality in osteosarcoma rely not in the primary disease but in the metastatic disease. The pursuit of novel molecular therapies is attractive due to their targeted ability to combat metastasis. Unlike traditional chemotherapy agents, which work by targeting rapidly dividing cells, targeted therapies may spare normal cells and decrease the adverse effects of chemotherapy by targeting specific pathways. Here, we discuss key molecular pathways in osteosarcoma and their ability to be modulated for the goal of eradication of primary and metastatic disease. We focus specifically on the aldehyde dehydrogenase (ALDH), epidermal growth factor receptor (EGFR), and insulin-like growth factor-1 receptor (IGF-1R) pathways.

Keywords: osteosarcoma, molecular inhibition, metastasis, ALDH, EGFR, IGF-1R

1. Introduction

Prior to the use of chemotherapeutics, the 5-year survival rate of osteosarcoma (OS) was approximately 20% [1]. Despite new surgical techniques and the adoption of neoadjuvant therapy, patients diagnosed with nonmetastatic OS have a 65.8% 10-year survival rate, while those diagnosed with metastatic disease have a 15–30% 5-year survival rate [2]. These statistics have not improved in a generation. This stagnation may reflect recurrent disease as well as the intrinsic resistance of OS to chemotherapy.

The pursuit of targeted molecular therapies to treat OS has increased in popularity over the past decade. The inhibition of specific molecular pathways critical to OS metabolism may decrease its metastatic potential, slow its rate of growth, and potentially eliminate the disease altogether. Unlike chemotherapeutics, which act on all rapidly dividing cells, targeted therapies may be mechanistically independent in their efficacy. By specifically targeting OS cells, we may save normal cells and decrease the risk of adverse clinical side effects [3].

Here, we examine the inhibition of specific molecular targets that are critical to the biologic pathways of OS, but may spare other critical organ systems from damage.

2. Aldehyde dehydrogenase (ALDH)

Aldehyde dehydrogenases (ALDHs) are a superfamily of nicotinamide adenine dinucleotide phosphate ($NADP^+$)-dependent tetrameric enzymes that participate in aldehyde metabolism via catalysis of exogenous and endogenous aldehydes into their corresponding carboxylic acids and the cell's resistance to oxidative stress [4–7]. Inhibition of ALDH can lead to a build-up of aldehydes that can lead to toxic side-effects, which include enzyme inactivation, DNA damage, impairment of cellular homeostasis, and cell death by forming adducts with various cellular targets [4, 8, 9].

Cancer stem cells (CSCs) comprise a small, distinct subpopulation of cancer cells that demonstrate robust self-renewal properties, enhanced differentiation capacity, the ability to propagate tumor growth, and increased resistance to chemotherapeutic drugs. ALDHs have been identified in numerous studies as elevated in highly malignant tumors and in CSCs [4, 10–12]. ALDHs exert their effects through cellular processes such as target gene expression, protein translation, signal transduction, and antioxidative mechanisms. ALDH has, therefore, been implicated as a potential CSC marker. Cells found to be high in ALDH have demonstrated enhanced tumorigenicity in multiple cancers [7].

Elevated ALDH levels have been associated with poor survival in patients with breast and ovarian cancers [13, 14]. ALDH expression also appears to be linked with metastatic potential. Semisolid matrigel matrix invasion assays showed a correlation between ALDH levels and increased invasiveness when comparing two murine OS cell lines [7]. OS cells treated with disulfiram, an ALDH-inhibitor, show reduced ALDH expression and altered cellular morphology, with fewer invadopodia and greater shape uniformity [6, 15, 16].

2.1. Pathophysiology

Reactive oxygen species (ROS) are a natural by-product of aerobic metabolism and can lead to DNA damage, protein degeneration, and lipid membrane destruction. Cancer cells often generate abnormally high levels of ROS because of the aberrant metabolism and protein translation typical of diseased cells [17]. ALDHs play a vital role in clearing ROS and reducing the oxidative stress caused by ultraviolet radiation and chemotherapeutic agents. Cells that have high levels of ALDH expression have consistently lower ROS than those incapable of such expression [18–20].

CSCs have relatively low levels of ROS, which may be because of elevated antioxidant enzyme levels [6, 21, 22]. The protective effects of ALDH for CSCs may also include the inhibition of downstream apoptosis-related pathways [18, 23, 24]. ALDH-positive CSCs have also demonstrated resistance to myriad chemotherapeutic agents such as anthracyclines and taxanes [25, 26], two classes of drugs commonly used in OS treatment. ALDH-positive cancer cells develop this drug resistance in part because of their increased ability to metabolize certain drugs into their nontoxic byproducts [27]. Once tumors are treated with chemotherapy or radiotherapy, the levels of CSCs with high ALDH expression tend to increase, increasing the cells' abilities to become drug-resistant [25, 28].

Retinoic acid (RA) signaling plays a pivotal role both in embryonic [29] and tumor cells [30]. This pathway in fact exerts an antitumor effect. This is due to activation of a series of cellular genetic programs that modulate cell differentiation, apoptosis, and growth involved in the classical RA pathway [4, 31] (**Figure 1**). In this pathway, retinol is absorbed by cells, oxidized to retinal, and then oxidized to RA by ALDH. RA then enters the nucleus and can induce the transcriptional activity of downstream effectors through activation of heterodimers of the RA

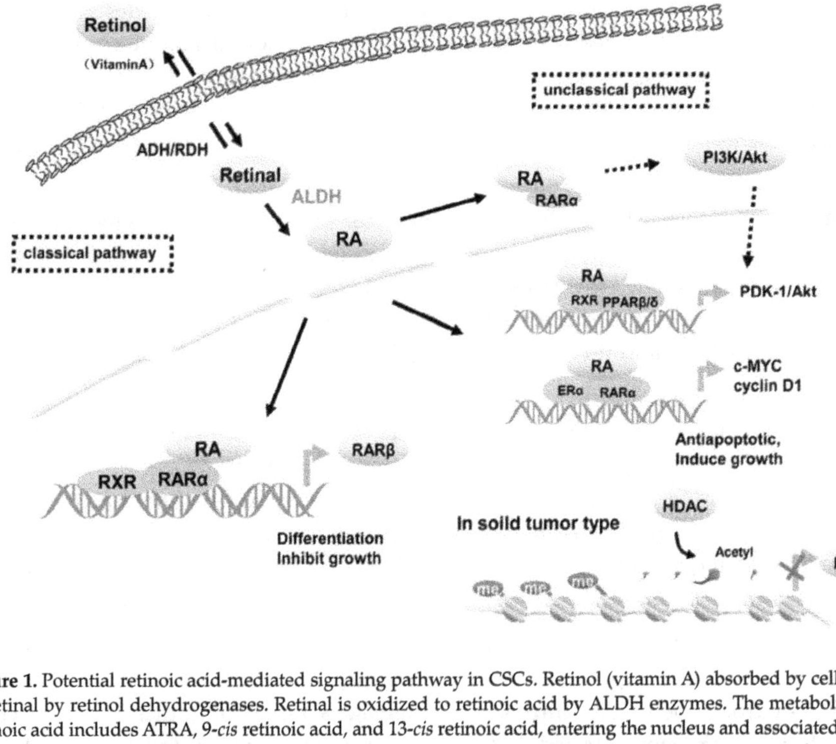

Figure 1. Potential retinoic acid-mediated signaling pathway in CSCs. Retinol (vitamin A) absorbed by cells is oxidized to retinal by retinol dehydrogenases. Retinal is oxidized to retinoic acid by ALDH enzymes. The metabolized product retinoic acid includes ATRA, 9-*cis* retinoic acid, and 13-*cis* retinoic acid, entering the nucleus and associated with RARα. In the classical pathway, retinoic acid binds to dimers of RARα and RXRs to induce the expression of its downstream target genes including RARβ. In the solid tumor type, RARβ promoter is methylated and/or the histones are significantly deacetylated, leading to low expression. In the nonclassical pathway, retinoic acid binds to dimers of RXRs and PPARβ/δ to induce the expression of its downstream target genes including PDK-1/Akt. In cells expressing ERα, retinoic acid can bind to dimers of RXRs and ERα as well as induce the expression of c-MYC and cyclin D1. Retinoic acid which extranuclearly binds with RARα can also induce the expression of c-MYC and cyclin D1 through the PI3K/Akt signaling pathway.

receptor and retinoic X receptors. RA binds its nuclear receptors and activates gene expression that affects loss of CSC markers, differentiation, cell cycle arrest, and morphology [32, 33]. The upregulation of these receptors generates a positive feedback loop for RA signaling. ALDH serves a paradoxical role in the RA pathway, by inducing differentiation of CSCs. The overall effect of this is antitumor, and thus exploiting this pathway is the goal for certain therapeutics.

2.2. Therapeutic applications

Disulfiram (DSF) has been shown to enhance the cytotoxicity of several anticancer drugs, as well as radiotherapy, which early on indicated its potential role as either a novel chemotherapeutic agent or a sensitizer for other treatments [34]. Theories of its mechanism include the induction of oxidative stress and inhibition of proteasome activity through c-Jun N-terminal kinase (JNK), NF-κB, and PI3K pathways [35–38].

In metastatic OS, the phenomenon of CSCs plays a large role in the ability of the disease to withstand a great amount of stress and remain invasive. ALDH is considered not only a surrogate marker for these cells but also a functionally important target [39]. The beauty of ALDH serving both roles is that the effects of DSF can be targeted to tumor cells exclusively due to their high ALDH content and additionally exert its antitumor effects. As described above, ALDH serves a pivotal role in reducing ROS to protect CSCs from oxidative stress and subsequent intracellular destruction. DSF as an inhibitor of this process has been shown to make the cancer cells more susceptible to oxidative stress and subsequently to improve survival in many cancer patients [40, 41].

DSF has also demonstrated efficacy in defeating the invasive nature of cancer by inhibiting matrix metalloproteinases (MMPs). In metastatic cancer physiology, the degradation of the extracellular matrix allows for primary tumor metastasis and distal site invasion. MMPs facilitate this process and are known to be closely associated with tumor growth and metastasis. In one study, nontoxic ranges of DSF successfully suppressed MMP-2 and MMP-9 activity and expression, producing a near complete growth inhibition at a 10 μM concentration of DSF [42].

Various studies have demonstrated that the cytotoxicity of DSF is copper dependent [38, 43, 44]. Copper plays an essential role in redox reactions and triggers generation of ROS in both normal and tumor cells [37, 44]. As a bivalent metal ion chelator, DSF forms a complex with copper and allows for Ctrl-transporter-independent transport of copper into tumor cells [43, 45]. For this reason, the DSF-copper complex is a much stronger inducer of ROS [46]. Furthermore, the abundance of copper in cancer cells enables DSF to specifically target cancer as opposed to normal tissues [47].

Copper ions promote ROS formation, which has been shown in multiple cancer cell lines [44]. Two forms of intracellular copper (cupric and cuprous) induce the formation of hydroxyl radicals from hydrogen peroxide, which serve to damage a variety of intracellular molecules [48]. Since studies have demonstrated that cytotoxicity of DSF appears to be copper dependent, the high concentration of copper in CSCs allows for an excellent substrate on which DSF can act in the treatment of cancer [43].

RA has been shown to inhibit proliferation of malignant tumors and induce apoptosis and differentiation [32, 49–53]. Most notably, all-*trans*-retinoic acid (ATRA) is an effective treatment for acute promyelocytic leukemia (APL) and has been shown to result in complete remission [50, 54]. RA is derived from ATRA by the action of ALDHs. Since ALDH is often specifically upregulated in CSCs, clever design can exploit this pathway for tumor suppression [49].

In mouse model studies, the highly metastatic K7M2 OS cells seem to be preferentially targeted by RA [49]. The role of retinal in decreasing cell proliferation and cell survival was demonstrated by exposing cells to oxidative stress in the form of hydrogen peroxide. ALDH-high K7M2 cells exhibited a greater increase in apoptosis compared to ALDH-low cells. Additionally, RT-PCR demonstrated that retinal treatment resulted in downregulation of various genes involved in cell proliferation and cell survival in a dose-dependent manner [49]. This would suggest that retinal can effectively be used as a cellular "Trojan Horse" of sorts to specifically target OS cells, as the very ALDH-rich nature that is crucial to their metastatic potential leads to their willful acceptance and rapid metabolism of retinal, leading ultimately to their demise.

3. Epidermal growth factor receptor (EGFR)

In order to obtain enough EGFR protein to biochemically purify and sequence, scientists initially used an epidermoid carcinoma cell line which was found to contain 100-fold higher levels of the receptor tyrosine kinase (TK). Since then, aberrant EGFR signaling has been implicated in the development and progression of many types of carcinomas including small cell lung, breast, stomach, prostate, ovarian, and glioblastoma. In the past decade, more attention has been placed on the role of EGFR signaling in OS.

3.1. Pathway physiology

Epidermal growth factor (EGF) was the first growth factor to be discovered and was found to have significant mitogenic effects of multiple cell types. Its receptor EGFR is a receptor tyrosine kinase (TK) which contains an extracellular domain where binding occurs to ligands of the EGF family such as, TGF-α, EGF, β-cellulin, epiregulin, and heparin-binding EGF. EGFR also contains a hydrophobic transmembrane region and a cytoplasmic TK domain [55]. Ligands bind to the cell surface domain and cause a conformational shift in the intracellular domain of the protein, which leads to dimerization and autophosphorylation. This phosphorylation then activates several other proteins downstream such as JNK, Akt, and mitogen-activated protein kinases (MAPK), which are responsible for normal cellular functions such as proliferation, apoptosis, adhesion, DNA synthesis, and migration. Signaling also occurs through other related TKs: HER2, HER3, and HER4. EGFR also has been shown to activate NFκB signaling, as well as being linked to certain G protein-coupled receptor signaling.

3.2. Pathophysiology

EGFR structure and function is closely related to erbB oncogene of avian erythroblastosis virus. The oncogene erbB is a part of a larger family of ErbB TKs including ErbB2 or HER2, HER3, and HER4. In addition, sequence anomalies found in the extracellular domain of EGFR were found to cause constitutive signal transduction independent of binding. Overexpressed

EGFR levels in cancer cells also cause EGFR to undergo ligand-independent firing due to spontaneous activation of TK activity [56].

Recently, more attention to the action and therapeutic intervention of aberrant EGFR signaling in OS has been studied. Immunohistochemistry demonstrated high EGFR protein expression in 57% of 37 established bone tumor-derived cell lines [57]. Additionally, 90% of 27 OS biopsy samples showed moderate-to-high EGFR protein levels, as well as in four established OS cell lines HOS, KHOS/NP, MG-63, and U-2 OS . EGFR expression was not found to correlate to response to preoperative chemotherapy or survival [58]. Another group demonstrated that OS cell lines, MG-63 and Saos-2 proliferative abilities, were decreased by natural flavonoid Icariside II. Treatment also inactivated EGFR/mTOR signaling pathway including PI3K, serine/threonine protein kinase (Akt), mitogen-activated protein kinase kinase (MEK), and Extracellular-Signal-Regulated Kinases (ERK) [59].

3.3. Therapeutic applications

3.3.1. Gefitinib (Gef)

This molecular inhibitor of EGFR acts by binding to the cytoplasmic adenosine triphosphate binding site of the TK domain [60]. Signaling dysfunction leads to an inhibition of downstream malignant phenotypes through Akt, MAPK, and Ras signal cascades. Gef is used clinically in non–small-cell lung cancer known to be harboring aberrant EGFR levels, typically used in combination with other chemotherapy regimens.

Researchers have shown under serum starvation, EGFR inhibition in OS cells by Gef was more pronounced compared to normal conditions, suggesting that aberrant EGFR signaling contributes to OS progression but is not the major driver for proliferation. The EGFR inhibitor Gef was found to moderately synergize with doxorubicin and methotrexate in attenuating the proliferative capabilities of OS cell lines U-2 OS, Saos-2, OS-9, and others. Gef EGFR inhibition antagonized the cytotoxic effects of cisplatin [61].

3.3.2. Erlotinib (Erl)

Erl is another molecular inhibitor of EGFR via the ATP binding site of the cytoplasmic domain [62]. Erl is used in treating advanced metastatic non–small-cell lung cancer and pancreatic cancer, usually in combination with other chemotherapies.

Canine OS cell lines treated with another selective EGFR inhibitor Erl did not inhibit downstream protein kinase B (PKB/Akt) activation, and vascular endothelial growth factor (VEGF) levels increased. Conversely, Erl enhanced the effects of radiation therapy on a subset of OS cell lines [63].

3.3.3. Trastuzumab (Tra)

As the name suggests, Tra is a monoclonal antibody which interferes with normal HER2 receptor functioning of EGFR [64]. It has been suggested that Tra does not alter receptor expression but instead causes inhibition of downstream Akt and MAPK proliferation signaling. A phase

II clinical trial of metastatic OS with EGFR2 overexpression showed that Tra can be safely delivered in combination with anthracycline-based chemotherapy [65].

Targeting one substrate of the receptor TK signaling cascade is likely insufficient to effectively abrogate downstream effects. Incremental improvements for the treatments of OS will depend on the novel chemotherapeutic interactions now being observed in the laboratory. BreAkthroughs will occur by further testing intricate combination therapies including sensitizers like EGFR inhibitors (Erl and Gef) with traditional chemotherapeutics such as doxorubicin, methotrexate, and cisplatin.

4. Insulin-like growth factor-1 receptor (IGFR-1R)

Insulin-like growth factor-1 receptor (IGF-1R) has been shown to play role in various cancers, including pediatric sarcomas. IGF-1R is just one cog in the complicated system of insulin-like growth factor (IGF) and insulin family of growth factors and is located in various tissues including bone. It plays an important role in regulating bone homeostasis, and activation of this unique TK receptor leads to several important downstream signaling cascades that play a crucial role in cell proliferation and protein synthesis. Aberrant signaling in the IGF-1R pathway may be implicated in the development of OS. Studying the basic physiology and pathophysiology in this pathway has been critical to the development of OS-targeted therapy. Here, we examine the basic biology of IGF-1R in relation to OS- and molecular-targeted therapies that exploit this signaling pathway.

4.1. Physiology

IGF-1R signaling is involved in normal osteogenesis and bone homeostasis [66]. IGF-1R is a type II receptor TK consisting of two α- and two β-subunits. The binding of IGF-1 to IGF-1R induces autophosphorylation of tyrosine residues in the kinase domain. This autophosphorylation leads to the downstream activation of insulin receptor substrate (IRS) proteins and Shc, an adapter protein between IGF-IR and the network of their signaling pathways [67, 68] (**Figure 2**). Phosphorylation of Shc and its binding to Grb2 is required for the activation of mitogen-activated protein kinases (MAPK)/extracellular-signal-regulated kinases (ERK), both important regulators of proliferation, invasion, angiogenesis, and inflammatory responses [69, 70].

There are four isomers of IRS, and of these isomers, IRS1 and IRS2 are expressed in osteoblasts. These adaptors are important in normal bone turnover. Furthermore, deficiencies in IRS1/2 impair osteoblast proliferation and differentiation and result in decreased bone mass [71, 72]. IRS1 is one of the many activators of phosphatidylinositol 3 kinase (PI3K). PI3K converts phosphatidylinositol 4,5-biphosphate (PIP2) into phosphatidylinositol 3,4,5-triphosphate (PIP3), which then recruits the signaling proteins PDK1 and Akt to the plasma membrane [73]. The PI3K/Akt pathway is implicated in the proliferation and invasion of malignant OS via multiple pathways, such as increasing the expression of cyclins and cyclin-dependent kinases that act as positive regulators of the cell cycle in OS [74]. The mammalian target of rapamycin (mTOR) is one of the most important downstream effectors of PI3K/Akt and controls cell cycling and protein synthesis by activation of its downstream targets p70S6K and 4E-BP [68].

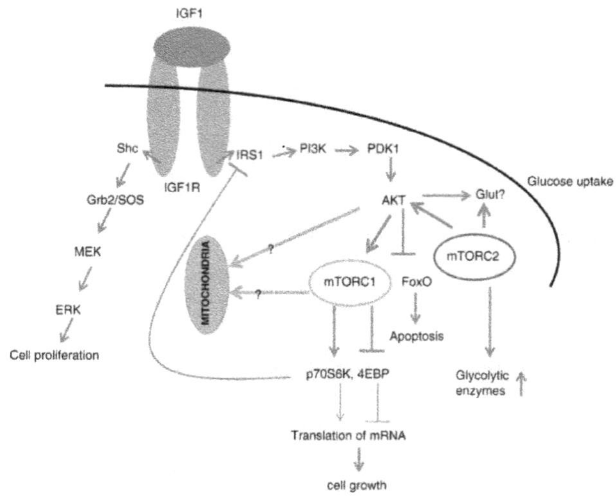

Figure 2. IGF-1 signaling pathway which can activate MAPK and PI3K signaling pathways.

Aside from regulating insulin's control of carbohydrate metabolism, the ligands IGF-1 and IGF2 may play a role in the neoplasticity of OS [75]. It has been demonstrated that there may be increased local IGF-1 levels in primary OS, which may affect survival, aggressiveness, and chemotherapeutic response [76]. Activation of IGF-1R by IGF-I stimulates OS cell growth *in vitro* and *in vivo* [77]. IGF-1 levels peak during adolescence, also the same age where OS incidences peak [78]. Interestingly, IGF-2 levels are increased in OS after chemotherapy treatment and may increase OS cell survival by inducing an autophagic state of dormancy, protecting OS against chemotherapy [79]. These ligands' influences in the tumorigenicity of OS have made them attractive targets in OS treatment. However, the only IGF-1 neutralizing antibody in clinical trials is MEDI-573 and is still in the early stages of development [80].

It is not completely clear yet whether mutations in IGF-1R contribute to cell growth, differentiation, apoptosis, and so on. Interestingly, mutations in IGF-1R are rare and produce growth retardation rather than neoplasia [81]. The recent discovery of somatic mutations in the IGF-1R kinase catalytic domain showed a small reduction in peptide phosphorylation. However, the mutant kinase domains were active, not hyper-activated relative to the wildtype [82]. Interactions between wildtype and mutant variants of the tumor suppressor gene, p53, and IGF-1R have also been studied. Normally, p53 suppresses the activity of IGF-1R, thus preventing cell proliferation. However, mutant variants of p53 derived from tumor have shown to enhance promotor activity and increase the transcription of IGF-1R, increasing the survivability of malignant cells [81, 83, 84].

4.2. Therapeutic applications

Currently, there are several IGF-1R inhibitors categorized into TK inhibitors, monoclonal antibodies, or microRNA targets of IGF-1R. Monoclonal antibodies against IGF-1R ligands have been studied but may be ineffective because of the redundancy in autocrine and paracrine secretion of this growth factor [85]. Several monoclonal antibodies against IGF-1R, such as Ganitumab or Dalotuzumab, are still being tested but tend to have a stronger inhibitory effect when combined with other therapies such as Rapamycin, an mTOR inhibitor [80]. Here, we focus on one small molecular IGF-1R inhibitor, OSI-906, and assess its current status in OS therapy.

The ATP-binding or substrate-binding site in the IGF-1R kinase domain can be targeted by small-molecule inhibitors, thus inhibiting IGF-1R signaling. An example of these inhibitors is OSI-906 (Linsitinib), a highly selective, small-molecule dual IGF-1R/IR kinase inhibitor given in an oral formulation that is in clinical trial. It has been shown that OSI-906 inhibits the downstream effectors of IGF-1R, ERK1/2 and Akt, thus affecting cell survival and proliferation [86]. One of the issues with molecular targeting of IGF-1R is the high degree of homology between the binding sites in IGF-1R and the insulin receptor. Molecular targets that cross-react with the insulin receptor may produce unwanted side effects such as dysregulating glucose metabolism [87]. Fortunately, OSI-906 exhibits a nine-fold selectivity for human IGF-1R over human insulin receptor [88]. The inhibitory effect of OSI-906 was tested on four unique OS cell lines and was found to inhibit phosphorylation of IRS-1 and proliferation in three of the four OS cell lines tested [89]. OSI-906 in combination with the EGFR inhibitor, Erl, has also been tested on human colorectal cancer cell lines and found to exhibit a synergistic inhibition of cell proliferation and survival [88]. Though OSI-906 has been somewhat successful as a single-agent for inhibiting IGF-1R in OS, further studies examining combination therapies with OSI-906 are necessary.

5. Conclusion

There is definitely hope and evidence to apply targeted molecular therapies to treat OS. As our understanding of the different molecular pathways that affect OS improves, we will be better equipped to attack this disease in ways that were not available before. Though numerous molecular pathways have been described here, it is important to understand that there are many more pathways that exist or are under investigation. Clearly, there is still much to learn about the biology of OS and its targeted therapies. The weight of evidence described above suggests that we are steadily moving forward in the right direction.

Author details

Adel Mahjoub[1], Jared A. Crasto[2], Jonathan Mandell[2], Mitchell S. Fourman[2], Rashmi Agarwal[2] and Kurt R. Weiss[2*]

*Address all correspondence to: weiskr@upmc.edu

1 School of Medicine, University of Pittsburgh, Pittsburgh, PA, USA

2 Department of Orthopaedic Surgery, University of Pittsburgh, Pittsburgh, PA, USA

References

[1] Guise TA, O'Keefe R, Randall RL, Terek RM: Molecular biology and therapeutics in musculoskeletal oncology. *J Bone Joint Surg Am* 2009, **91**(3):724–732.

[2] Duchman KR, Gao Y, Miller BJ: Prognostic factors for survival in patients with high-grade osteosarcoma using the Surveillance, Epidemiology, and End Results (SEER) Program database. *Cancer Epidemiol* 2015, **39**(4):593–599.

[3] Oeffinger KC, Mertens AC, Sklar CA, Kawashima T, Hudson MM, Meadows AT, Friedman DL, Marina N, Hobbie W, Kadan-Lottick NS *et al*: Chronic health conditions in adult survivors of childhood cancer. *N Engl J Med* 2006, **355**(15):1572–1582.

[4] Xu X, Chai S, Wang P, Zhang C, Yang Y, Yang Y, Wang K: Aldehyde dehydrogenases and cancer stem cells. *Cancer Lett* 2015, **369**(1):50–57.

[5] Marchitti SA, Brocker C, Stagos D, Vasiliou V: Non-P450 aldehyde oxidizing enzymes: the aldehyde dehydrogenase superfamily. *Expert Opin Drug Metab Toxicol* 2008, **4**(6): 697–720.

[6] Shi X, Zhang Y, Zheng J, Pan J: Reactive oxygen species in cancer stem cells. *Antioxid Redox Signal* 2012, **16**(11):1215–1228.

[7] Greco N, Schott T, Mu X, Rothenberg A, Voigt C, McGough Iii RL, Goodman M, Huard J, Weiss KR: ALDH activity correlates with metastatic potential in primary sarcomas of bone. *J Cancer Ther* 2014, **5**(4):331–338.

[8] Theruvathu JA, Nath RG, Brooks PJ: Polyamines facilitate the formation of the mutagenic DNA adduct 1, N-2-PropanodG from acetaldehyde and DNA: implications for the mechanism of alcohol-related carcinogenesis. In*: 2004*: Wiley-Liss Div John Wiley & Sons Inc, Hoboken, NJ: 231.

[9] Brooks PJ, Theruvathu JA: DNA adducts from acetaldehyde: implications for alcohol-related carcinogenesis. *Alcohol* 2005, **35**:187–193.

[10] Croker AK, Goodale D, Chu J, Postenka C, Hedley BD: High aldehyde dehydrogenase and expression of cancer stem cell markers selects for breast cancer cells with enhanced malignant and metastatic ability. *J Cell Mol Med* 2009, **13**(8B):2236–2252.

[11] Su Y, Qiu Q, Zhang X, Jiang Z, Leng Q, Liu Z, Stass SA, Jiang F: Aldehyde Dehydrogenase 1 A1–Positive Cell Population Is Enriched in Tumor-Initiating Cells and Associated with Progression of Bladder Cancer. *Cancer Epidemiol Biomarkers Prev* 2010, **19**(2):327–338.

[12] Douville J, Beaulieu R, Balicki D: ALDH1 as a functional marker of cancer stem and progenitor cells. *Stem Cells Dev* 2009, **18**(1):17–25.

[13] Bortolomai I, Canevari S, Facetti I, Cecco LD, Zacchetti A, Alison MR, Miotti S, Bortolomai I, Canevari S, Facetti I *et al*: Tumor initiating cells: development and critical

characterization of a model derived from the A431 carcinoma cell line forming spheres in suspension. *Cell Cycle* 2010, **9**(6):1194–1206.

[14] Ginestier C, Hur MH, Charafe-jauffret E, Monville F, Dutcher J, Brown M, Jacquemier J, Viens P, Kleer CG, Liu S *et al*: ALDH1 is a marker of normal and malignant human mammary stem cells and a predictor of poor clinical outcome. *Cell Stem Cell* 2007, **1**:555–567.

[15] Mu X, Isaac C, Greco N, Huard J, Weiss K: Notch signaling is associated with ALDH activity and an aggressive metastatic phenotype in murine osteosarcoma cells. *Front Oncol* 2013, **3**(June):1–10.

[16] Mu X, Isaac C, Schott T, Huard J, Weiss K: Rapamycin inhibits ALDH activity, resistance to oxidative stress, and metastatic potential in murine osteosarcoma cells. *Sarcoma* 2013, **2013**:1–11.

[17] Gorrini C, Harris IS, Mak TW: Modulation of oxidative stress as an anticancer strategy. *Nat Rev* 2013, **12**(12):931–947.

[18] Singh S, Brocker C, Koppaka V, Ying C, Jackson B, Thompson DC, Vasiliou V: Aldehyde dehydrogenases in cellular responses to oxidative/electrophilic stress. *Free Radic Biol Med* 2013, **56**:89–101.

[19] Ikeda J-i, Mamat S, Tian T, Wang Y, Luo W, Rahadiani N, Aozasa K, Morii E: Reactive oxygen species and aldehyde dehydrogenase activity in Hodgkin lymphoma cells. *Lab Invest* 2012, **92**(4):606–614.

[20] Mizuno T, Suzuki N, Makino H, Furui T, Morii E, Aoki H, Kunisada T, Yano M, Kuji S, Hirashima Y *et al*: Cancer stem-like cells of ovarian clear cell carcinoma are enriched in the ALDH-high population associated with an accelerated scavenging system in reactive oxygen species. *Gynecol Oncol* 2015, **137**(2):299–305.

[21] Ye X-q, Li Q, Wang G-h, Sun F-f, Huang G-j, Bian X-w, Yu S-c, Qian G-S: Mitochondrial and energy metabolism-related properties as novel indicators of lung cancer stem cells. *Int J Cancer* 2011, **129**:820–831.

[22] Diehn M, Cho RW, Lobo NA, Kalisky T, Dorie MJ, Kulp AN, Qian D, Lam JS, Ailles LE, Wong M *et al*: Association of reactive oxygen species levels and radioresistance in cancer stem cells. *Nature* 2009, **458**:6–11.

[23] Allensworth JL, Evans MK, Aldrich J, Festa RA, Finetti P, Ueno NT, Safi R, McDonnell DP, Thiele DJ, Laere SV *et al*: Disulfiram (DSF) acts as a copper ionophore to induce copper-dependent oxidative stress and mediate anti-tumor efficacy in inflammatory breast cancer. *Mol Oncol* 2015, **9**:1155–1168.

[24] Chiba T, Suzuki E, Yuki K, Zen Y, Oshima M, Miyagi S, Tawada A, Nakatsura T, Hayashi T, Yamashita T *et al*: Disulfiram eradicates tumor-initiating hepatocellular carcinoma cells in ROS-p38 MAPK pathway-dependent and -independent manners. *PLoS ONE* 2014, **9**(1):1–11.

[25] Croker AK, Allan AL: Inhibition of aldehyde dehydrogenase (ALDH) activity reduces chemotherapy and radiation resistance of stem-like ALDH hi CD44 + human breast cancer cells. *Breast Cancer Res Treat* 2012, **133**:75–87.

[26] Brennan SK, Meade B, Wang Q, Merchant AA, Kowalski J, Matsui W: Mantle cell lymphoma activation enhances bortezomib sensitivity. *Blood* 2010, **116**(20):4185–4191.

[27] Magni M, Shammah S, Schiro R, Mellado W, Dalla-Favera R, Gianni AM: Induction of cyclophosphamide-resistance by aldehyde-dehydrogenase gene transfer. *Blood* 1996, **8**(3):1097–1103.

[28] Dylla SJ, Beviglia L, Park I-k, Chartier C, Raval J, Ngan L, Aguilar J, Lazetic S, Smith-berdan S, Clarke MF *et al*: Colorectal cancer stem cells are enriched in xenogeneic tumors following chemotherapy. *PLoS ONE* 2008, **3**(6):e2428–e2428.

[29] Chanda B, Ditadi A, Iscove NN, Keller G: Retinoic acid signaling is essential for embryonic hematopoietic stem cell development. *Cell* 2013, **155**(1):215–227.

[30] Qiu JJ, Zeisig BB, Li S, Liu W, Chu H, Song Y, Giordano A, Schwaller J, Gronemeyer H, Dong S *et al*: Critical role of retinoid/rexinoid signaling in mediating transformation and therapeutic response of NUP98-RARG leukemia. *Leukemia* 2015, **29**:1153–1162.

[31] Dragnev KH, Petty WJ, Dmitrovsky E: Retinoid targets in cancer therapy and chemoprevention. *Cancer Biol Ther* 2003, **2**(4):S150–S156.

[32] Ginestier C, Wicinski J, Cervera N, Monville F, Finetti P, Bertucci F, Wicha MS, Birnbaum D, Ginestier C, Wicinski J *et al*: Retinoid signaling regulates breast cancer stem cell differentiation. *Cell Cycle* 2009, **8**(20):3297–3302.

[33] Ying M, Wang S, Sang Y, Sun P, Lal B, Goodwin CR, Laterra J, Xia S: Regulation of glioblastoma stem cells by retinoic acid: role for Notch pathway inhibition. *Oncogene* 2011, **30**:3454–3467.

[34] Rae C, Tesson M, Babich JW, Boyd M, Sorensen A, Mairs RJ: The role of copper in disulfiram-induced toxicity and radiosensitization of cancer cells. *J Nucl Med* 2013, **54**(6):953–960.

[35] Zhang H, Chen D, Ringler J, Chen W, Cui QC, Ethier SP, Dou QP, Wu G: Disulfiram treatment facilitates phosphoinositide 3-kinase inhibition in human breast cancer cells in vitro and in vivo. *Cancer Res* 2010, **70**(10):3996–4004.

[36] Paranjpe A, Srivenugopal KS: Degradation of NF-κB, p53 and other regulatory redox-sensitive proteins by thiol-conjugating and-nitrosylating drugs in human tumor cells. *Carcinogenesis* 2013:bgt032–bgt032.

[37] Yip NC, Fombon IS, Liu P, Brown S, Kannappan V, Armesilla AL, Xu B, Cassidy J, Darling JL, Wang W: Disulfiram modulated ROS–MAPK and NFκB pathways and targeted breast cancer cells with cancer stem cell-like properties. *Br J Cancer* 2011, **104**(10):1564–1574.

[38] Xu B, Shi P, Fombon IS, Zhang Y, Huang F, Wang W, Zhou S: Disulfiram/copper complex activated JNK/c-jun pathway and sensitized cytotoxicity of doxorubicin in doxorubicin resistant leukemia HL60 cells. *Blood Cells Mol Dis* 2011, **47**(4):264–269.

[39] Tirino V, Desiderio V, Paino F, De Rosa A, Papaccio F, La Noce M, Laino L, De Francesco F, Papaccio G: Cancer stem cells in solid tumors: an overview and new approaches for their isolation and characterization. *FASEB J* 2013, **27**(1):13–24.

[40] Triscott J, Lee C, Hu K, Fotovati A, Berns R, Pambid M, Luk M, Kast RE, Kong E, Toyota E: Disulfiram, a drug widely used to control alcoholism, suppresses the self-renewal of glioblastoma and over-rides resistance to temozolomide. *Oncotarget* 2012, **3**(10):1112–1123.

[41] Liu P, Kumar IS, Brown S, Kannappan V, Tawari PE, Tang JZ, Jiang W, Armesilla AL, Darling JL, Wang W: Disulfiram targets cancer stem-like cells and reverses resistance and cross-resistance in acquired paclitaxel-resistant triple-negative breast cancer cells. *Br J Cancer* 2013, **109**:1876–1885.

[42] Cho H-j, Lee T-s, Park J-b, Park K-k, Choe J-y, Sin D-i, Park Y-y, Moon Y-s, Lee K-g, Yeo J-h *et al*: Disulfiram suppresses invasive ability of osteosarcoma cells via the inhibition of MMP-2 and MMP-9 expression. *J Biochem Mol Biol* 2007, **40**(6):1069–1076.

[43] Liu P, Brown S, Goktug T, Channathodiyil P, Kannappan V, Hugnot JP, Guichet PO, Bian X, Armesilla AL, Darling JL: Cytotoxic effect of disulfiram/copper on human glioblastoma cell lines and ALDH-positive cancer-stem-like cells. *Br J Cancer* 2012, **107**(9):1488–1497.

[44] Tardito S, Bassanetti I, Bignardi C, Elviri L, Tegoni M, Mucchino C, Bussolati O, Franchi-Gazzola R, Marchiò L: Copper binding agents acting as copper ionophores lead to caspase inhibition and paraptotic cell death in human cancer cells. *J Am Chem Soc* 2011, **133**(16):6235–6242.

[45] Duan L, Shen H, Zhao G, Yang R, Cai X, Zhang L, Jin C, Huang Y: Inhibitory effect of disulfiram/copper complex on non-small cell lung cancer cells. *Biochem Biophys Res Commun* 2014, **446**(4):1010–1016.

[46] Nagai M, Vo NH, Ogawa LS, Chimmanamada D, Inoue T, Chu J, Beaudette-Zlatanova BC, Lu R, Blackman RK, Barsoum J: The oncology drug elesclomol selectively transports copper to the mitochondria to induce oxidative stress in cancer cells. *Free Radic Biol Med* 2012, **52**(10):2142–2150.

[47] Wang F, Jiao P, Qi M, Frezza M, Dou QP, Yan B: Turning tumor-promoting copper into an anti-cancer weapon via high-throughput chemistry. *Curr Med Chem* 2010, **17**(25):2685–2698.

[48] Eguchi H, Ikeda Y, Koyota S, Honke K, Suzuki K, Gutteridge JMC, Taniguchi N: Oxidative damage due to copper ion and hydrogen peroxide induces GlcNAc-specific cleavage of an Asn-linked oligosaccharide. *J Biochem* 2002, **131**(3):477–484.

[49] Mu X, Patel S, Mektepbayeva D, Mahjoub A, Huard J, Weiss K: Retinal targets ALDH positive cancer stem cell and alters the phenotype of highly metastatic osteosarcoma **cells**. *Sarcoma* 2015, **2015**:14–16.

[50] Tang X-h, Gudas LJ: Retinoids, retinoic acid receptors, and cancer. *Annu Rev Pathol Mech Dis* 2011, **6**:345–364.

[51] Schenk T, Stengel S, Zelent A: Unlocking the potential of retinoic acid in anticancer therapy. *Br J Cancer* 2014, **111**:2039–2045.

[52] Chen M-c, Huang C-y, Hsu S-l, Lin E, Ku C-t, Lin H, Chen C-m: Retinoic acid induces apoptosis of prostate cancer DU145 cells through Cdk5 overactivation. *Evid Based Complement Alternat Med* 2012:1–11.

[53] Huss WJ, Lai L, Barrios RJ, Hirschi KK, Greenberg NM: Retinoic acid slows progression and promotes apoptosis of spontaneous prostate cancer. *The Prostate* 2004, **9999**:1–11.

[54] Huang M-e, Ye Y-c, Chen S-r, Chai J-r, Lu J-X, Zhao L, Gu L-j, Wang Z-y: Use of all-trans retinoic acid in the treatment of acute promyelocytic leukemia. *Blood* 1988, **72**(2):567–572.

[55] Yufen X, Binbin S, Wenyu C, Jialiang L, Xinmei Y: The role of EGFR-TKI for leptomeningeal metastases from non-small cell lung cancer. *Springerplus* 2016, **5**(1):1244.

[56] Normanno N, De Luca A, Bianco C, Strizzi L, Mancino M, Maiello MR, Carotenuto A, De Feo G, Caponigro F, Salomon DS: Epidermal growth factor receptor (EGFR) signaling in cancer. *Gene* 2006, **366**(1):2–16.

[57] Wen YH, Koeppen H, Garcia R, Chiriboga L, Tarlow BD, Peters BA, Eigenbrot C, Yee H, Steiner G, Greco MA: Epidermal growth factor receptor in osteosarcoma: expression and mutational analysis. *Hum Pathol* 2007, **38**(8):1184–1191.

[58] Lee JA, Ko Y, Kim DH, Lim JS, Kong CB, Cho WH, Jeon DG, Lee SY, Koh JS: Epidermal growth factor receptor: is it a feasible target for the treatment of osteosarcoma? *Cancer Res Treat* 2012, **44**(3):202–209.

[59] Geng YD, Yang L, Zhang C, Kong LY: Blockade of epidermal growth factor receptor/mammalian target of rapamycin pathway by Icariside II results in reduced cell proliferation of osteosarcoma cells. *Food Chem Toxicol* 2014, **73**:7–16.

[60] Lynch TJ, Bell DW, Sordella R, Gurubhagavatula S, Okimoto RA, Brannigan BW, Harris PL, Haserlat SM, Supko JG, Haluska FG *et al*: Activating mutations in the epidermal growth factor receptor underlying responsiveness of non-small-cell lung cancer to gefitinib. *N Engl J Med* 2004, **350**(21):2129–2139.

[61] Mok TS, Wu YL, Thongprasert S, Yang CH, Chu DT, Saijo N, Sunpaweravong P, Han B, Margono B, Ichinose Y *et al*: Gefitinib or carboplatin-paclitaxel in pulmonary adenocarcinoma. *N Engl J Med* 2009, **361**(10):947–957.

[62] Raymond E, Faivre S, Armand JP: Epidermal growth factor receptor tyrosine kinase as a target for anticancer therapy. *Drugs* 2000, **60 Suppl 1**:15–23; discussion 41–12.

[63] Mantovani FB, Morrison JA, Mutsaers AJ: Effects of epidermal growth factor receptor kinase inhibition on radiation response in canine osteosarcoma cells. *BMC Vet Res* 2016, **12**:82.

[64] Hudis CA: Trastuzumab—mechanism of action and use in clinical practice. *N Engl J Med* 2007, **357**(1):39–51.

[65] Ebb D, Meyers P, Grier H, Bernstein M, Gorlick R, Lipshultz SE, Krailo M, Devidas M, Barkauskas DA, Siegal GP *et al*: Phase II trial of trastuzumab in combination with cytotoxic chemotherapy for treatment of metastatic osteosarcoma with human epidermal growth factor receptor 2 overexpression: a report from the children's oncology group. *J Clin Oncol* 2012, **30**(20):2545–2551.

[66] McCarthy TL, Centrella M: Local IGF-I expression and bone formation. *Growth Horm IGF Res* 2001, **11**(4):213–219.

[67] Hernandez-Sanchez C, Blakesley V, Kalebic T, Helman L, LeRoith D: The role of the tyrosine kinase domain of the insulin-like growth factor-I receptor in intracellular signaling, cellular proliferation, and tumorigenesis. *J Biol Chem* 1995, **270**(49):29176–29181.

[68] Guntur AR, Rosen CJ: IGF-1 regulation of key signaling pathways in bone. *Bonekey Rep* 2013, **2**:437.

[69] Chandhanayingyong C, Kim Y, Staples JR, Hahn C, Lee FY: MAPK/ERK signaling in osteosarcomas, ewing sarcomas and chondrosarcomas: therapeutic implications and future directions. *Sarcoma* 2012, **2012**:404810.

[70] Ling Y, Maile LA, Lieskovska J, Badley-Clarke J, Clemmons DR: Role of SHPS-1 in the regulation of insulin-like growth factor I-stimulated Shc and mitogen-activated protein kinase activation in vascular smooth muscle cells. *Mol Biol Cell* 2005, **16**(7):3353–3364.

[71] Akune T, Ogata N, Hoshi K, Kubota N, Terauchi Y, Tobe K, Takagi H, Azuma Y, Kadowaki T, Nakamura K *et al*: Insulin receptor substrate-2 maintains predominance of anabolic function over catabolic function of osteoblasts. *J Cell Biol* 2002, **159**(1):147–156.

[72] Ogata N, Chikazu D, Kubota N, Terauchi Y, Tobe K, Azuma Y, Ohta T, Kadowaki T, Nakamura K, Kawaguchi H: Insulin receptor substrate-1 in osteoblast is indispensable for maintaining bone turnover. *J Clin Invest* 2000, **105**(7):935–943.

[73] Rubashkin MG, Cassereau L, Bainer R, DuFort CC, Yui Y, Ou G, Paszek MJ, Davidson MW, Chen YY, Weaver VM: Force engages vinculin and promotes tumor progression by enhancing PI3K activation of phosphatidylinositol (3,4,5)-triphosphate. *Cancer Res* 2014, **74**(17):4597–4611.

[74] Zhang J, Yu XH, Yan YG, Wang C, Wang WJ: PI3K/Akt signaling in osteosarcoma. *Clin Chim Acta* 2015, **444**:182–192.

[75] Burrow S, Andrulis IL, Pollak M, Bell RS: Expression of insulin-like growth factor receptor, IGF-1, and IGF-2 in primary and metastatic osteosarcoma. *J Surg Oncol* 1998, **69**(1):21–27.

[76] Jentzsch T, Robl B, Husmann M, Bode-Lesniewska B, Fuchs B: Worse prognosis of osteosarcoma patients expressing IGF-1 on a tissue microarray. *Anticancer Res* 2014, **34**(8):3881–3889.

[77] Rikhof B, de Jong S, Suurmeijer AJ, Meijer C, van der Graaf WT: The insulin-like growth factor system and sarcomas. *J Pathol* 2009, **217**(4):469–482.

[78] Duan Z, Choy E, Harmon D, Yang C, Ryu K, Schwab J, Mankin H, Hornicek FJ: Insulin-like growth factor-I receptor tyrosine kinase inhibitor cyclolignan picropodophyllin inhibits proliferation and induces apoptosis in multidrug resistant osteosarcoma cell lines. *Mol Cancer Ther* 2009, **8**(8):2122–2130.

[79] Shimizu T, Sugihara E, Yamaguchi-Iwai S, Tamaki S, Koyama Y, Kamel W, Ueki A, Ishikawa T, Chiyoda T, Osuka S *et al*: IGF2 preserves osteosarcoma cell survival by creating an autophagic state of dormancy that protects cells against chemotherapeutic stress. *Cancer Res* 2014, **74**(22):6531–6541.

[80] Chen HX, Sharon E: IGF-1R as an anti-cancer target—trials and tribulations. *Chin J Cancer* 2013, **32**(5):242–252.

[81] Werner H: Tumor suppressors govern insulin-like growth factor signaling pathways: implications in metabolism and cancer. *Oncogene* 2012, **31**(22):2703–2714.

[82] Craddock BP, Miller WT: Effects of somatic mutations in the C-terminus of insulin-like growth factor 1 receptor on activity and signaling. *J Signal Transduct* 2012, **2012**:804801.

[83] Werner H, Karnieli E, Rauscher FJ, LeRoith D: Wild-type and mutant p53 differentially regulate transcription of the insulin-like growth factor I receptor gene. *Proc Natl Acad Sci U S A* 1996, **93**(16):8318–8323.

[84] Idelman G, Glaser T, Roberts CT, Jr., Werner H: WT1-p53 interactions in insulin-like growth factor-I receptor gene regulation. *J Biol Chem* 2003, **278**(5):3474–3482.

[85] Benini S, Baldini N, Manara MC, Chano T, Serra M, Rizzi S, Lollini PL, Picci P, Scotlandi K: Redundancy of autocrine loops in human osteosarcoma cells. *Int J Cancer* 1999, **80**(4):581–588.

[86] Mulvihill MJ, Cooke A, Rosenfeld-Franklin M, Buck E, Foreman K, Landfair D, O'Connor M, Pirritt C, Sun Y, Yao Y *et al*: Discovery of OSI-906: a selective and orally efficacious dual inhibitor of the IGF-1 receptor and insulin receptor. *Future Med Chem* 2009, **1**(6):1153–1171.

[87] Sachdev D, Yee D: Disrupting insulin-like growth factor signaling as a potential cancer therapy. *Mol Cancer Ther* 2007, **6**(1):1–12.

[88] Ji QS, Mulvihil MJ, Rosenfeld-Franklin M, Buck E, Cooke A, Eyzaguirrel A, Mak G, O'Connor M, Pirritt C, Yao Y *et al*: Preclinical characterization of OSI-906: A novel IGF-1R kinase inhibitor in clinical trials. *Molecular Cancer Therapeutics* 2007, **6**(12):3590s–3590s.

[89] Kuijjer ML, Peterse EF, van den Akker BE, Briaire-de Bruijn IH, Serra M, Meza-Zepeda LA, Myklebost O, Hassan AB, Hogendoorn PC, Cleton-Jansen AM: IR/IGF1R signaling as potential target for treatment of high-grade osteosarcoma. *BMC Cancer* 2013, **13**:245.

Chapter 4

Osteosarcoma: From Molecular Biology to Mesenchymal Stem Cells

Matthew L. Broadhead, Saumiyar Sivaji,
Zsolt Balogh and Peter F.M. Choong

Additional information is available at the end of the chapter

http://dx.doi.org/10.5772/67371

Abstract

Osteosarcoma is the most common primary malignant tumour of bone. Currently, despite treatment with multi-agent chemotherapy and limb salvage surgery, the five-year survival rate for osteosarcoma remains at 70%. The pathogenesis of osteosarcoma is complex and involves alterations in cellular apoptosis, adhesion, migration, invasion and molecular signalling. Research most recently has focused on the molecular basis of the disease with the goal of identifying novel therapeutic targets. To this end, mesenchymal stem cells (MSCs) have been identified to play a role in sarcomagenesis. MSC transformation may give rise to tumours, whereas interactions of MSCs with osteosarcoma cells in the tumour microenvironment may cause increased cell proliferation. This is in stark contrast to the role of MSCs as a promising source for tissue repair and regeneration. In order to utilize MSCs for biological reconstruction in the setting of osteosarcoma, further research is necessary to delineate the role of MSCs in osteosarcoma transformation and progression.

Keywords: osteosarcoma, pathogenesis, mediators, mesenchymal stem cell, MSC

1. Introduction

Osteosarcoma is the most common primary malignancy that arises from bone. While relatively rare, with an annual incidence of 1–3 cases per million [1], it is fatal if left untreated. Osteosarcoma has a bimodal distribution affecting patients in the 2nd and 3rd decade of life and those after the 6th decade of life [2]. It is the sixth most common paediatric cancer and is the second-highest cause of cancer-related death in this age group [3, 4].

Current treatment protocols for osteosarcoma combine neoadjuvant chemotherapy, surgery and adjuvant chemotherapy. The five-year survival rate for patients diagnosed with osteosarcoma remains at 60–75% [5]. The medical and surgical treatments of osteosarcoma can cause significant morbidity for the patient. Chemotherapy agents are systemically toxic and surgery, in the form of amputation or limb salvage, require a prolonged period of rehabilitation. Despite the advent of multi-agent chemotherapeutic regimens, the prognosis for osteosarcoma has not significantly improved; hence, there is a real need to optimize current strategies and to develop novel approaches for treatment.

Our understanding of osteosarcoma has traditionally been based upon anatomical and histological principles. Primary osteosarcoma arises in the metaphysis of long bones, most commonly, within the medullary cavity. The most common sites for osteosarcoma are the distal femur, proximal tibia and proximal humerus. The occurrence of osteosarcoma in sites other than long bones increases with age. The tumour typically breaks through the cortex of the bone into surrounding soft tissues, around which a pseudocapsule forms [6].

Histologically, osteosarcoma is a malignant mesenchymal cell tumour, characterized by pleomorphic spindle-shaped cells, capable of producing an osteoid matrix. Tumour cells metastasize primarily via the haematogenous route. There are various subtypes of osteosarcoma, including the intramedullary 'classic' osteosarcoma already described, periosteal osteosarcoma, parosteal osteosarcoma, small cell osteosarcoma and telangiectatic osteosarcoma.

Current standards for staging and surgical resection of osteosarcoma rely on this anatomical knowledge [1]. However, recent advances in molecular biology have provided insight into the molecular pathogenesis of the disease. Through the identification of specific mediators of osteosarcoma progression and tumour pathways, novel approaches for targeting osteosarcoma are being developed.

This chapter will outline our current understanding of the molecular pathogenesis of osteosarcoma with some reference to the development of novel treatment agents. The environmental, genetic and molecular alterations that underlie osteosarcomagenesis will be discussed with further emphasis on the role of mesenchymal stem cells (MSCs). MSCs have been identified as playing a role in not only sarcomagenesis but also the progression of disease. This role of MSCs in osteosarcoma contrasts with their ability to differentiate into the various cell types of connective tissue for tissue repair. This chapter discusses MSC origin, differentiation and transformation in sarcomagenesis. The interactions between MSCs and osteosarcoma cells are outlined. A number of research models that utilize MSCs in order to replicate the human condition will be discussed along with the potential use of MSCs in biologic reconstruction.

2. Pathogenesis of osteosarcoma

The pathogenesis of osteosarcoma is a complex process, which is not completely understood and involves tumorigenesis from mesenchymal cells, alterations in cellular apoptosis, adhesion, migration and invasion, as well as tumour-induced osteolysis and angiogenesis. Various genetic and molecular alterations underlie these processes. It is hoped that by targeting the deranged molecular signalling of these pathways that novel treatment agents could be developed that enhance the efficacy of conventional chemotherapeutics and possibly reduce patient morbidity.

2.1. Environmental factors

Physical, biological and chemical agents have been implicated in osteosarcoma pathogenesis. There is a well-documented risk of osteosarcoma following exposure to ultraviolet and ionizing radiation, which occurs in 2-3% of cases. The first identified case of radiation exposure association with osteosarcoma was found in female watch-makers working with radium [7]. Nevertheless, only 2% of osteosarcoma cases are associated with radiation exposure [8] and it is not thought to contribute significantly to paediatric disease. Samartiz et al., have identified that radiation-related-sarcoma formation can even occur in those with low-level radiation exposure. Of children who received radiotherapy for treatment of a solid tumour, 5.4% develop a secondary neoplasm and only 25% of these are sarcomas [9]. A latent period of 10–20 years between radiation exposure and osteosarcoma formation has been observed [10]. Methylcholanthrene and chromium salts [11], beryllium oxide [12], zinc beryllium silicate [13], asbestos and aniline dyes [14] are among the chemical agents associated with osteosarcoma formation.

2.2. Familial and chromosomal abnormalities

Amplifications of chromosomes 6p21, 8q24 and 12q14, and loss of heterozygosity of 10q21.1, are among the most common genomic alterations in osteosarcoma [15]. Numerical chromosomal abnormalities associated with osteosarcoma include loss of chromosomes 9, 10, 13 and 17, as well as gain of chromosome 1 [4]. Osteosarcoma has been reported in patients with Werner syndrome, Rothmund-Thompson syndrome, Bloom syndrome, Li-Fraumeni syndrome, and hereditary retinoblastoma [14]. In particular, Werner, Rothmund-Thompson and Bloom [16] syndromes are characterized by genetic defects in the RecQ helicase family. DNA-helicases separate double stranded DNA prior to replication [17, 18].

Pagetic osteosarcoma occurs in approximately 1% of patients with Paget's disease [19]. These tumours are characteristically high grade pleiomorphic intramedullary tumours. Loss of heterozygosity of chromosome 18q is a recognized genetic anomaly contributing to tumorigenesis: the specific region located between loci D18S60 and D18S42 contains the tumour suppressor locus [20]. This region also encodes for receptor activator of nuclear factor kappa B (RANK), a peptide which is a mediator of osteoclastic activity [21].

2.3. Tumour suppressor gene dysfunction

The p53 mutation is the most common genetic aberrancy in malignancy, and is a causative factor in the transformation and proliferation of osteosarcoma cells [22]. Here, it is found to be mutated in 22% of cases [4]. The presence of p53 mutation in osteosarcoma was initially identified in the autosomal dominant Li-Fraumeni syndrome, which is a syndrome characterised by a predisposition to forming multiple malignancies, such as osteosarcoma, rhabdomyosarcoma and breast cancer.

Normally, p53 is a vital protein in cell cycle arrest, cellular senescence and DNA damage response and repair [23]. It is regulated by mouse double minute 2 homolog (MDM2), a protein that inhibits p53 activation via multiple methods including the ubiquitin degradation pathway and competitively binding to the amino terminus of p53 (instead of transcriptional co-activators) [24]. Transcriptional activation of p21 (cyclin-dependent kinase inhibitor) mediates p53 activity, where its expression results in cellular arrest in either the G1 or G2 phase. This can be either temporary, until the source of the cellular stress has been removed or subsided, or can be irreversible, which is known as cellular senescence. Cellular senescence is stimulated by the presence of oncogene activation or presence of DNA damage. Its ability to arrest the cell cycle in the G1/G2 phase is dependent on its response to stressful stimuli [25].

Mutation in the retinoblastoma gene (Rb1) is the most common mutation found in osteosarcomas whereby greater than 70% of cases are associated with an alteration in Rb gene. The association between hereditary retinoblastoma and osteosarcoma has been localised to this mutation, where it acts as a dysfunctional tumour suppressor. Normally, Rb1 is found on chromosome 13, which encodes for a nuclear protein allowing sequestration of transcription factors and acts as a tumour suppressor. This protein is vital in regulation of cell cycle progression from the G1 to S phase of the cell cycle. Hypophosphorylation of Rb protein allows it to bind to E2F transcription factor which inhibits cellular progression from G1 into the S phase. Once pRb is phosphorylated, it releases E2F, allowing continuation of the cell cycle. Additional biological characteristics include regulating DNA replication, apoptosis, cellular differentiation, as well as DNA damage response and repair [26–28].

2.4. Transcription and growth factors

Osteosarcoma cells produce a number of transcription and growth factors that contribute towards continued tumour cell growth and proliferation. During transcription single-stranded messenger RNA (mRNA) is formed from double-stranded DNA. Transcription factors bind to promoter sequences for specific genes to initiate the process. Transcription is usually a tightly regulated process and deregulation can lead tumour formation. Growth factors may act via both autocrine and paracrine mechanisms and overexpression or constitutive activation may lead to accelerated osteosarcoma cell proliferation.

The activator protein 1 complex (AP-1) is a regulator of transcription that controls cell proliferation, differentiation and bone metabolism. AP-1 is comprised of Fos and Jun proteins, products of the c-fos and c-jun proto-oncogenes, respectively. Upregulation of Fos and Jun is seen in high-grade osteosarcomas [29, 30] and is also associated with a propensity to develop metastatic lesions [31].

Myc is a transcription factor that acts in the nucleus to stimulate cell growth and division. Myc amplification has been implicated in osteosarcoma pathogenesis and resistance to chemotherapeutics. Overexpression of Myc in bone marrow stromal cells leads to osteosarcoma development and loss of adipogenesis [32]. This factor is amplified in U2OS osteosarcoma cell line variants with the highest resistance to doxorubicin and gain of Myc was found in SaOS-2 methotrexate-resistant variants [33].

http://dx.doi.org/10.5772/67371

In addition to Myc, transforming growth factor beta 1 (TGF-β1) has been shown to be overexpressed in high grade osteosarcomas [34]. Smad activation was implicated downstream of TGF-β with an inability to phosphorylate the Rb protein.

Insulin-like growth factor (IGF)-I and IGF-II are overexpressed by osteosarcomas. Activation of the IGF-1R receptor leads to the activation of phosphoinositide 3-kinase (PI3K) and mitogen-activated protein kinase (MAPK) pathways. This leads to accelerated cell proliferation and inhibition of apoptosis [35].

Connective tissue growth factor (CTGF) is a potent stimulator for the proliferation of osteosarcoma cells, leading to increased expression of type I collagen, alkaline phosphatase, osteopontin and osteocalcin, markers for bone cell differentiation and maturation [36]. CCN3, a related protein, is overexpressed in osteosarcoma and is associated with a worse prognosis [37].

The wingless-type (Wnt) canonical pathway, is a specific cascade that occurs within the Wnt family of glycoproteins and has been identified in the molecular basis of osteosarcoma formation. The Wnt family is essential in cellular differentiation and cell fate determination, and in the context of osteosarcomas, directing mesenchymal stem cells down the osteogenic lineage. Through this pathway, bone morphogenic protein 2 (BMP-2) is the key factor in osteogenesis. Another factor has been identified to inhibit the Wnt cascade, and histologically has been identified at the peripheries of osteosarcomas, Dickkopf 1 (DKK1). A secreted antagonist of Wnt pathway is low density lipoprotein receptor related protein 5 (LRP-5) which has been correlated with metastatic disease in osteosarcoma, independent of the histological type. When LRP-5 is expressed, the Wnt pathway is activated resulting in the up-regulation of a number of genetic factors including matrix metalloproteinases (MMP) which have been known to be involved in metastatic activity of cancers. Hoang et al. have analysed osteosarcoma patients expressing LRP-5, who were metastases free at time of diagnosis to have a lower probability of an event-free survival [38].

Stromal cell derived factor-1 (SDF-1), also known as C-X-C motif chemokine 12 (CXCL-12), [39] is a ligand for CXCR-4 and a part of the cxc chemokine family, where CXCR-4 has been implicated in various cancer types. SDF-1/CXCL-12 is a chemokine that has a paracrine effect within the interstitial space stimulation migration of pluripotent cells as well as tumour cells. The interaction between CXCR-4 and SDF-1/CXCL-12 has an important role in cancer progression as it promotes osteosarcoma cell migration and angiogenesis [40]. Within osteosarcoma the level of CXCR-4 mRNA is low however the SDF-1/CXCL-12/CXCR4 combination is required in osteosarcoma cell proliferation. Tumour promotion occurs by SDF-1/CXCL-12 in a paracrine manner, stimulating cellular growth and survival. Besides tumour promotion CXCR-4 is involved in metastatic spread of tumour cells into areas where SDF-1/CXCL-12 is expressed. This factor is important in angiogenesis as it promotes endothelial cells into the tumour microenvironment [39].

2.5. Osteosarcoma invasion

Degradation of the extracellular matrix by osteosarcoma cells allows for invasion of surrounding tissues by the primary tumour mass. Matrix metalloproteinases (MMPs) and the urokinase plasminogen activator (uPA) system are the effectors of this matrix breakdown.

The MMPs include collagenases, gelatinases and stromelysins. Collagenases break down collagen types I, II and III. Gelatinases break down collagen type IV, while stromelysins break down collagen types III, IV and V as well proteoglycans [41].

The urokinase plasminogen activator (uPA) system has been studied extensively with relation to osteosarcoma invasion. When uPA binds to its receptor uPAR it becomes active. Activated uPA then cleaves plasminogen to form plasmin. Plasmin is both responsible for direct breakdown of the extracellular matrix but also for further activation of pro-MMPs [42, 43].

uPA levels possess prognostic significance in osteosarcoma. An inverse relationship exists between survival time and uPA levels in osteosarcoma [44]. The downregulation of uPAR in a clinically relevant murine model of osteosarcoma resulted in limited primary tumour growth and inhibited metastatic spread [45].

2.6. Osteoclasts and osteosarcoma-induced osteolysis

Substantial osteolysis may result from osteosarcoma growth. This osteolysis at the tumour site is the result of interactions between osteosarcoma cells, osteoclasts, osteoblasts and the bone matrix. Growth factors such as transforming growth factor beta (TGF-β) are released from degraded bone matrix and stimulate the release of tumoral cytokines that induce osteoclastic resorption of bone. Among the osteoclast-stimulating cytokines are parathyroid hormone-related protein (PTHrP), interleukin-6 (IL-6) and interleukin-11 (IL-11) [46, 47]. Further growth factors are then released from the bone matrix, leading to a cycle of osteolysis, osteoclast activation and osteosarcoma invasion.

The critical involvement of osteoblasts in the osteolytic process is a surprising finding. Among the other factors that osteosarcoma cells release are the osteoblast-stimulating factors endothelin-1 (ET-1), vascular endothelial growth factor (VEGF), and platelet-derived growth factor (PDGF) [48, 49]. Osteoblast stimulation by these factors leads to increased expression of receptor activator of nuclear factor κB ligand (RANKL). RANKL is a key regulator of osteoclast differentiation and activity. Osteosarcoma cells have been noted to produce RANKL independently also [50].

2.7. Osteosarcoma angiogenesis

Tumour neovascularization is required for continued osteosarcoma growth and progression. Osteosarcoma cells obtain the necessary oxygen and nutrients for cellular proliferation from the neovasculature and gain access to these vessels in order to metastasize.

The process of angiogenesis is regulated by a balance between pro-angiogenic and anti-angiogenic regulators. Loss of tumour suppressor gene function and oncogene activation pushes this balance toward neoangiogenesis. The hypoxic and acidotic environment that surrounds the primary tumour also promotes vascular proliferation. Such conditions lead to de-ubiquitination of the von Hippel Lindau protein. Von Hippel Lindau protein releases hypoxia-inducible factor-1α (HIF-1α). HIF-1α upregulates vascular endothelial growth factor (VEGF) [51]. VEGF is pro-angiogenic through stimulation of the processes of endothelial cell proliferation, migration and maturation. An immature, irregular and leaky vasculature is thus formed in and around the tumour.

Anti-angiogenic factors are downregulated in osteosarcoma. These include thrombospondin 2, transforming growth factor beta (TGF-β) [52], troponin I, reversion-inducing cysteine rich protein with Kazal motifs (RECK) [53] and pigment epithelial derived factor (PEDF) [54]. Downregulation of such molecules may lead to increased invasion through predominately avascular zones, such as the growth plate [55, 56].

Osteosarcoma is a particularly vascular tumour. However, the true significance of vascular density is yet to be fully elucidated. While vascular tumours may be more likely to lead to increased rated of metastasis, increased osteosarcoma microvascular density may offer a survival advantage attributed to improved tumour penetration by intravenously delivered chemotherapeutics [57].

3. Mesenchymal stem cell origin and differentiation

The defining features that characterise stem cells as a group are the ability to self-renew and the ability to differentiate into distinctive cell line types. Stem cells, broadly speaking, may fall into one of four main categories:

1. Embryonic stem cells
2. Pluripotent stem cells
3. Cancer stem cells
4. Tissue specific stem cells

Various tissue specific stem cells have been identified and mesenchymal stem cells (MSCs) are but one of these. Other tissue specific stem cells include cord blood stem cells, neural stem cells, gut stem cells, amniotic fluid stem cells and others. MSCs are multipotent cells that are able to differentiate into bone, cartilage, fat and muscle. Due to this ability they represent a promising source for tissue repair and regeneration. Research has focused on the cellular and molecular pathways that direct differentiation towards a particular cell type and aberrant differentiation of MSCs may contribute to sarcomagenesis. Prior to understanding the interactions between MSCs and osteosarcoma cells, an understanding of the biological factors that characterize MSCs is essential.

The initial work of identifying and characterising MSCs can be largely credited to the work of Friedenstein, Cohnheim and Caplan [58–61]. Cohnheim hypothesised that certain fibroblastic cells originating from bone marrow were a key factor in wound healing. In the 1970s and 1980s, Friedenstein isolated a population of plastic adherent stromal cells from bone marrow, which had the capacity to differentiate into certain colony forming units (CFU). These CFUs possessed the capacity to give rise to osteoblasts, chondrocytes, adipocytes, muscle and haematopoietic tissue. Beyond this, Kopen et al. [62] have demonstrated that not only are MSCs able to differentiate into mesoderm-derived cells but they are also able to undergo transdifferentiation, forming endoderm-derived cells.

Since these early studies, MSCs have been identified and isolated from tissues other than bone marrow, including adipose tissue, muscle, peripheral blood, placenta, umbilical cord and amniotic fluid. Irrespective of the tissue of origin of MSCs are able to adhere to plastic and differentiate along mesenchymal cell lines. The expression of specific surface antigens has also been used to identify MSCs. The International Society for Cellular Therapy use the following characteristics to identify and standardize isolated human MSCs [63]:

1. Plastic adherence – *in vitro* under standard culture conditions (1–5 days);
2. Tri-lineage differentiation into cells of mesodermal lineage (osteoblasts, chondroblasts and adipocytes);
3. Surface antigens:

a. Expression of CD105, CD73, CD 90

b. Absence of CD45, CD 34, CD 14, CD 11b, CD79b, CD 19, HLA-DR (haematopoietic markers)

Most relevant in the setting of translational research, however, is that significant variation exists in the expression at surface antigens across species. MSCs of murine origin may be identified by the expression of CD106 and Sca-1, and the absence of CD31, CD45 and CD11b. Studies have demonstrated significant variability in surface antigen expression which changes once MSCs undergo expansion and ex-plantation [64].

3.1. Sources of MSCs

MSCs are found in nearly all tissues, including adult bone marrow, peripheral blood and adipose tissues. MSCs are derived from pericytes (cells surrounding blood vessels) and exist in a perivascular niche. This explains the presence of adult MSCs in a number of different tissue types [65], including:

- Bone marrow
- Synovium and synovial fluid
- Periosteum
- Peripheral blood
- Adipocytes
- Liver
- Brain
- Kidney

- Lung
- Spleen
- Blood vessels

While MSCs may be obtained from a variety of different tissue types, the concentration of MSCs in these tissues varies widely. Pittenger et al. [66] isolated MSCs from bone marrow, adipocyte and peripheral blood. 0.001-0.01% of bone marrow cells were MSCs in comparison to ~5000 cells of 1g of adipose were MSCs. Furthermore, in addition to the variable concentration of the stem cells sourced from different tissues, it has been demonstrated that there is altered capacity to form osteocytes in vivo dependent on the tissue of origin of MSCs. Cosimo De Bari showed that periosteal derived MSCs have a greater potential to form osteocytes than those derived from synovium [67].

Mesenchymal stem cells can also be obtained from birth associated tissues [65], including:

- Placenta
- Human amnion membrane
- Umbilical cord
- Cord blood
- Chorionic villi and chorion membrane
- Wharton's jelly

The major advantages of MSCs derived from birth associated tissue, over those obtained from bone marrow, are the availability of the tissue, as well as the greater proliferative and differentiation capacity of these cells. The rate of expansion varies between adult and birth associated tissue derived MSCs. The mean doubling time for umbilical cord MSCs is approximately 24 hours whilst it is 40 hours for bone marrow MSCs. Additionally, umbilical cord MSCs proliferate with multi-layering, while bone marrow MSCs demonstrate contact inhibition. Bone marrow MSCs are multipotent, while birth associated tissue MSCs are pluripotent and are able to differentiate into all three germinal layers.

3.2. Multi-lineage potential and transdifferentiation of MSCs

Friedenstiein et al. initially demonstrated that bone marrow derived MSCs differentiated exclusively into cells of mesodermal lineage, namely osteocytes, adipocytes and chondrocytes [59]. More recently, however, MSCs have been shown to also possess the ability to differentiate along endodermal and neuroectodermal lines. In vitro studies have shown formation of neural tissue from bone marrow derived MSCs. This has propagated multiple studies determining the factors that stimulate MSCs to differentiate into cell lineages.

Pittenger et al. [66] highlighted that in vitro mesenchymal stem cells can maintain a stable and undifferentiated state, however when exposed to certain cues or cultured in certain media they are able to differentiate into diverse cell types. MSCs that have undergone 20 cumulative population doublings maintain this multipotent ability.

The osteogenic potential of MSCs has been observed *in vitro*, however this ability *in vivo* is still incompletely defined. Osteoblasts may stimulate the expansion of MSCs and regulate differentiation down the osteogenic pathway, however this may be secondary to the role of osteocytes in stimulating differentiation toward osteogenesis.

Huang et al. demonstrated the process of osteogenic differentiation in vitro, through multiple stages [68, 69]:

1. Day 1–4
    a. Peak number of cells
2. Day 5–14
    a. Early cell differentiation
    b. Deposition of type 1 collagen early in this phase
    c. Expression of alkaline phosphatase (ALP), however the level of ALP decreases at the end of the second phase
3. Day 14–28
    a. Expression of fibroblast growth factor 2 (FGF-2) and bone morphogenetic protein 2 (BMP-2)
    b. Expression of osteocalcin and osteopontin
    c. Calcium and phosphate deposition

The early response growth factors were distinguished from the growth factors present in late cycle. The early response factors include transforming growth factor beta, insulin-like growth factor and vascular endothelial growth factor. The later phase growth factors include platelet derived growth factor, bone morphogenetic protein 2 (BMP-2) and fibroblast growth factor 2 (FGF-2)

Transforming growth factor beta (TGF-beta) administration stimulates osteoblast activity as well as cell proliferation, alkaline phosphatase activity and calcium deposition. BMP-2 is a notable cytokine which is osteoinductive, and has been shown to commit cells into either a chondrogenic or osteogenic lineage depending on its culture medium. When these two factors co-exist in an environment, there is approximately five-fold greater osteogenic potential.

Other groups of factors are important for adipogenic and chondrogenic differentiation. Factors favouring adipogenic differentiation include 1-methyl-3-isobutylxanthine, dexamethasone, insulin and indomethacin, whereby the adipocytes expressed lipoprotein lipase, fatty acid-binding protein (Ap2) and peroxisome proliferation-activated receptor gamma 2 (PPAR-2) [66, 68]. Factors for chondrogenic potential include glutamine, linoleic acid, dexamethasone, ascorbic acid, proline and sodium pyruvate. Dexamethasone is required as it promotes TGF-beta1 upregulation of type II collagen. The potent factors which were found to be important in chondrocyte formation are BMP-2 and BMP-7, with TGF-beta being a weaker factor. The effect of BMP-2 is dose-dependent, whereby it stimulates the production of mRNA for type II collagen and aggrecan [70, 71].

There are two main pathways important in differentiation. One discussed previously is through TGF-beta, involved in the formation of chondrocytes. This occurs through multiple intra-cellular cascades (mitogen activated protein, JNK, p38). The other pathway is the Wnt canonical pathway, where soluble glycoproteins stimulate and regulate cellular differentiation and expansion. Like the TGF-beta pathway, the binding of Wnt to receptors on cells trigger an intracellular cascade, however, this pathway has an osteogenic potential.

4. Transformation of mesenchymal stem cells

Transformation is the sequential accumulation of genetic changes in a cell that may lead to altered behaviour and function of the subsequent cell lineage. Transformation causes cells to both acquire new and lose certain characteristics of the original cell type. This may be reflected as changes in the morphology of the cells, altered expression of surface antigens, changes in the growth characteristics, as well as increased tumorigenicity. Differentiation of MSCs at a variety of stages may underlie sarcomagenesis. Sarcomas may arise from cells already committed to a particular differentiation pathway, or alternatively, from multipotent cells that are pushed towards a particular sarcoma subtype. Alterations in oncogenes, tumour suppressor genes, growth factors and transcription factors may underlie the transformation of MSCs.

Studies that have utilised MSCs of both murine and human origins have supported the concept of transformation of MSCs for tumorigenesis. The findings of human studies have been conflicting, however, and warrant further evaluation. Transformed murine MSCs demonstrate altered morphology and growth characteristics. Transformed murine MSCs exhibit a compact morphology, demonstrate anchorage-independent growth, lack contact inhibition and form multiple layers in culture. This is in contrast to the spindle-shaped single layer growth characteristics of MSCs [72–75]. The proliferation rates of transformed murine MSCs have been shown to be increased and genetic and molecular signalling alterations underlie these changes [72, 76, 77]. Increased chromosome number beyond the usual 40 acrocentric chromosomes have been demonstrated in transformed murine MSCs by multiple authors [72, 73, 78]. Additionally, Matushansky et al. [79] showed that inactivation of the Wnt pathway in transformed MSCs gave rise to a cell population with a similar appearance to that of malignant fibrous histiocytoma.

Human models require MSCs that are able to undergo ex vivo expansion prior to its clinical application and through this process some cells undergo spontaneous transformation. This is particularly concerning when considering the potential therapeutic use of MSCs for tissue repair and regeneration. There are also pharmacological agents that mobilise MSCs into the bloodstream. However, there has been some variability in studies using human MSCs. Some studies have shown spontaneous transformation of human MSCs in culture [80, 81] while other research groups have demonstrated that human MSCs are not able to spontaneously transform into malignant cells and with prolonged *in vitro* culturing become senescent [82–85]. These conflicting studies have been further confounded by Torsvik et al. [86] and de la Fuente et al. [87] that demonstrated previously considered transformed MSCs were tainted by contamination. Pan et al. [88] have subsequently shown MSCs to undergo transformation and have eliminated the possibility of contamination. In this study, 46 cultures of MSCs were studied and 4 of these cultures showed characteristics of transformation, including morphological changes and increased proliferation rates. Increased tumorigenicity was demonstrated when these cells were introduced into immunodeficient mice.

In addition to the cellular, molecular and genetic changes underlying osteosarcoma pathogenesis, the transformation of MSCs have also been implicated in the tumorigenesis of osteosarcoma. Wang et al. [89] were among the first to hypothesise that a subpopulation of cancer stem cells existed in human osteosarcoma. In order to demonstrate such a subpopulation of tumorigenic cells, Wang et al. characterised cells with high aldehyde dehydrogenase (ALDH) in 4 human osteosarcoma cell lines. Of these, the OS99-1 cell line, which was derived from an aggressive primary human osteosarcoma, had significantly higher ALDH activity. When OS99-1 cells were introduced into a murine xenograft model, 3% of tumour cells demonstrated high ALDH activity and these cells demonstrated the characteristics of MSCs, namely self-renewal, tri-lineage differentiation and the expression of typical cell surface antigens.

Since then, Adhikari et al. [90] have further characterised a subpopulation of cancer stem cells in osteosarcoma using cell surface antigens. This study took the concept of tumour-initiating cells further by identifying a possible role of cancer stem cells in highly metastatic and resistant osteosarcoma. Mouse and human osteosarcoma stem cells were identified using the MSC markers CD117 and Stro-1. Expression of these markers were largely in spheres and doxorubicin-resistant cells. Cells that were positive for both CD117 and Stro-1 were serially transplantable and gave rise to more aggressive metastatic disease when applied to an orthotopic murine model. CD117 and Stro-1 positive tumours in the model were highly invasive and demonstrated drug resistance.

Alterations in oncogenes, tumour suppressor genes, growth factors and transcription factors may underlie the transformation of MSCs for osteosarcoma tumorigenesis. In one study, Mohseny et al. [74] examined the pre-malignant stages of osteosarcoma using murine mesenchymal cells. A functional and phenotypical analysis of MSCs, transformed MSCs and osteosarcoma cells was performed in parallel using. Aneuploidization, translocations, homozygous loss of the cyclin-dependent kinase inhibitor (cdkn2) region, and alterations in sarcoma amplified sequence (SAS), retinoblastoma 1 (Rb1), mouse double minute 2 homolog (Mdm2), c-myc, p53 and p16 have all been implicated in the transformation of MSCs for osteosarcoma formation [74, 91].

Tao et al. [92] identified the transformation of immature osteoblasts as a potential source for osteosarcoma transformation. Using a murine model of osteosarcoma with conditional overexpression of intracellular domain of Notch1 (NICD), expression of NICD in osteoblast stem cells caused the formation of bone tumours including osteosarcoma. These tumours demonstrated histopathological, metastatic and genetic features of human osteosarcoma. Additionally, when overexpression of NICD and loss of p53 were combined in the murine model, osteosarcoma development and progression was accelerated.

5. Interactions between mesenchymal stem cells and osteosarcoma cells

The interaction between MSCs and tumour cells is an evolving area of current research. MSCs have been shown to be capable of migrating to not only sites of inflammation and injury but also to tumours and sites of metastasis. Once at these tumour sites, cellular interactions may cause progression of both primary and metastatic lesions. While these interactions between MSCs and osteosarcoma cells in the tumour microenvironment have been demonstrated, some studies show that MSCs may cause increased proliferation of tumour cells while others show reduced proliferation and pro-differentiation. Khakoo et al. [93] showed that systemically injected MSCs inhibit the growth of Kaposi sarcoma using a xenotransplant model.

Yu et al. [40] characterised the interaction between MSCs and osteosarcoma cells in vitro and showed that bone marrow derived MSCs had the potential to promote osteosarcoma cell proliferation and invasion. In this study bone marrow MSCs were cultured with osteosarcoma cells. Osteosarcoma cells were also cultured with conditioned media from MSCs. Cellular proliferation was measured by cell counting kit 8 (CCK-8) assay and a matrigel assay was used to evaluate tumour cell invasion. Tumour cell proliferation and invasion were promoted under these conditions with the implication of stromal derived factor-1 (SDF-1). SDF-1 is a cytokine that controls tumour neoangiogenesis, apoptosis, migration and invasion through binding to the CXCR4 receptor.

Tsukamoto et al. [94] showed that MSCs may provide a favourable environment for osteosarcoma growth and metastasis in a rat osteosarcoma model. In this study, rat COS1NR osteosarcoma cells were injected along with rat bone marrow derived MSCs. Injections were performed subcutaneously and intravenously. Osteosarcoma tumour formation and growth was increased significantly prior to 5 weeks using the subcutaneous injection model. When injected intravenously there was increased pulmonary lesion formation in the group that received co-injections of COS1NR and MSCs. The expression of genes by MSCs involved in cellular adhesion and extracellular matrix receptors were suggested as possible explanations for this tumour behaviour.

6. Mesenchymal stem cell utilization for biological reconstruction

MSCs are being portrayed in the literature as the key to biological reconstruction, however, studies are few and results are varied. There are significant challenges to be overcome if we are to utilise MSCs in biological reconstruction after tumour resection. Much of the concern relates to the yet to be fully characterised ability of MSCs to transform into sarcomas and the interactions between MSCs and tumours that cause increased tumorigenesis and disease progression. In order to apply MSCs to clinical reconstruction the cells require prior in vitro expansion. As has been discussed above, there are concerns of chromosomal instability and malignant transformation during this process of expansion.

A number of attempts at utilizing MSCs in the reconstruction process after tumour resection have been made. Perrot et al. [95] raised concern of osteosarcoma recurrence after autologous fat grafting, reporting a case of late recurrent osteosarcoma 13 years after the use of a lipofilling procedure. Following this they utilised a pre-clinical murine model of osteosarcoma to show that injection of fat grafts and MSCs promoted tumour growth.

Since then, Centeno et al. [96, 97] has published two papers with results for 339 patients that were treated following orthopaedic procedures with *in vitro* expanded, autologous bone marrow derived MSC implantation. Follow up by general observation and MRI tracking beyond 3 years post-operatively did not demonstrate tumour formation at the sites of injection. 2 patients were diagnosed with cancer during the follow up period, however these cases were assessed not to be related to the MSC therapy and the rate of neoplasm development was comparable to that of the general population. While the results presented by Centano et al. [96, 97] appear reassuring with regards to the safety of MSCs for reconstruction, further studies, particularly in the setting of reconstruction after treatment for malignancy are required. There are hundreds of clinical trials currently underway evaluating the therapeutic safety and efficacy of MSC based treatments.

7. Conclusions

While the advent of multi-agent chemotherapeutic regimes dramatically improved the prognosis for patients with osteosarcoma, novel treatment agents are required in order to reduce morbidity and improve function following surgical reconstruction. The pathogenesis of osteosarcoma is complex and current research is focusing on defining the deranged cell behaviours and molecular signalling pathways that underpin tumorigenesis and disease progression. Mesenchymal stem cells have attracted great interest over recent years due to their ability to expand into mesodermal tissues including bone, cartilage, fat and muscle; however, pre-clinical studies have highlighted possible roles in the processes of sarcomogenesis through transformation and interactions with the tumour cells themselves. Further studies defining the role of MSCs in osteosarcoma pathogenesis are required prior to studies of therapeutic safety and efficacy

Author details

Matthew L. Broadhead[1]*, Saumiyar Sivaji[1], Zsolt Balogh[1] and Peter F.M. Choong[2]

*Address all correspondence to: matthewbroadhead@me.com

1 John Hunter Hospital, University of Newcastle, New Lambton Heights NSW, Australia

2 St Vincent's Hospital Melbourne, University of Melbourne, Fitzroy VIC, Australia

References

[1] Canale ST, Beaty JH. Campbell's Operative Orthopaedics. 11th ed: Philadelphia Mosby Elsvier; 2008.

[2] Geller DS, Gorlick R. Osteosarcoma: a review of diagnosis, management, and treatment strategies. Clin Adv Hematol Oncol. 2010;8(10):705-18.

[3] Longhi A, Errani C, De Paolis M, Mercuri M, Bacci G. Primary bone osteosarcoma in the pediatric age: state of the art. Cancer treatment reviews. 2006;32(6):423-36.

[4] Ta HT, Dass CR, Choong PF, Dunstan DE. Osteosarcoma treatment: state of the art. Cancer Metastasis Rev. 2009;28(1-2):247-63.

[5] Bielack SS, Kempf-Bielack B, Delling G, Exner GU, Flege S, Helmke K, et al. Prognostic factors in high-grade osteosarcoma of the extremities or trunk: an analysis of 1,702 patients treated on neoadjuvant cooperative osteosarcoma study group protocols. Journal of clinical oncology : official journal of the American Society of Clinical Oncology. 2002;20(3):776-90.

[6] Vigorita VJ, editor. Orthopaedic Pathology. 2nd ed. Philadelphia, PA: Lippincott, Williams and Wilkins; 2008.

[7] Polednak AP. Bone cancer among female radium dial workers. Latency periods and incidence rates by time after exposure: brief communication. Journal of the National Cancer Institute. 1978;60(1):77-82.

[8] Picci P. Osteosarcoma (osteogenic sarcoma). Orphanet J Rare Dis. 2007;2:6.

[9] Paulino AC, Fowler BZ. Secondary neoplasms after radiotherapy for a childhood solid tumor. Pediatric hematology and oncology. 2005;22(2):89-101.

[10] Longhi A, Barbieri E, Fabbri N, Macchiagodena M, Favale L, Lippo C, et al. Radiation-induced osteosarcoma arising 20 years after the treatment of Ewing's sarcoma. Tumori. 2003;89(5):569-72.

[11] Rani AS, Kumar S. Transformation of non-tumorigenic osteoblast-like human osteosarcoma cells by hexavalent chromates: alteration of morphology, induction of anchorage-independence and proteolytic function. Carcinogenesis. 1992;13(11):2021-7.

[12] Dutra FR, Largent EJ. Osteosarcoma induced by beryllium oxide. The American journal of pathology. 1950;26(2):197-209.

[13] Mazabraud A. [Experimental production of bone sarcomas in the rabbit by a single local injection of beryllium]. Bulletin du cancer. 1975;62(1):49-58.

[14] Romagnoli S, Fasoli E, Vaira V, Falleni M, Pellegrini C, Catania A, et al. Identification of potential therapeutic targets in malignant mesothelioma using cell-cycle gene expression analysis. Am J Pathol. 2009;174(3):762-70.

[15] Smida J, Baumhoer D, Rosemann M, Walch A, Bielack S, Poremba C, et al. Genomic alterations and allelic imbalances are strong prognostic predictors in osteosarcoma. Clin Cancer Res.16(16):4256-67.

[16] Greenspan A, Jundt G, Remagen W. Differential diagnosis in orthopaedic oncology. Philadelphia: Lippincott Williams ' Wilkins; 2007. xi, 529 p. p.

[17] German J, Crippa LP, Bloom D. Bloom's syndrome. III. Analysis of the chromosome aberration characteristic of this disorder. Chromosoma. 1974;48(4):361-6.

[18] Fukuchi K, Martin GM, Monnat RJ, Jr. Mutator phenotype of Werner syndrome is characterized by extensive deletions. Proceedings of the National Academy of Sciences of the United States of America. 1989;86(15):5893-7.

[19] Hansen MF, Seton M, Merchant A. Osteosarcoma in Paget's disease of bone. J Bone Miner Res. 2006;21 Suppl 2:P58-63.

[20] Hansen MF, Nellissery MJ, Bhatia P. Common mechanisms of osteosarcoma and Paget's disease. J Bone Miner Res. 1999;14 Suppl 2:39-44.

[21] HUGO Gene Nomenclature Committee. TNFRSF11A TNF receptor superfamily member 11a [Homo sapiens (human)] [Internet]. 2016 [cited 01/08/2016]. Available from: http://www.ncbi.nlm.nih.gov/gene/8792.

[22] Guo W, Wang X, Feng C. P53 gene abnormalities in osteosarcoma. Chinese medical journal. 1996;109(10):752-5.

[23] Tongyuan Li NK, 1 Le Jiang,1 Minjia Tan,2 Thomas Ludwig,1 Yingming Zhao,2 Richard Baer,1 and Wei Gu1,, *. Tumor Suppression in the Absence of p53-Mediated Cell-Cycle Arrest, Apoptosis, and Senescence. Cell. 2012(149):1269 - 83.

[24] Balint EE, Vousden KH. Activation and activities of the p53 tumour suppressor protein. British journal of cancer. 2001;85(12):1813-23.

[25] Shaw PH. The role of p53 in cell cycle regulation. Pathology, research and practice. 1996;192(7):669-75.

[26] Kumaramanickavel G, InTech Open Access Books. Retinoblastoma An Update on Clinical, Genetic Counseling, Epidemiology and Molecular Tumor Biology. S.l.: InTech,; 2012. Available from: http://www.intechopen.com/books/retinoblastoma-an-update-on-clinical-genetic-counseling-epidemiology-and-molecular-tumor-biology.

[27] Weinberg RA. The Retinoblastoma Protein and Cell Cycle Control Cell. 1995;81(3):320-30.

[28] C Giacinti AG. RB and cell cycle progression. Oncogene. 2006(25):5220-7.

[29] Wu JX, Carpenter PM, Gresens C, Keh R, Niman H, Morris JW, et al. The proto-oncogene c-fos is over-expressed in the majority of human osteosarcomas. Oncogene. 1990;5(7):989-1000.

[30] Franchi A, Calzolari A, Zampi G. Immunohistochemical detection of c-fos and c-jun expression in osseous and cartilaginous tumours of the skeleton. Virchows Arch. 1998;432(6):515-9.

[31] Gamberi G, Benassi MS, Bohling T, Ragazzini P, Molendini L, Sollazzo MR, et al. C-myc and c-fos in human osteosarcoma: prognostic value of mRNA and protein expression. Oncology. 1998;55(6):556-63.

[32] Shimizu T, Ishikawa T, Sugihara E, Kuninaka S, Miyamoto T, Mabuchi Y, et al. c-MYC overexpression with loss of Ink4a/Arf transforms bone marrow stromal cells into osteosarcoma accompanied by loss of adipogenesis. Oncogene. 2010, 29 (42) 5687-5699

[33] Hattinger CM, Stoico G, Michelacci F, Pasello M, Scionti I, Remondini D, et al. Mechanisms of gene amplification and evidence of coamplification in drug-resistant human osteosarcoma cell lines. Genes Chromosomes Cancer. 2009;48(4):289-309.

[34] Franchi A, Arganini L, Baroni G, Calzolari A, Capanna R, Campanacci D, et al. Expression of transforming growth factor beta isoforms in osteosarcoma variants: association of TGF beta 1 with high-grade osteosarcomas. J Pathol. 1998;185(3):284-9.

[35] Rikhof B, de Jong S, Suurmeijer AJ, Meijer C, van der Graaf WT. The insulin-like growth factor system and sarcomas. J Pathol. 2009;217(4):469-82.

[36] Nishida T, Nakanishi T, Asano M, Shimo T, Takigawa M. Effects of CTGF/Hcs24, a hypertrophic chondrocyte-specific gene product, on the proliferation and differentiation of osteoblastic cells in vitro. J Cell Physiol. 2000;184(2):197-206.

[37] Perbal B, Zuntini M, Zambelli D, Serra M, Sciandra M, Cantiani L, et al. Prognostic value of CCN3 in osteosarcoma. Clin Cancer Res. 2008;14(3):701-9.

[38] Hoang BH, Kubo T, Healey JH, Sowers R, Mazza B, Yang R, et al. Expression of LDL receptor-related protein 5 (LRP5) as a novel marker for disease progression in high-grade osteosarcoma. International journal of cancer Journal international du cancer. 2004;109(1):106-11.

[39] Jan A. Burger TJK. CXCR4: a key receptor in the crosstalk between tumor cells and their microenvironment. Blood. 2006;107:1751-67.

[40] Yu FX, Hu WJ, He B, Zheng YH, Zhang QY, Chen L. Bone marrow mesenchymal stem cells promote osteosarcoma cell proliferation and invasion. World journal of surgical oncology. 2015;13:52.

[41] Chakraborti S, Mandal M, Das S, Mandal A, Chakraborti T. Regulation of matrix metalloproteinases: an overview. Mol Cell Biochem. 2003;253(1-2):269-85.

[42] Choong PF, Nadesapillai AP. Urokinase plasminogen activator system: a multifunctional role in tumor progression and metastasis. Clin Orthop Relat Res. 2003(415 Suppl):S46-58.

[43] Pillay V, Dass CR, Choong PF. The urokinase plasminogen activator receptor as a gene therapy target for cancer. Trends Biotechnol. 2007;25(1):33-9.

[44] Choong PF, Fernö M, Akerman M, Willén H, Långström E, Gustafson P, et al. Urokinase-plasminogen-activator levels and prognosis in 69 soft-tissue sarcomas. Int J Cancer. 1996;69(4):268-72.

[45] Dass CR, Nadesapillai AP, Robin D, Howard ML, Fisher JL, Zhou H, et al. Downregulation of uPAR confirms link in growth and metastasis of osteosarcoma. Clin Exp Metastasis. 2005;22(8):643-52.

[46] Guise TA, Chirgwin JM. Transforming growth factor-beta in osteolytic breast cancer bone metastases. Clin Orthop Relat Res. 2003(415 Suppl):S32-8.

[47] Quinn JM, Itoh K, Udagawa N, Hausler K, Yasuda H, Shima N, et al. Transforming growth factor beta affects osteoclast differentiation via direct and indirect actions. J Bone Miner Res. 2001;16(10):1787-94.

[48] Kingsley LA, Fournier PG, Chirgwin JM, Guise TA. Molecular biology of bone metastasis. Mol Cancer Ther. 2007;6(10):2609-17.

[49] Chirgwin JM, Guise TA. Skeletal metastases: decreasing tumor burden by targeting the bone microenvironment. J Cell Biochem. 2007;102(6):1333-42.

[50] Kinpara K, Mogi M, Kuzushima M, Togari A. Osteoclast differentiation factor in human osteosarcoma cell line. J Immunoassay. 2000;21(4):327-40.

[51] Hicklin DJ, Ellis LM. Role of the vascular endothelial growth factor pathway in tumor growth and angiogenesis. J Clin Oncol. 2005;23(5):1011-27.

[52] Ren B, Yee KO, Lawler J, Khosravi-Far R. Regulation of tumor angiogenesis by thrombospondin-1. Biochim Biophys Acta. 2006;1765(2):178-88.

[53] Clark JC, Thomas DM, Choong PF, Dass CR. RECK--a newly discovered inhibitor of metastasis with prognostic significance in multiple forms of cancer. Cancer Metastasis Rev. 2007;26(3-4):675-83.

[54] Cai J, Parr C, Watkins G, Jiang WG, Boulton M. Decreased pigment epithelium-derived factor expression in human breast cancer progression. Clin Cancer Res. 2006;12(11 Pt 1):3510-7.

[55] Quan GM, Ojaimi J, Li Y, Kartsogiannis V, Zhou H, Choong PF. Localization of pigment epithelium-derived factor in growing mouse bone. Calcif Tissue Int. 2005;76(2):146-53.

[56] Moses MA, Wiederschain D, Wu I, Fernandez CA, Ghazizadeh V, Lane WS, et al. Troponin I is present in human cartilage and inhibits angiogenesis. Proceedings of the National Academy of Sciences of the United States of America. 1999;96(6):2645-50.

[57] Kreuter M, Bieker R, Bielack SS, Auras T, Buerger H, Gosheger G, et al. Prognostic relevance of increased angiogenesis in osteosarcoma. Clin Cancer Res. 2004;10(24):8531-7.

[58] Friedenstein AJ, Piatetzky S, II, Petrakova KV. Osteogenesis in transplants of bone marrow cells. J Embryol Exp Morphol. 1966;16(3):381-90.

[59] Bianco P, Robey PG, Simmons PJ. Mesenchymal stem cells: revisiting history, concepts, and assays. Cell Stem Cell. 2008;2(4):313-9.

[60] Friedenstein AJ, Chailakhyan RK, Gerasimov UV. Bone marrow osteogenic stem cells: in vitro cultivation and transplantation in diffusion chambers. Cell Tissue Kinet. 1987;20(3):263-72.

[61] Caplan AI. Mesenchymal stem cells. J Orthop Res. 1991;9(5):641-50.

[62] Kopen GC, Prockop DJ, Phinney DG. Marrow stromal cells migrate throughout forebrain and cerebellum, and they differentiate into astrocytes after injection into neonatal mouse brains. Proceedings of the National Academy of Sciences of the United States of America. 1999;96(19):10711-6.

[63] Dominici M, Le Blanc K, Mueller I, Slaper-Cortenbach I, Marini F, Krause D, et al. Minimal criteria for defining multipotent mesenchymal stromal cells. The International Society for Cellular Therapy position statement. Cytotherapy. 2006;8(4):315-7.

[64] Adam R. Williams JMH. Mesenchymal Stem Cells Biology, Pathophysiology, Translational Findings, and Therapeutic Implications for Cardiac Disease. Circulation research. 2011(109):923-40.

[65] Hass R, Kasper C, Bohm S, Jacobs R. Different populations and sources of human mesenchymal stem cells (MSC): A comparison of adult and neonatal tissue-derived MSC. Cell Commun Signal. 2011;9:12.

[66] Pittenger MF, Mackay AM, Beck SC, Jaiswal RK, Douglas R, Mosca JD, et al. Multilineage potential of adult human mesenchymal stem cells. Science. 1999;284(5411):143-7.

[67] Alan Tyndall UAW, Andrew Cope, Francesco Dazzi, Cosimo De Bari, Willem Fibbe, Serena Guiducci, Simon Jones, Christian Jorgensen, Katarina Le Blanc, Frank Luyten, Dennis McGonagle, Ivan Martin, Chiara Bocelli-Tyndall, Giuseppina Pennesi, Vito Pistoia, Constantino Pitzalis, Antonio Uccelli, Nico Wulffraat and Marc Feldmann. Immunomodulatory properties of mesenchymal stem cells: a review based on an interdisciplinary meeting held at the Kennedy Institute of Rheumatology Division, London, UK, 31 October 2005. Arthritis Research ' Therapy. 2007(9):301.

[68] Huang Z1 NE, Smith RL, Goodman SB. The sequential expression profiles of growth factors from osteoprogenitors [correction of osteroprogenitors] to osteoblasts in vitro. Tissue Engineering. 2007;13(9):2311-20.

[69] Hanumantha Rao Balaji Raghavendran SP, Sepehr Talebian, Malliga Raman Murali, Sangeetha Vasudevaraj Naveen, G. Krishnamurithy, Robert McKean, and Tunku Kamarul. A Comparative Study on In Vitro Osteogenic Priming Potential of Electron Spun Scaffold PLLA/HA/Col, PLLA/HA, and PLLA/Col for Tissue Engineering Application. PLOS 2014;9(8):e104389.

[70] Grunder T, Gaissmaier C, Fritz J, Stoop R, Hortschansky P, Mollenhauer J, et al. Bone morphogenetic protein (BMP)-2 enhances the expression of type II collagen and aggrecan in chondrocytes embedded in alginate beads. Osteoarthritis Cartilage. 2004;12(7):559-67.

[71] Kurth T, Hedbom E, Shintani N, Sugimoto M, Chen FH, Haspl M, et al. Chondrogenic potential of human synovial mesenchymal stem cells in alginate. Osteoarthritis Cartilage. 2007;15(10):1178-89.

[72] Furlani D, Li W, Pittermann E, Klopsch C, Wang L, Knopp A, et al. A transformed cell population derived from cultured mesenchymal stem cells has no functional effect after transplantation into the injured heart. Cell Transplant. 2009;18(3):319-31.

[73] Ren Z, Wang J, Zhu W, Guan Y, Zou C, Chen Z, et al. Spontaneous transformation of adult mesenchymal stem cells from cynomolgus macaques in vitro. Exp Cell Res. 2011;317(20):2950-7.

[74] Mohseny AB, Szuhai K, Romeo S, Buddingh EP, Briaire-de Bruijn I, de Jong D, et al. Osteosarcoma originates from mesenchymal stem cells in consequence of aneuploidization and genomic loss of Cdkn2. J Pathol. 2009;219(3):294-305.

[75] Tolar J, Nauta AJ, Osborn MJ, Panoskaltsis Mortari A, McElmurry RT, Bell S, et al. Sarcoma derived from cultured mesenchymal stem cells. Stem Cells. 2007;25(2):371-9.

[76] Zheng Y, He L, Wan Y, Song J. H3K9me-enhanced DNA hypermethylation of the p16INK4a gene: an epigenetic signature for spontaneous transformation of rat mesenchymal stem cells. Stem Cells Dev. 2013;22(2):256-67.

[77] Zhou YF, Bosch-Marce M, Okuyama H, Krishnamachary B, Kimura H, Zhang L, et al. Spontaneous transformation of cultured mouse bone marrow-derived stromal cells. Cancer Res. 2006;66(22):10849-54.

[78] Miura M, Miura Y, Padilla-Nash HM, Molinolo AA, Fu B, Patel V, et al. Accumulated chromosomal instability in murine bone marrow mesenchymal stem cells leads to malignant transformation. Stem Cells. 2006;24(4):1095-103.

[79] Matushansky I, Hernando E, Socci ND, Mills JE, Matos TA, Edgar MA, et al. Derivation of sarcomas from mesenchymal stem cells via inactivation of the Wnt pathway. J Clin Invest. 2007;117(11):3248-57.

[80] Rosland GV, Svendsen A, Torsvik A, Sobala E, McCormack E, Immervoll H, et al. Long-term cultures of bone marrow-derived human mesenchymal stem cells frequently undergo spontaneous malignant transformation. Cancer Res. 2009;69(13):5331-9.

[81] Rubio D, Garcia-Castro J, Martin MC, de la Fuente R, Cigudosa JC, Lloyd AC, et al. Spontaneous human adult stem cell transformation. Cancer Res. 2005;65(8):3035-9.

[82] Bernardo ME, Zaffaroni N, Novara F, Cometa AM, Avanzini MA, Moretta A, et al. Human bone marrow derived mesenchymal stem cells do not undergo transformation after long-term in vitro culture and do not exhibit telomere maintenance mechanisms. Cancer Res. 2007;67(19):9142-9.

[83] Choumerianou DM, Dimitriou H, Perdikogianni C, Martimianaki G, Riminucci M, Kalmanti M. Study of oncogenic transformation in ex vivo expanded mesenchymal cells, from paediatric bone marrow. Cell Prolif. 2008;41(6):909-22.

[84] Wang Y, Huso DL, Harrington J, Kellner J, Jeong DK, Turney J, et al. Outgrowth of a transformed cell population derived from normal human BM mesenchymal stem cell culture. Cytotherapy. 2005;7(6):509-19.

[85] Aguilar S, Nye E, Chan J, Loebinger M, Spencer-Dene B, Fisk N, et al. Murine but not human mesenchymal stem cells generate osteosarcoma-like lesions in the lung. Stem Cells. 2007;25(6):1586-94.

[86] Torsvik A, Rosland GV, Svendsen A, Molven A, Immervoll H, McCormack E, et al. Spontaneous malignant transformation of human mesenchymal stem cells reflects cross-contamination: putting the research field on track - letter. Cancer Res. 2010;70(15):6393-6.

[87] de la Fuente R, Bernad A, Garcia-Castro J, Martin MC, Cigudosa JC. Retraction: Spontaneous human adult stem cell transformation. Cancer Res. 2010;70(16):6682.

[88] Pan Q, Fouraschen SM, de Ruiter PE, Dinjens WN, Kwekkeboom J, Tilanus HW, et al. Detection of spontaneous tumorigenic transformation during culture expansion of human mesenchymal stromal cells. Exp Biol Med (Maywood). 2014;239(1):105-15.

[89] Wang L, Park P, Zhang H, La Marca F, Lin CY. Prospective identification of tumorigenic osteosarcoma cancer stem cells in OS99-1 cells based on high aldehyde dehydrogenase activity. Int J Cancer. 2011;128(2):294-303.

[90] Adhikari AS, Agarwal N, Wood BM, Porretta C, Ruiz B, Pochampally RR, et al. CD117 and Stro-1 identify osteosarcoma tumor-initiating cells associated with metastasis and drug resistance. Cancer Res. 2010;70(11):4602-12.

[91] He JP, Hao Y, Wang XL, Yang XJ, Shao JF, Guo FJ, et al. Review of the molecular pathogenesis of osteosarcoma. Asian Pac J Cancer Prev. 2014;15(15):5967-76.

[92] Tao J, Jiang MM, Jiang L, Salvo JS, Zeng HC, Dawson B, et al. Notch activation as a driver of osteogenic sarcoma. Cancer Cell. 2014;26(3):390-401.

[93] Khakoo AY, Pati S, Anderson SA, Reid W, Elshal MF, Rovira, II, et al. Human mesenchymal stem cells exert potent antitumorigenic effects in a model of Kaposi's sarcoma. J Exp Med. 2006;203(5):1235-47.

[94] Tsukamoto S, Honoki K, Fujii H, Tohma Y, Kido A, Mori T, et al. Mesenchymal stem cells promote tumor engraftment and metastatic colonization in rat osteosarcoma model. Int J Oncol. 2012;40(1):163-9.

[95] Perrot P, Rousseau J, Bouffaut AL, Redini F, Cassagnau E, Deschaseaux F, et al. Safety concern between autologous fat graft, mesenchymal stem cell and osteosarcoma recurrence. PLoS One. 2010;5(6):e10999.

[96] Centeno CJ, Schultz JR, Cheever M, Freeman M, Faulkner S, Robinson B, et al. Safety and complications reporting update on the re-implantation of culture-expanded mesenchymal stem cells using autologous platelet lysate technique. Curr Stem Cell Res Ther. 2011;6(4):368-78.

[97] Centeno CJ, Schultz JR, Cheever M, Robinson B, Freeman M, Marasco W. Safety and complications reporting on the re-implantation of culture-expanded mesenchymal stem cells using autologous platelet lysate technique. Curr Stem Cell Res Ther. 2010;5(1):81-93.

Chapter 5

Microenvironment Signals and Mechanisms in the Regulation of Osteosarcoma

Yu Zhang, Qing Mai, Xiaowen Zhang,
Chunyuan Xie and Yan Zhang

Additional information is available at the end of the chapter

http://dx.doi.org/10.5772/67068

Abstract

Osteosarcoma (OS) is the most common malignant primary bone tumor in children and adolescents and features rapid development, strong metastatic ability, and poor prognosis. It has been well established that diverse genetic aberrations and metabolic alterations confer the tumorigenesis and development of OS. The intricate metabolism and vascularization that contributes to the nutrient and structural support for tumor progression should be thoroughly clarified to help us gain novel insights into OS and its clinical diagnoses and treatments. With regard to the complex bone extracellular matrix (ECM) and local cell populations, we intend to illustrate the interrelationship between various microenvironmental signals and the different stages of OS evolution. Solid evidence has noted two crucial factors of the OS microenvironment in the acquisition of stem cell phenotypes - transforming growth factor-β1 (TGF-β1) signaling and hypoxia. Different cell subtypes in the local environment might also serve as unique contributors that interact with each other and communicate with distant cells, thus participating in local invasion and metastasis. Proper models have been established and improved to reveal the evolutionary footsteps of how normal cells transform into a neoplastic state and progress toward malignancy.

Keywords: microenvironment, genetic aberrations, vasculogenesis, niches, models

1. Introduction

Osteosarcoma (OS) is the second highest cause of cancer-related death in children and adolescents. Unfortunately, complete surgical resection fails to eliminate OS due to the early hematogenous spread of pulmonary metastases. Despite advanced multi-agent neoadjuvant and adjuvant chemotherapies, the clinical outcome for patients with OS unfortunately remains discouraging, and the long-term survival rate for high-grade OS remains poor [1]. It is urgent to identify innovative diagnostic and prognostic markers as well as effective therapeutic targets.

The vast majority of OS arises in the metaphyseal regions adjacent to physes with a strong capacity of proliferation, including the distal femur, proximal tibia, and proximal humerus [2]. Evidence has elucidated that the complex etiology of OS is characterized by genomic instability, highly abnormal karyotypes, and multiple genomic aberrations with copy number variations occurring in multiple chromosomes [3, 4]. The story of how OS originates and develops is mysterious and is still the subject of exploration on many fronts.

In addition to the complexity of OS cells, the microenvironment of OS is also dynamic and variable with a complex bone extracellular matrix (ECM) and diverse populations of localized cells. Regulating various microenvironmental signals and different niches in OS warrant attention. Importantly, the OS microenvironment is characterized by abundant transforming growth factor-β1 (TGF-β1) and hypoxia. These conditions induce non-stem-like OS cells to adopt cancer stem cell characteristics, which in turn promote tumorigenesis and chemoresistance [5]. In addition, identifying distinct metabolic patterns and vascularization in OS should be considered in more detail and could provide a potential framework for clinical applications.

By reviewing the literature on classical and cutting-edge studies, we will discuss the regulation of microenvironmental signals during OS development and illustrate novel models for the study of OS.

2. Cells of origin: tumorigenesis

When a normal cell acquires the first cancer-promoting mutation(s) and initiates neoplasm, it is termed as cell of origin. As more information is gathered on the characteristic features of cell of origin, it is not difficult to create a clear assessment and better understanding on tumor evolution, which may remarkably lead to clinical improvements.

OS was believed to originate from bone mesenchymal stem cells (MSCs) or osteoprogenitors [6]. The deficiency of p53 alone or in combination with pRb in undifferentiated adipose-derived MSCs (ASCs) or bone marrow-derived MSCs (BM-MSCs) promotes metastatic osteoblastic OS development upon intrabone (i.b.) or periosteal (p.) orthotopic inoculation in immunodeficient mice [7]. In addition, the protein expression of cyclin-dependent kinase inhibitor 2A (CDKN2A)/p16 was identified as a sensitive prognostic marker in OS patients. Aneuploidy, translocations, and homozygous loss of the Cdkn2 region might have caused the malignant transformation of MSCs, which eventually evolved to OS in xenografted mice [8]. These findings proved that MSCs with genetic mutations might eventually develop into OS. Moreover, excision of p53-floxed alleles, which are p53 genes flanked by loxP sites that could be edited, in the osteoblastic lineage mediated by an osterix (OSX)-Cre transgene would cause spontaneous OS in mice. This model traced the cells of origin to osteoprogenitors because the excision was driven by the osterix promoter expressed in osteoprogenitor cells [6].

Nonetheless, there have been some other disputes as to the cell of origin for OS (**Figure 1**). Induced pluripotent stem cells (iPSCs) were generated from fibroblasts obtained from a family with Li-Fraumeni syndrome (LFS), a rare autosomal dominant syndrome characterized by the occurrence of diverse mesenchymal and epithelial neoplasms at multiple sites. LFS iPSC-derived osteoblasts (OBs) from these individuals have provided a sophisticated model system to study the early stages of OS development and elucidate the pathological mechanism of p53 mutant-associated OS development [9]. Recent research has provided evidence that pericytes, a mesenchymal cell population surrounding endothelial cells, could be a cell of origin for benign and malignant mesenchymal neoplasms [10]. Lineage-tracing studies in mice were accomplished to reveal sarcomas that are driven by the deletion of p53, and desmoid tumors that are driven by a mutation in adenoma polyposis coli (Apc) could be derived from neuron-glial antigen 2/chondroitin sulfate proteoglycan 4 (Ng2/Cspg)-expressing pericytes. They also determined the role of β-catenin dysregulation in the neoplastic phenotype.

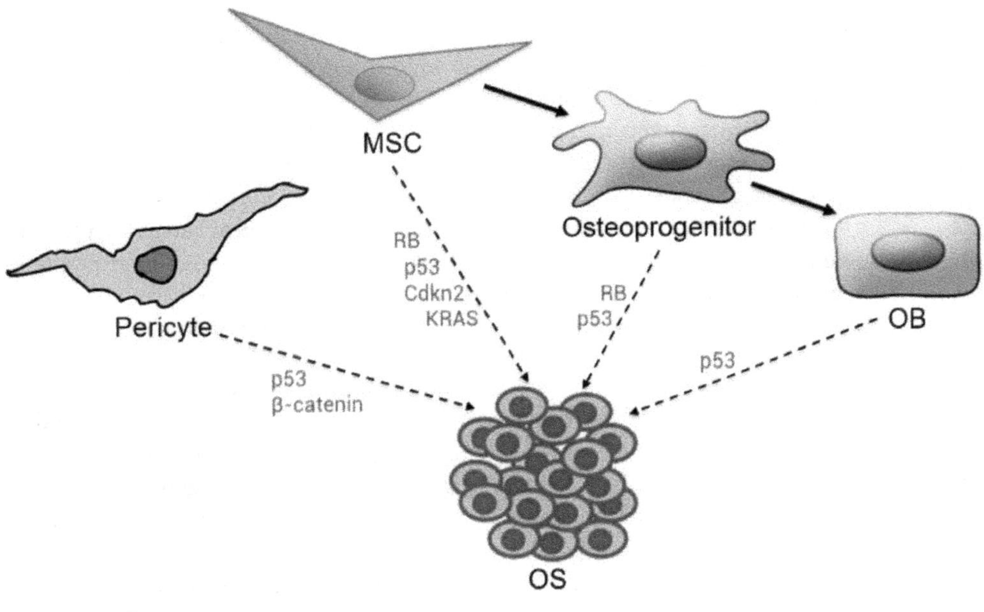

Figure 1. Cells of origin in OS. OS initiation is promoted by multiple genetic alterations (e.g., activation of oncogenes or inactivation of tumor suppressor genes).

The etiology of OS is still vague, while its pathogenesis remains mysterious. Generally, tumorigenesis is closely associated with inherited gene defects or mutations and exposure to exogenous carcinogens. These factors will affect the mutation rate and continually play a role in tumor evolution [11]. In the most likely scenario, the unique properties of OS might be related to either the genetic or epigenetic aberrations generated from either the cell of origin or components in the bone marrow microenvironment, such as the elevated levels of TGF-β1 and low oxygen tension. Uncovering the relationship between cytogenetic changes and microenvironmental signals in tumorigenesis will provide solutions for tumor eradication.

2.1. Tumor suppressor genes and oncogenes

OS results from multiple factors and gene aberrations. During the initiation and progression of OS, diverse oncogenes or tumor suppressor genes cause aberrant expression and hence dysregulate cell proliferation, apoptosis, and angiogenesis. Currently, the etiology and pathogenesis research on OS mainly focus on these oncogenes, tumor suppressor genes, and multidrug-resistant genes.

OS is a malignant bone cancer with severe chromosomal abnormalities and often has mutations of p53 and pRb. Up to 22% of OS patients carry an abnormal TP53 gene, and the allelic loss on chromosome 17p13 was confirmed in 75% of patients by a detection of mutation in the germ line [12, 13]. Strong evidence also suggested that p53 could regulate the genomic stability, proliferation, and immune properties of MSCs. p53 loss of function in MSCs compromises osteogenic differentiation and affects bone tumor microenvironment, both of which influence the development of OS [14].

A German group generated the first porcine model of OS by introducing oncogenic $TP53^{R167H}$ and $KRAS^{G12D}$ mutations as well as overexpressing Myc in porcine MSCs. These transformed porcine MSCs, with genomic instability and complex karyotypes, had the ability to develop into sarcomas upon transplantation into immunodeficient mice [15]. Other models also indicated that intrabone or periosteal inoculation of p53−/− or p53−/−RB−/− BM-MSCs or ASCs originated metastatic osteoblastic osteosarcoma (OS). Moreover, the subcutaneous (s.c.) coinfusion of p53−/−RB−/− MSCs together with BMP-2 resulted in appearance of tumoral osteoid areas [7]. pRb and p16(INK4a) are crucial G1-checkpoint proteins that maintain the balance of cellular proliferation. Deletion of p16 expression is significantly associated with decreased survival in a univariate analysis. The loss of pRb activation permits the hyper-proliferation of aberrant cells [16].

The progression of health informatics and the comprehensive study of "big data" have brought about new insights of genomic research. OS gene expression was first compared in gene expression omnibus (GEO) datasets and genomic aberrations in the International Cancer Genome Consortium (ICGC) database to identify differentially expressed genes (DEGs) and correlate these with both single-nucleotide polymorphisms (SNPs) and copy number variants (CNVs) in OS. The functional annotation of SNP- or CNV-associated DEGs was accomplished in accordance with gene ontology analysis, pathway analysis, and protein-protein interactions (PPIs). The PPI network analysis showed that chaperonin containing TCP subunit 3 (CCT3), COP9 signalosome subunit 3 (COPS3), and WW domain-containing E3 ubiquitin-protein ligase 1 (WWP1) could be candidate driver genes in OS tumorigenesis [17].

Another study performed a microarray-based comparative genomic hybridization (array-CGH) analysis on genomic DNA isolated from 41 patients with p53 +/− OS and 10 rhabdomyosarcoma samples. Results showed either gains or losses in the recurrent copy number, and the regions indicated known candidate oncogenes on mouse chromosomes 9 and 15. Furthermore, functional assays proved that the matrix metalloproteinase 13 (MMP13) gene, the antiapoptoticgenes Birc2 (cIAP1) and Birc3 (cIAP2) are potential oncogenic drivers in the chromosome 9A1 amplicon [18].

2.2. MicroRNAs and their target genes

MicroRNAs (miRNAs) are a class of small, single-stranded RNA molecules ranging from 18 to 25 nucleotides in length. miRNAs play important roles in proliferation, differentiation, apoptosis, and other cellular activities through posttranscriptional regulation of genes [19, 20]. miRNA signatures are detected in diverse types of cancers such as sarcoma, breast and prostate cancer [21–23]. Emerging evidence suggests that miRNAs are involved in the pathogenesis of OS and could potentially be developed for use as diagnostic biomarkers and therapeutic strategies.

Expression profiling of 723 human miRNAs was performed in seven OS specimens. Of the miRNAs tested, 38 were differentially expressed ≥ 10-fold (28 under- and 10 overexpressed) as shown in **Figure 2A**. In this analysis, miRNA-mRNA pairings were identified along with copy number changes of their corresponding target genes (**Figure 2B**). Many of the predicted gene targets of differentially expressed miRNAs are involved in intracellular signaling pathways important for OS, which include the c-Met, Notch, RAS/p21, mitogen-activated protein kinase (MAPK), Wnt, and Jun/Fos pathways [24]. For example, GADD45A, a putative target of miR-148a, could promote DNA repair and cell cycle arrest via the p38 MAPK and c-Jun N-terminal kinase (JNK) pathways. Overexpression of miR-148a contributed to the downregulation of GADD45A in OS, which was associated with multidrug resistance [25]. In this set of OS specimens, miR-126 was overexpressed and reported to downregulate the expression of polo-like kinase 2 (PLK2). PLK2 was proven to undergo transcriptional silencing via methylation in various cancer types, thus acting as a presumptive tumor suppressor gene [26]. Furthermore, miR-126 could stimulate developmental angiogenesis via vascular endothelial growth factor (VEGF) signaling [27].

The expression and either genetic or epigenetic alterations of the miR-34 family were examined in 117 primary OS samples. The miR-34 family was found to be decreased and undergo minimal deletions and epigenetic inactivation in OS cells [28]. Mutations in the TP53 gene sequence, functional inhibition of p53 protein, and hypermethylation of the miR-34a promoter are all associated with the loss of miR-34a expression in tumors [29]. miR-34a was proven to be involved in the drug resistance, proliferation, and metastasis of OS [30, 31]. Sarcomas occur at a high frequency in p53-deficient mice and patients with Li-Fraumeni syndrome (LFS). The overexpression of c-Met in these tumors suggested that the miR-34-p53-c-Met axis could comprise a regulatory gene network that cooperatively controls tumor progression in OS [32].

As one of the common target of miR-34a, c-Met is encoded by the MET oncogene, which is the receptor for hepatocyte growth factor (HGF). This receptor is overexpressed in a variety of human malignancies and stimulates cell proliferation, local invasion, and distant migration [33]. Researchers transformed OBs into malignant cells characterized with OS properties via overexpression of MET [34]. HGF-c-Met signals can activate the downstream signals of RAS/MAPK and PI3K-Akt, which enhances the drug resistance of OS and promotes the motility and proliferation of sarcoma cells [35, 36].

A

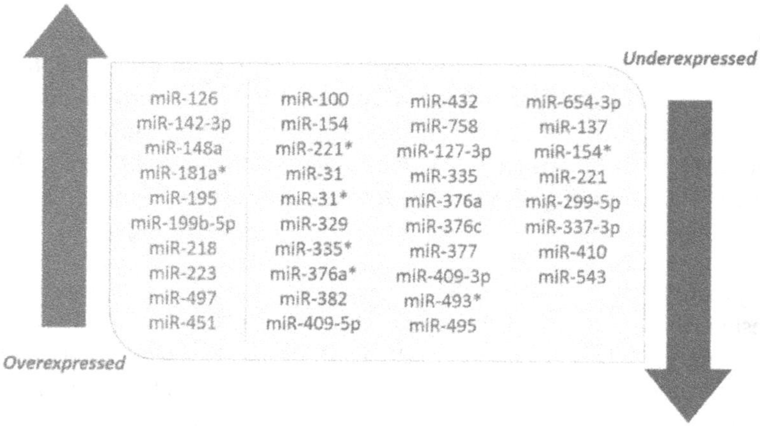

B

Mature miRNA	Target gene	Number of samples		
		Normal	Loss	Gain
Overexpressed				
hsa-miR-223	RBPJ		1	6
hsa-miR-148a	GADD45A		1	6
hsa-miR-218	RELN	1	2	4
hsa-miR-195	HSPA4L	1	2	4
hsa-miR-223	RASA1	2	4	1
hsa-miR-126	PLK2	2	5	0
Underexpressed				
hsa-miR-335	WWP1		1	6
hsa-miR-31	CD48		2	5
hsa-miR-137	FXYD6	1	4	2
hsa-miR-382	NDRG2	1	3	3
hsa-miR-335	E1F4A2	2	3	2

Figure 2. miRNA signature and relevant target genes in OS. (A) Differentially expressed miRNAs more than 10-fold in OSs relative to OBs in at least four tumor samples are listed. (B) Genomic status and relative expression of relevant target genes.

3. Osteosarcoma stem cells and dedifferentiation

Cancer stem cells (CSCs) are characterized by self-renewal, pluripotency, and increased cell plasticity. Some OS cells expressed specific surface markers of MSCs such as Stro-1, CD105, and CD44 [37]. Other evidences suggested that single-cell suspensions were able to form sarcospheres in anchorage-independent and serum-free conditions. These spheroids showed increased expression of the pluripotency-associated genes OCT4, NANOG, and SOX2 compared with adherent cells [38].

The currently embraced notion assumes that CSCs are critical for the recurrence and metastasis of malignancies, and common chemo- and radiotherapies are ineffective at killing CSCs. Thus, there is a need to explore the characteristics of CSCs in OS. CSCs isolated from OS are able to self-renew, sustain tumor generation, and confer metastatic potential and drug resistance [39]. The enhanced chemoresistance of the CSC subpopulation appears to be related to a more tolerant DNA repair ability [40] as well as an increased drug efflux capacity due to the high expression of ATP-binding cassette (ABC) transporters such as P-glycoprotein (MDR-1) and the breast cancer-resistant protein (BCRP/ABCG2) [41]. Developing CSC-targeted therapies could yield exciting new approaches for clinical application. The inhibition of ABC transporters is able to sensitize OS-derived sarcospheres to doxorubicin [42]. The nuclear factor κB (NF-κB) inhibitor BRM270 can specifically target the SaOS-2 stemlike cell population to undergo apoptosis [43].

Normal cells and cancer cells can acquire stem-like properties by several dedifferentiation inducers, including transcriptional networks involving key transcription factors (e.g., Oct4, Sox2, Nanog), miRNAs (e.g., let-7, miR-200 family), microenvironmental signals (e.g., hypoxia, inflammation, autocrine/paracrine oncogenic signaling pathways), epigenetic modifications (e.g., DNA demethylation, histone acetylation/methylation), and metabolic reprogramming [44].

Our group has demonstrated the role of the microenvironment and the intracellular context of OS on dedifferentiation. TGF-β1 and hypoxia are crucial factors that induce OS cells toward a CSC phenotype, which is characterized by the ability to self-renew and pluripotency. The dedifferentiated cells induced by TGF-β1 and hypoxia could differentiate into vascular endothelial-like cells (CD31 positive) in either a 3D culture system or xenografts. These cells could also form lipid droplets in an adipogenic differentiation medium. Gene set enrichment analysis (GSEA) revealed that gene alterations during the process of dedifferentiation are closely correlated with chemoresistance and metastasis in OS patients [5].

3.1. TGF-β1

The expression level of TGF-β1 is related to the metastatic potential of OS patients [45]. TGF-β1 suppressed miR-143 expression through a SMAD2/3-dependent mechanism and collaboratively upregulated the expression of versican to promote OS cell migration and invasion in vitro [46]. Blockage of the TGF-β1 autocrine loop inhibited OS cell proliferation and enhanced chemotherapy sensitivity, which might serve as a viable clinical treatment [47]. The tumor suppressor p16(INK4) inhibited the paracrine pro-migratory effect on OS stromal fibroblasts through the inhibition of TGF-β1 expression/secretion via an ERK1/2-dependent pathway [48].

OS cells can secrete factors that initiate osteoclast-mediated bone destruction, which coincides with TGF-β1 release from the bone matrix. It was suggested that OS cells might secrete TGF-β1 to maintain the stemness of MSCs and promote the production of pro-tumorigenic cytokines [49]. Elevated secretion of TGF-β1 by MSCs under hypoxic conditions could promote the growth, motility, and invasiveness of breast cancer cells [50]. This result indicated a possible link between TGF-β1 signaling and hypoxia.

High TGF-β1 expression occurs in many other types of cancer and is related to the state of ECM, angiogenesis, and immune escape [51]. The activation of TGF-β1 signaling triggers the epithelial-mesenchymal transition (EMT) and ensures that the transformed cancer cells possess a stronger capacity of self-renewal, tumorigenesis, and chemo-/radioresistance [52]. In OS or other tumor types, solid evidence suggests that TGF-β1 is responsible for promoting stemness [5, 53]. The TGF-β1 inhibitor SB525334 significantly inhibited the migration and invasion of sphere-forming stemlike cells [54]. In an OS mouse model, either overexpression of the natural TGF-β/SMAD signaling inhibitor SMAD7 in OS cells or treatment with the TGF-β receptor inhibitor SD208 affected the microarchitectural parameters of the bone and inhibited lung metastasis [55]. The natural alkaloid halofuginone, an inhibitor of the TGF-β/Smad3 cascade, specifically hindered OS progression against lung metastatic dissemination [56]. All of these studies revealed that blocking TGF-β resulted in the repression of the tumorigenic potential of OS cell lines, tumor-associated bone remodeling, and the development of metastasis, highlighting TGF-β1 as a promising therapeutic target.

3.2. Hypoxia

The hypoxic niche plays a vital role in regulating tumor cell behavior. During tumor proliferation, oxygen is unable to diffuse completely throughout the tumor. On the other hand, if newly formed blood vessels cannot reach the tumor region, these results in an imbalance between oxygen consumption and acquisition and creates a hypoxic microenvironment. Hypoxia-inducible factors (HIFs) are associated with the maintenance of cellular oxygen equilibrium and hypoxia adaptation when oxygen levels cannot meet the demand [57]. Hypoxic signaling promotes the expression and function of HIF-1α and HIF-2α.

It has been reported that in OS, HIF-1α is associated with drug resistance and/or radioresistance via either activation of Bcl-2 proapoptotic family-induced AMP-activated protein kinase (AMPK) signaling or an autophagy mechanism [58]. The downregulation of HIF-1α suppresses OS cell growth by inducing apoptosis [59], and the HIF-1α/CXCR4 pathways contribute to metastasis in human OS cells [60]. A recent meta-analysis has suggested that overexpression of HIF-1α is a predictive factor for poor outcomes in OS and could serve as a promising prognostic biomarker to predict the outcome of OS patients [61, 62].

HIF-2α plays a role in the maintenance of stem cell properties in both normal and cancer stem cells [63, 64]. It has been indicated that the long noncoding RNA (lncRNA) TCONS_00004241, also known as HIF-2α promoter upstream transcript (HIF2PUT), was associated with the sphere-forming capacity of CD133-positive OS stem cells. Overexpression of HIF2PUT markedly decreased the percentage of CD133-expressing cells in the MG-63 OS cell line and impaired their proliferation, migration, and self-renewal capacities [65]. These results suggest that HIF2PUT and the HIF-2α axis could provide a hypoxia-mediated therapeutic strategy to targeting stemlike cells in OS.

HIF is highly expressed in CSCs in various types of cancer, and blockade of either HIF-1α or HIF-2α activity would significantly attenuate the proliferation and self-renewal of CSCs [66]. Targeting the hypoxic microenvironment could be a possible therapeutic strategy to eradicate the CSC population in malignant tumors including OS. Researchers exposed highly metastatic mouse OS cells to hyperbaric oxygen and measured the cell viability. Cell proliferation was significantly suppressed under hyperbaric oxygen conditions, and a hyperbaric oxygen treatment in combination with carboplatin exhibited significant synergy in the suppression of cell proliferation. Concomitant hyperbaric oxygen enhanced the chemotherapeutic effects of carboplatin on both tumor growth and lung metastasis and reduced the mortality of OS-bearing mice. These findings suggested that the concomitant treatment of hyperbaric oxygen plus carboplatin could be an efficient therapeutic strategy for OS treatment [67].

4. Glycolysis in osteosarcoma

Metabolic reprogramming is considered to be a prominent hallmark in cancer [68]. In the 1920s, Otto Warburg found that cancer cells were prone to glycolysis even under aerobic conditions, while most of the surrounding normal cells underwent oxidative phosphorylation. This phenomenon, known as the "Warburg effect," has been confirmed in cancers from different tissues [69]. Although ATP productivity via glycolysis is lower than that via oxidative phosphorylation, glycolysis provides tumor cells with a stronger adaptability to a hypoxic environment caused by the lack of vasculature. Furthermore, glycolysis intermediates can provide precursors such as lipids, proteins, and nucleotides for the synthesis of macromolecules needed for proliferation [70].

The oxidative phosphorylation levels in different OS cell lines (LM7, 143B, SaOS-2, and HOS) were evaluated compared with those in noncancerous counterpart osteoblastic hFOB cells. The results showed that two of the OS cell lines (SaOS-2 and HOS) were actively respiring, whereas LM7 and 143B were highly glycolytic. Further analysis of the mitochondrion in the latter cell lines indicated mitochondrial swelling, depolarization, and membrane permeabilization, all of which could explain their reliance on glycolysis [13].

In OS, glycolysis might be caused by either gene mutation or a hyperactivated metabolic pathway. For example, the tumor suppressor p53, which is well characterized in safeguarding the body from developing OS [71], is important in the maintenance of the cytochrome C oxidase complex. The dysfunction of p53 can lead to reduced oxygen consumption from mitochondrial respiration and enhanced glycolysis [72]. The PI3K-Akt-mTOR pathway, a key oncogenic pathway in multiple human cancers that promotes glucose metabolism and cell proliferation, is frequently hyperactivated in OS and leads to glycolysis [73, 74].

Although the significance of glycolysis in OS is still under investigation, its value regarding clinical diagnosis and treatment has already been proven. 18F-Fluorodeoxyglucose (FDG)-positron emission tomography/computed tomography (PET/CT) has emerged as a promising tool for the diagnosis and prognosis for OS based on its ability to quantify glucose consumption. In several studies, patients with OS had undergone 18F-FDG PET/CT scans to measure imaging parameters such as the maximum standardized uptake value, metabolic tumor volume, and total lesion glycolysis both before and after chemotherapy. Significant differences between nonresponding tumors and responding lesions were observed and therefore could be used as predictors of the histological response to chemotherapy and patient survival [75, 76].

Lactate dehydrogenase A (LDHA) is a key enzyme involved in anaerobic glycolysis and converts pyruvate into lactate. It is upregulated in OS compared to normal OB cells (hFOB1.19). LDHA inhibition could decrease lactate production, inhibit cell proliferation and invasion in vitro, and compromise tumorigenesis in vivo [77]. 2-Deoxy-D-glucose (2DG), a glucose analogue, can be used as a glycolysis inhibitor which decreases lactate production, enhances oxidative phosphorylation, inhibits the metastatic phenotype in vitro, and delays metastasis in an orthotopic post-surgical model [78]. 2-DG is also used in combination with either adriamycin (ADR) or paclitaxel in animal models for the treatment of human OS and non-small-cell lung cancer [79].

As a heterogeneous entity with multicomponent interactions, the progression of OS depends upon reciprocal interactions between the neoplastic cells and the dynamic microenvironment. Tumor microenvironments include ECM, immune cells, endothelial cells, pericytes, fibroblasts, MSCs, adipocytes, and other components [80, 81]. Recent studies have described metabolic coupling among stromal cells such as cancer-associated fibroblasts (CAFs), adipocytes, immune cells, and neoplastic cells [82–90]. Glycolytic CAFs can provide nutrients such as lactates and ketones as fuel for tumor cells [82–84]. Adipocytes produce free fatty acids and promote fatty acid oxidation in tumor cells [85]. MSCs cocultured with OS cells can lead to metabolic reprogramming in both MSCs and neoplastic cells as described by the Warburg effect. After coculturing, MSCs underwent a metabolic shift toward aerobic glycolysis with increased lactate production and efflux due to the upregulation of monocarboxylate transporter-4 (MCT-4). In the meantime, OS cells would utilize lactate by increasing MCT-1 expression to enhance mitochondrial biogenesis and oxidative phosphorylation. Interestingly, these MSC-activated SaOS-2 and HOS cells also acquired an increased migratory capacity [91].

5. Angiogenesis and vasculogenic mimicry

Vascularization plays an important role in tumor survival and progression. Angiogenesis and vasculogenic mimicry (VM) have been demonstrated to be the two major processes in the development of tumor vascularization system, which supplies cancer cells with blood.

The growth, invasion, and metastasis of solid tumors require an adequate blood supply to transport nutrition and oxygen as well as metabolic waste and carbon dioxide [68, 92]. Tumors have their own vascular system, which is, however, highly abnormal and different from the normal vasculature with respect to organization, structure, and function.

OS is a type of malignant bone tumor with abundant blood vessels, indicating the prominent functions of the vasculature in OS progression. Increased vasculature could be a poor prognostic factor in human OS [93]. Similarly, a decrease in the number of vessels was shown to significantly reduce primary OS growth in a mouse model [94]. Here, we intend to summarize the theoretical and clinical findings in OS angiogenesis and VM.

5.1. Angiogenesis in OS

Angiogenesis is a dynamic and programmed process in which new capillaries sprout from preexisting vessels, and is induced by different triggers (e.g., hypoxia) that modulate a broad range of molecular mechanisms manipulating tip cells and stalk cells [95]. Angiogenesis firstly demonstrated its correlation to tumor growth by inserting a transparent chamber into mouse ears [96]. Subsequently, in vitro tumor-induced angiogenesis was established with a wound chamber [97].

Clinical studies on OS angiogenesis are highly controversial. The first clinical discussion on the relationship between angiogenesis and long-term outcomes of patients with OS was published in 2001 [98]. A retrospective immunohistochemical study was performed on biopsy specimens from non-metastatic OS patients with CD34 antibody staining and quantified the average intratumoral microvessel density (MVD) per field, but results showed no correlation with long-term outcome in patients with non-metastatic OS. Additionally, angiogenesis was correlated with the overall and disease-free survival as well as the metastasis rates because patients with a higher MVD had a shorter survival time and a higher metastatic rate [99]. However, the quantification and analysis have been hampered by heterogeneous OS vascularization and non-standardized methods in detecting microvessels and small study cohorts. Recent study applied highly standardized whole-slide imaging to overcome these limitations. Intratumoral vascularization was quantified at the time of diagnosis in whole sections from a multicenter cohort of 131 osteosarcoma patients. The results suggested that patients with low OS vascularization have a prolonged survival and good response to neoadjuvant chemotherapy [100]. Moreover, inhibition of angiogenesis in murine OS by the angiogenic inhibitor TNP470 indicated an antitumor ability with higher cancer cell death rate and an effective suppression of pulmonary metastasis in an OS mouse model [101].

Vascular endothelial growth factor (VEGF), a homo-dimeric protein also known as VEGFA, is a key trigger to induce either physiological or pathological angiogenesis including OS [102]. Elevated expression of VEGF in primary OS notably promotes angiogenesis, increases the local MVD and perimeter, and subsequently leads to a prominently higher rate ($p < 0.05$) of pulmonary metastasis. These findings correlate with a worse outcome in terms of the disease-free survival and overall survival in untreated patients [103, 104]. Furthermore, patients with serum VEGF > 1000 pg/ml had significantly worse survival than patients with levels < 1000 pg/ml ($p = 0.002$) despite the lack of a link between serum VEGF levels and the tumor volume as well as the sensitivity to preoperative chemotherapy [105]. The transcription level of VEGF isoform variants and VEGF receptors (Flt-1 and KDR) was detected in 30 OS samples. Interestingly, the cell-retained VEGF isoforms VEGF165 and VEGF189 might be critical for neovascularization in OS, while the soluble VEGF121 isoform is insufficient to stimulate neovascularization in this type of neoplasm [106]. This also indicated that only specific types of VEGF isoforms have the ability to induce OS angiogenesis. Orthotopic injection of human OS cells with either high or low VEGF expression into severe combined immunodeficient mice uncovered that high VEGF-expressing OS cells developed more malignant xenografts with earlier neoplasm formation, larger tumor size, more frequent invasion to the peritumoral tissue, and a higher rate of lung metastasis [107]. VEGF blockade by sFlt1 in a murine model partially abrogated the angiogenesis and delayed VEGF-promoted tumor growth [108]. In view of the substantial influence of VEGF in OS progression, molecular regulation of VEGF in tumorigenesis and progression of OS has been studied in recent years. STAT3 has been determined as an important upstream regulator in VEGF expression, while the

PI3K-Akt pathway has been suggested as the main signaling cascade downstream of VEGF that mediates OS angiogenesis [109, 110]. Several studies also showed that members of the interleukin (IL) family, such as IL-6 and IL-17, could induce VEGF expression and promote angiogenesis in OS [111, 112]. The CXCL12-CXCR4 axis has additionally been demonstrated to be involved in promoting VEGF expression [113]. As opposed to the factors mentioned above, miR-145 targets VEGF and inhibits angiogenesis as well as the invasion and metastasis of OS cells [114].

Endostatin, a 20 kDa fragment of collagen XVIII, is a member of a group of endogenous anti-angiogenic proteins activated by proteolytic processing. Endostatin inhibits endothelial cell proliferation, migration, and invasion by modifying 12% of the human genome to downregulate pathological angiogenesis without exerting side effects, which makes this protein a broad-spectrum angiogenesis inhibitor. Anti-angiogenic therapy by endostatin was performed in OS-burdened mice models [115, 116]. Notably, the number of pulmonary metastatic lesions was lower, and the size of the pulmonary metastatic lesions was smaller in the group treated with endostatin compared to control group. Thus, anti-angiogenic therapy might be a potential treatment for OS because it provides patients with a promising improvement to their prognosis, although anti-angiogenic therapies cannot thoroughly cure OS [117].

5.2. Vasculogenic mimicry

Apart from the important role of angiogenesis in OS vessel network formation, VM has emerged as another effective pathway in OS vascular development. VM is defined as a type of vasculature-like lumen formed by tumor cells and the extracellular matrix instead of by endothelial cells and becomes incorporated into the tumor blood microcirculation. It was first reported in melanoma and identified by CD34-negative and periodic acid-Schiff (PAS)-positive staining in which red blood cells could be detected [118].

VM also has been detected in OS in vivo and in vitro. Immunohistochemical staining for endothelial cell marker CD34, OB-related marker osteocalcin, and PAS was performed on OS clinical samples. VM channels were confirmed in OS specimens in which the channel wall was positive for osteocalcin and PAS but negative for CD34 [119]. Further investigation by using the Kaplan-Meier survival analysis found that the present rate of VM in OS patients after preoperative chemotherapy was correlated with both the overall survival ($p = 0.011$ and 0.040) and metastasis-free survival ($p = 0.002$ and 0.045). Additionally, as a strong mediating factor in vascular formation, inhibition of VEGF by siRNA in the human OS cell line MG-63 could suppress VM formation in vitro [103]. Furthermore, vascular endothelial-cadherin (VE-cadherin) seems to be critical in the formation of VM. After knocking down VE-cadherin, OS cells could not form OS-generated endothelial-like networks in vitro [120].

Notably, unlike the typical $CD31^-/CD34^-/PAS^+$ VM, our group found that osteosarcoma stem cells (OSCs) had the capability to construct a CD31-positive vascular network de novo either under hypoxia or upon VEGFA induction [5]. This neo-VM subtype was formed by a type of vascular endothelial cell-like cells that transdifferentiated from OSCs as shown in **Figure 3**.

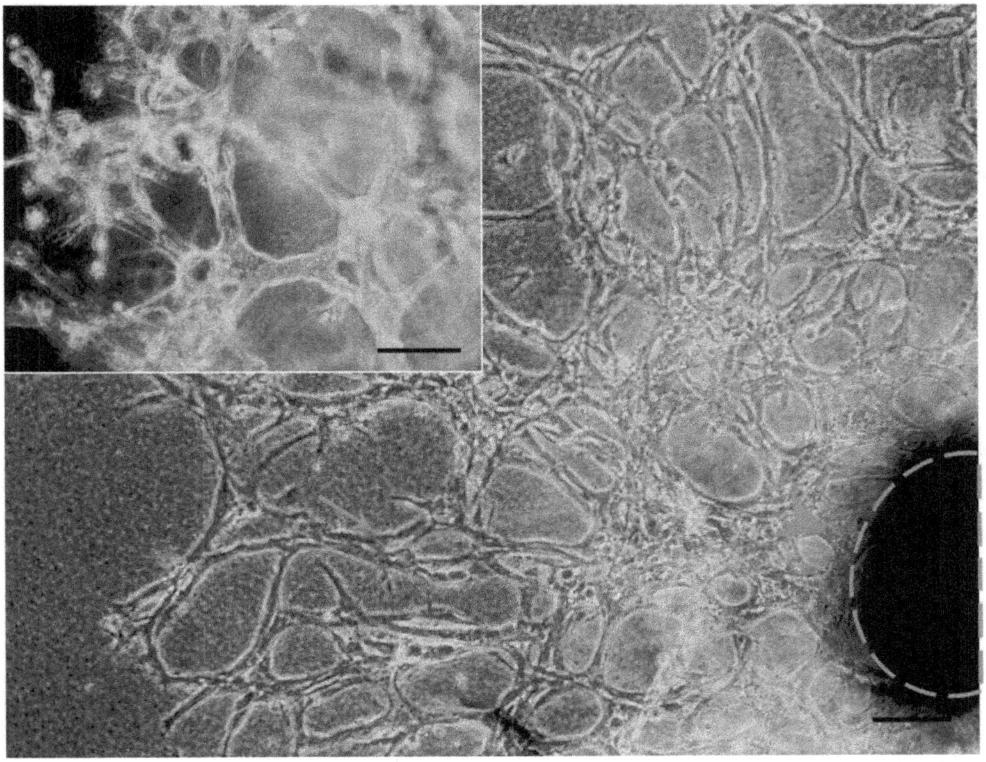

Figure 3. Differentiation potential of OSCs into vascular endothelial-like cells and formed vasculature-like network. During the transdifferentiation, vessel-like sprouts appeared around the outermost region of the OSCs (*arrowhead*), followed by the appearance of numerous branches (*arrow*). These branches extended out from the spheres and eventually formed a vasculature-like network. The *dotted line* and *arrowhead* show the region of the OSCs. The arrow indicates the vasculature-like network which is formed by vascular endothelial-like cells. High magnification image of the vasculature-like network is shown as an inset. Scale bar = 100 μm.

6. Stromal niche: bone marrow mesenchymal stem cell

OS is more often found in the distal femur and proximal tibia, which are also the major milieu of bone marrow MSCs. MSCs are a heterogeneous subpopulation of adult stem cells with immunomodulatory properties and a potential to differentiate into several tissue-specific cells such as OBs, adipocytes, and chondrocytes [121].

It is widely accepted that the tumor microenvironment is correlated with tumorigenesis and cancer progression. Since MSCs are one of the important components in the OS microenvironment, many studies have investigated the contribution of bone marrow MSCs to OS growth and progression. MSCs isolated from primary OS tissue, which show no neoplastic features, are similar to their bone marrow counterparts with regard to morphology, specific gene expression, and differentiation potential. Exogenous MSCs could target the OS site and promote OS growth and progression in a mouse xenograft model [122]. Similar results were also found in a rat model [123]. IL-6 secreted by MSCs could activate STAT3 signaling in OS cells, which in turn augment cell proliferation, migration, invasion, and pulmonary metastasis [124]. Interestingly, IL-6/STAT3 signaling could also respond to MSCs to enhance drug resistance. MSC-conditioned medium could improve the survival of U-2 OS and SaOS-2 cells and reduce apoptosis in the presence of therapeutic concentrations of either doxorubicin or cisplatin via the IL-6/STAT3 signaling pathway by increasing the expression of multidrug-resistant protein (MRP) and MDR-1 and decreasing the expression of caspase 3/7 activity and annexin V binding. Furthermore, the proliferation and progression of neoplastic cells need to be initiated and induced by certain pro-tumor cytokines secreted by MSCs. Therefore, OS cells could inhibit MSC differentiation into OBs via the TGF-β/Smad2/3 signaling pathway to promote the secretion of cytokines from MSCs [49].

Basic helix-loop-helix (bHLH) transcription factors belong to the third largest family of recognized transcription factors in the human genome and are essential regulators of development and differentiation via DNA-binding elements known as E boxes. DNA binding of bHLH proteins is restricted by heterodimerization with inhibitors of DNA binding (IDs). ID ubiquitination by ubiquitin-specific peptidase 1 (USP1) has been demonstrated to not only be necessary for the proliferation of several OS cell lines but also sufficient to prevent normal mesenchymal cell differentiation and sustain the cells in a stemlike state [125]. Meanwhile, a recent study uncovered a phenomenon of functional mitochondrial transfer from bone marrow stromal cells to acute myeloid leukemia (AML) cells during chemotherapy, which confers survival advantages for AML cells [126]. Altogether, preventing the differentiation of MSCs into OBs might remodel the bone microenvironment and provide OS cells with a more suitable survival niche.

As a vital component of the OS environment, MSCs might play a critical role in OS malignancy and could be a potential target in cancer therapy.

7. Emerging role: exosomes

Tumor cell function not only depends on self-regulation but also requires a significant assistance from the microenvironment to support growth and help with immune escape and motility through the local area. Approximately 15–20% of patients diagnosed with OS are observed as having detectable metastasis via X-ray examination. Additionally, more than 30% of patients will develop metachronous lung metastases, which makes clinical treatment more challenging [127, 128]. There is an urgent need for more studies on the early diagnosis of distant metastasis of OS. In recent years, more researchers have focused their concentration on an emerging role of extracellular vesicles, also referred to as exosomes, in cancer metastasis.

Exosomes are extracellular vesicles that originate within microvesicular bodies and are shed from plasma membrane with sizes in the range from 30 to 100 nm [129, 130]. Exosomes are unilamellar vesicles composed of a lipid bilayer and have a homogenous cup-shaped appearance based on scanning electron microscopy [131, 132]. The contents of exosomes are varied and heavily depend on the originating cells, but these are broadly considered to include proteins, mRNAs, miRNAs, lipids, and carbohydrates [133]. Exosomes have been recognized as important to intercellular communication among tumor cells [134]. However, related papers focusing on exosomes in OS are scarce and limited.

Exosomes isolated from the multidrug-resistant human OS cell line MG-63DXR30 by differential centrifugation of the culture media could be taken up into secondary cells and induce a doxorubicin-resistant phenotype, suggesting that exosomes play a potential critical role in transferring the multidrug-resistant phenotype [135]. A systematic comparison of the proteomes, exosomes, and exosome-free fractions was performed in MG-63, U-2 OS, and SaOS-2 cells. The results showed that OS cells can secrete different exosomes involved in angiogenesis, cell adhesion, and migration [136]. Additionally, it has been indicated that Notch-activating factors can be delivered to the murine muscle cells by exosomes from the murine OS cell line K7M2 and specifically increase Notch signaling pathway activation [137]. The urokinase plasminogen activator (uPA) is a serine protease involved in ECM degradation and plays a significant role in the progression and metastasis of various solid tumors including the breast, lung, prostate, pancreas, ovary, kidney, and colon [138]. The levels of uPA and the uPA receptor (uPAR) were exclusively elevated in metastatic OS cells. These metastatic OS cells secrete both an active soluble form and an exosome-encapsulated form of uPA to drive the migration or metastatic conversion of OS cells [139]. Other research demonstrated that exosomes secreted by human MSCs could exhibit antiapoptotic function or cell-protective function to increase OS survival under serum starvation conditions [140]. Exosomes may also be a neo-drug vector for OS treatment. For example, synthetic miR-143 can be enveloped in exosomes and transferred to OS cells exhibiting that the delivery of miR-143 via exosomes could significantly reduce the migration of OS cells [141].

In the future, research of the effects of exosome should be focused on its constituents in OS. As these microvesicles are involved in tumor progression, they might be the promising targets for cancer therapy. We could possibly identify tumor antigens to improve the diagnosis and prognosis of OS if exosome contents are associated to different levels of aggressiveness. Importantly, exosomes are easily isolated from the peripheral blood and other bodily fluids and could be used as a noninvasive diagnostic tool [142–144].

8. Mimicking the bone microenvironment

To reveal the process in detail that normal cells take to evolve to a neoplastic state and their subsequent progression to metastasis, proper research models need to be established. Establishment of an OS research model has always been challenging. Researchers initially used transgenic technology to reedit key genes in mice [145], but since then great strides have been made for the establishment and improvement of various OS animal models [6–10, 15, 146]. Despite all this, animal models and patient tissues are often limited by the availability of test subjects, feasibility of the testing procedure, and maintaining viable tissue. Furthermore, there are important ethical concerns regarding the compassion for experimental animals that may suffer pain or discomfort during the study. In vitro models have the advantage of easier availability and operability as well as reducing time and monetary costs.

Traditional two-dimensional cultures are most commonly used for the in vitro study of mammalian cells and have made remarkable contributions to scientific discovery. Even so, cultivation either on plastic dishes or in flasks rarely recapitulates the conditions of cell activities in vivo. The limitations of flat culturing regarding the cellular microenvironment have prompted the use of three-dimensional (3D) cultures [147]. The advantages of 3D cell culture include better mimicry of the cell-cell interactions and of the intricate microenvironment. In recent years, zebrafish models have been generated as a comprehensive stand-in for malignancy research and are especially appealing for OS because of their similarities to human osteogenesis [148–152]. More high-tech models are being created with the rapid development of engineering techniques. It is promising that these novel technologies could be applied in drug testing as well as other physiological and biochemical studies with the goal of replacing animal models to reduce the use of experimental animals.

8.1. Extracellular matrix

ECM is a collection of extracellular molecules that provides structural and biochemical support to the surrounding cells and therefore plays a vital role in cell adhesion, cell communication, and maintenance of function. In the case of the bone, the organic portion of ECM primarily comprises type I collagen secreted by OB lineage cells, while calcium phosphate in the form of hydroxyapatite composes its mineralized portion. Bone ECM provides a scaffold for mineral storage and regulates OB lineage and osteoclast lineage cell function and differentiation of MSCs to OBs [153]. The usage of bone ECM in tissue engineering and biological studies has attracted attention [154, 155]. Porcine cartilage was decellularized, solubilized, and then methacrylated, and ultraviolet (UV) photocrosslinked to create methacrylated solubilized decellularized cartilage hydrogels. These hydrogels were characteristically similar to native cartilage tissue and could support ECM production. Additionally, these hydrogels supported the growth of rat bone marrow-derived MSCs that were encapsulated in the gel networks and caused significant upregulation of chondrogenic genes [156]. Bone-like ECM synthesized by OBs was used to enhance the osteoblastic differentiation of MSCs in vitro [157], and decellularized cartilage ECM was applied as a treatment for osteochondral defects [158].

Our group has generated tissue-derived bone ECM from humans, mice, and rats and established an OS model that could mimic an intact OS environment in vitro by injecting OS cells into bone ECM. Bone ECM is soaked in cell-cultured medium after decalcification and decellularization, and OS cells are injected into ECM and cultured under complete medium. As shown in **Figure 4**, bone ECM provides a scaffold for OS cell proliferation and shows amazing biocompatibility.

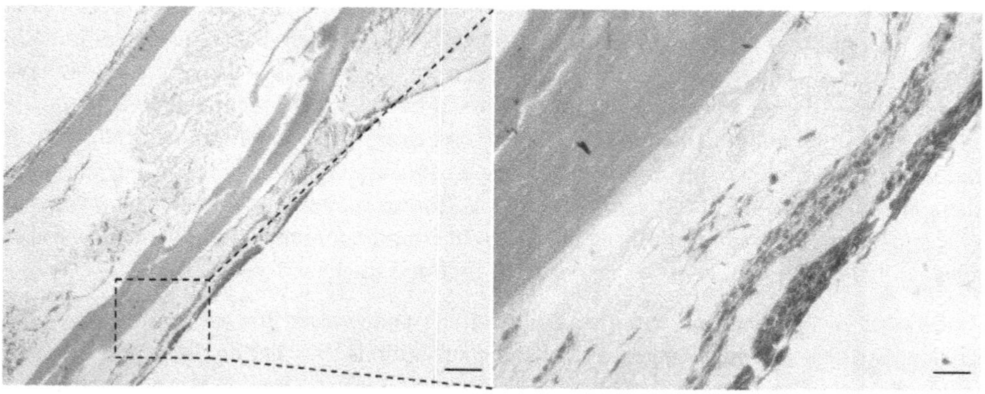

Figure 4. HE staining of mouse bone ECM after injecting MNNG/HOS (unpublished data). Scale bar = 100 μm.

8.2. Zebrafish: an in vivo model for OS research

Zebrafish is an important and widely used vertebrate model in scientific research. In recent years, they have become a useful model for cancer and other diseases due to their straightforward genome information with abundantly conserved regions homologous with those in human beings, their small size and ease of manipulation, and their transparent bodies which make observation of organ systems easy. Compared to the 3D model, zebrafish can address the issue of maturation, which is a virtually insurmountable barrier of in vitro development.

As a multifunctional model, zebrafish with genetic modifications have been used in a large number of experiments. Transgenic zebrafish with a GFP-tagged vasculature provide an advanced approach for the study of angiogenesis and cancer metastasis and can easily be observed by either light microscopy (**Figure 5**) or laser confocal microscopy. Furthermore, leukemia, melanoma, pancreatic adenocarcinoma, intestinal hyperplasia, and other types of solid tumor have been studied in zebrafish models, which are stable and effective assay method for investigating pathogenesis.

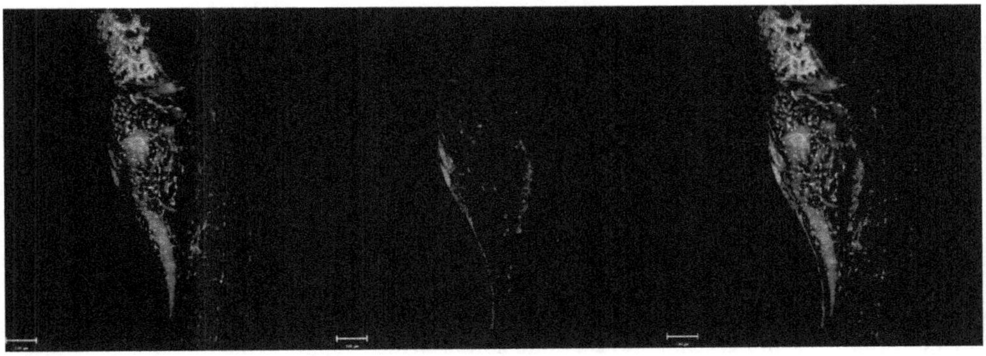

Figure 5. The FLK^{+}-GFP zebrafish showed a green vasculature system photographed by light sheet microscopy (unpublished data). Scale bar = 100 μm.

An OS xenograft zebrafish model has also been reported recently [159]. Since OS probably originates from MSCs mutated in the process of differentiation toward OBs, one group injected two MSC cell lines, after 8 months of culturing, and found that the cells gained a malignant transformation. The results found that transformed MSCs formed an OS mass, induced angiogenesis, and migrated through the bodies of the embryos of zebrafish, which was not observed in the normal MSC controls. Whole-genome analysis indicated higher expression of matrix metalloproteinase 19 (MMP-19) and erythroblastosis virus E26 oncogene homologue 1 (Ets-1) in the mutated cells compared to normal cells. Furthermore, upon investigation the host response, zebrafish embryos injected with transformed MSCs showed decreased expression of immune response-related genes, especially major histocompatibility complex class I (MHC-I), compared to embryos injected with normal MSCs. The above experiments also reproduced tumorigenesis, progression of OS, including angiogenesis, migration, and metastasis in vivo and identified potential molecular regulators by using a zebrafish model.

Zebrafish is also a useful tool for screening for OS therapeutic drugs. The development of metastases is still the major cause of death of patients with OS as well as other cancers. Ezrin, the prototypical ezrin/radixin/moesin (ERM) protein family member, is associated with the actin cytoskeleton and the plasma membrane. Ezrin has been demonstrated to be a vital protein related to cancer metastasis. Microinjection of ezrin small-molecule inhibitors, NSC305787 and NSC668394, into zebrafish embryos prominently inhibited cell mobility during embryonic development. The results supported an approach using ezrin protein as a putative target molecule in OS therapy [160].

8.3. Other novel OS models

With their advantages of in vivo vascularization and an immune system, animal models can be instrumental for executing drug screens and studying the etiology of OS. Apart from the cell-of-origin transgenic models and the zebrafish models mentioned above, there are more novel therapeutic interventions in various models that have already been reported or are in current veterinary clinical trials [161].

OS is an aggressive primary bone cancer with highly metastatic capacity, and the development of pulmonary metastases is the most common reason for treatment failure. K7M3 cells were injected into the tibia of wild-type BALB/c mice to induce a primary bone tumor or into the tail vein of wild-type BALB/c and gld mice to form pulmonary metastases [162]. To assess the importance of Fas in the process of OS lung metastasis, two animal models for lung metastases were generated through intravenous injection or subcutaneous injection in mice, and those proved the efficacy of aerosol gemcitabine (GCB) which targets Fas pathway [163].

The assessment of the safety issue of a regional aerosol GCB delivery and evaluation of the effect of GCB on Fas pathway in lung metastasis of OS-bearing dogs further confirmed clinical and pathological findings in mice [164]. The clinical and pathological findings in mice were further confirmed and extended in a canine model, which supports the notion that aerosolized gemcitabine may be useful against the pulmonary metastasis of OS and can allay patient tolerability concerns to a certain extent.

9. Conclusion

Multiple genomic aberrations together with abnormal activation of receptor kinases greatly contribute to the complex etiology of OS. There is no escaping the fact that in many respects, microenvironmental signals can either support or interrelate with tumor cells to regulate the biological behavior of OS. Although the remodeling systems established heretofore still require more precise characterization in vivo with respect to the extent of recapitulation, the utilization of physiological and biochemical studies can eventually be applied to clinical pharmacokinetic studies and evaluations of therapeutic efficiency. To gain exact and further insight on the cross talk between tumor cells and the microenvironment, both in vivo and in vitro novel models should be created and applied in research.

Author details

Yu Zhang, Qing Mai, Xiaowen Zhang, Chunyuan Xie and Yan Zhang*

*Address all correspondence to: zhang39@mail.sysu.edu.cn

Key Laboratory of Gene Engineering of the Ministry of Education, State Key Laboratory of Biocontrol, School of Life Sciences, Sun Yat-sen University, Guangzhou, China

References

[1] Berman SD, Calo E, Landman AS, et al. Metastatic osteosarcoma induced by inactivation of Rb and p53 in the osteoblast lineage. Proc Natl Acad Sci U S A. 2008 Aug 19;105(33):11851–11856. DOI: 10.1073/pnas.0805462105.

[2] Bielack SS, Kempf-Bielack B, Delling G, et al. Prognostic factors in high-grade osteosarcoma of the extremities or trunk: an analysis of 1702 patients treated on neoadjuvant cooperative osteosarcoma study group protocols. J Clin Oncol. 20:776–790. DOI: 10.1200/JCO.20.3.776.

[3] Overholtzer M, Rao PH, Favis R, et al. The presence of p53 mutations in human osteosarcomas correlates with high levels of genomic instability. Proc Natl Acad Sci U S A. 2003 Nov 25;100(24):14511. DOI: 10.1073/pnas.1934852100.

[4] Selvarajah S, Yoshimoto M, Maire G, et al. Identification of cryptic microaberrations in osteosarcoma by high-definition oligonucleotide array comparative genomic hybridization. Cancer Genet Cytogenet. 2007 Nov;179(1):52–61. DOI: 10.1016/j.cancergencyto.2007.08.003.

[5] Zhang H, Wu H, Zheng J, et al. Transforming growth factor β1 signal is crucial for dedifferentiation of cancer cells to cancer stem cells in osteosarcoma. Stem Cells. 2013 Mar;31(3):433–446. DOI: 10.1002/stem.1298.

[6] Basu-Roy U, Basilico C, Mansukhani A. Perspectives on cancer stem cells in osteosarcoma. Cancer Lett. 2013 Sep 10;338(1):158–167. DOI: 10.1016/j.canlet.2012.05.028.

[7] Rubio R, Abarrategi A, Garcia-Castro J, et al. Bone environment is essential for osteosarcoma development from transformed mesenchymal stem cells. Stem Cells. 2014 May;32(5):1136–1148. DOI: 10.1002/stem.1647.

[8] Mohseny AB, Szuhai K, Romeo S, et al. Osteosarcoma originates from mesenchymal stem cells in consequence of aneuploidization and genomic loss of Cdkn2. J Pathol. 2009 Nov;219(3):294–305. DOI: 10.1002/path.2603.

[9] Dung-Fang Lee, Jie Su, Huen Suk, et al. Modeling familial cancer with induced pluripotent stem cells. Cell. 2015 Apr 9;161(2):240–254. DOI: 10.1016/j.cell.2015.02.045.

[10] Sato S, Tang YJ, Wei Q, et al. Mesenchymal tumors can derive from Ng2/Cspg4-expressing pericytes with β-catenin modulating the neoplastic phenotype. Cell Rep. 2016 Jul 13. DOI: 10.1016/j.celrep.2016.06.058.

[11] Nowell PC. The clonal evolution of tumor cell populations. Science. 1976 Oct 1;194(4260):23–28. DOI: 10.1126/science.959840.

[12] Varley JM. Germline TP53 mutations and Li-Fraumeni syndrome. Hum Mutat. 2003 Mar;21(3):313–320. DOI:10.1002/humu.10185.

[13] Velletri T, Xie N, Wang Y, et al. P53 functional abnormality in mesenchymal stem cells promotes osteosarcoma development. Cell Death Dis. 2016 Jan 21;7:e2015. DOI: 10.1038/cddis.2015.367.

[14] Chen X, Bahrami A, Pappo A, et al. Recurrent somatic structural variations contribute to tumorigenesis in pediatric osteosarcoma. Cell Rep. 2014 Apr 10;7(1):104–112. DOI: 10.1016/j.celrep.2014.03.003.

[15] Saalfrank A, Janssen KP, Ravon M, et al. A porcine model of osteosarcoma. Oncogenesis. 2016 Mar;5(3):e210. DOI: 10.1038/oncsis.2016.19.

[16] Maitra A, Roberts H, Weinberg AG, Geradts J. Loss of p16INK4a expression correlates with decreased survival in pediatric osteosarcomas. Int J Cancer. 95:34–38. DOI: 10.1002/1097-0215(20010120)95:1<34::AID-IJC1006>3.0.CO;2-V.

[17] Xiong Y, Wu S, Du Q, et al. Integrated analysis of gene expression and genomic aberration data in osteosarcoma (OS). Cancer Gene Ther. 2015 Nov;22(11):524–529. DOI: 10.1038/cgt.2015.48.

[18] Ma O, Cai WW, Zender L, et al. MMP13, Birc2 (cIAP1), and Birc3 (cIAP2), amplified on chromosome 9, collaborate with p53 deficiency in mouse osteosarcoma progression. Cancer Res. 2009 Mar 15;69(6):2559–2567. DOI: 10.1158/0008-5472.CAN-08-2929.

[19] Ambros V. The functions of animal microRNAs. Nature. 2004 Sep 16;431(7006):350–355. DOI: 10.1038/nature02871.

[20] Bartel DP. microRNAs: genomics, biogenesis, mechanism, and function. Cell. 2004 Jan 23;116(2):281–297. DOI:10.1016/S0092-8674(04)00045-5.

[21] Subramanian S, Lui WO, Lee CH, et al. MicroRNA expression signature of human sarcomas. Oncogene. 2008;27:2015–2026. DOI: 10.1038/sj.onc.1210836.

[22] Israel A, Sharan R, Ruppin E, Galun E. Increased microRNA activity in human cancers. PLoS One. 2009;4:e6045. DOI: 10.1371/journal.pone.0006045.

[23] Ambs S, Prueitt RL, Yi M, et al. Genomic profiling of microRNA and messenger RNA reveals deregulated microRNA expression in prostate cancer. Cancer Res. 2008; 68:6162–6170. DOI: 10.1158/0008-5472.CAN-08-0144.

[24] Maire G, Martin JW, Yoshimoto M, et al. Analysis of miRNA-gene expression-genomic profiles reveals complex mechanisms of microRNA deregulation in osteosarcoma. Cancer Genet. 2011 Mar;204(3):138–146. DOI: 10.1016/j.cancergen.2010.12.012.

[25] Yang C, Yang S, Wood KB, et al. Multidrug resistant osteosarcoma cell lines exhibit deficiency of GADD45alpha expression. Apoptosis. 2009 Jan;14(1):124–133. DOI: 10.1007/s10495-008-0282-x.

[26] Pellegrino R, Calvisi DF, Ladu S, et al. Oncogenic and tumor suppressive roles of polo-like kinases in human hepatocellular carcinoma. Hepatology. 2010 Mar;51(3):857–868. DOI: 10.1002/hep.23467.

[27] Wang S, Aurora AB, Johnson BA, et al. The endothelial-specific microRNA miR-126 governs vascular integrity and angiogenesis. Dev Cell. 2008 Aug;15(2):261–271. DOI: 10.1016/j.devcel.2008.07.002.

[28] He C, Xiong J, Xu X, et al. Functional elucidation of miR-34 in osteosarcoma cells and primary tumor samples. Biochem Biophys Res Commun. 2009 Oct 9;388(1):35–40. DOI: 10.1016/j.bbrc.2009.07.101.

[29] Lodygin D, Tarasov V, Epanchintsev A, et al. Inactivation of miR-34a by aberrant CpG methylation in multiple types of cancer. Cell Cycle. 2008 Aug 15;7(16):2591–2600. DOI:10.4161/cc.7.16.6533.

[30] Pu Y, Zhao F, Wang H, et al. MiR-34a-5p promotes the multi-drug resistance of osteosarcoma by targeting the CD117 gene. Oncotarget. 2016 Apr 1. DOI: 10.18632/oncotarget.8546.

[31] Yan K, Gao J, Yang T, et al. MicroRNA-34a inhibits the proliferation and metastasis of osteosarcoma cells both *in vitro* and *in vivo*. PLoS One. 2012;7(3):e33778. DOI: 10.1371/journal.pone.0033778.

[32] Rong S, Donehower LA, Hansen MF, et al. Met proto-oncogene product is overexpressed in tumors of p53-deficient mice and tumors of Li-Fraumeni patients. Cancer Res. 1995 May 1;55(9):1963–1970.

[33] Maroun CR, Rowlands T. The Met receptor tyrosine kinase: a key player in oncogenesis and drug resistance. Pharmacol Ther. 2014 Jun;142(3):316–338. doi: 10.1016/j.pharmthera.2013.12.014.

[34] Patanè S, Avnet S, Coltella N, et al. MET overexpression turns human primary osteoblasts into osteosarcomas. Cancer Res. 2006, 1;66(9):4750–4757. DOI: 10.1158/0008-5472.CAN-05-4422.

[35] Wang K, Zhuang Y, Liu C, Li Y. Inhibition of c-Met activation sensitizes osteosarcoma cells to cisplatin via suppression of the PI3K-Akt signaling. Arch Biochem Biophys. 2012 Oct 1;526(1):38–43. doi: 10.1016/j.abb.2012.07.003.

[36] Baldanzi G, Pietronave S, Locarno D, et al. Diacylglycerol kinases are essential for hepatocyte growth factor-dependent proliferation and motility of Kaposi's sarcoma cells. Cancer Sci. 2011 Jul;102(7):1329–1336. DOI: 10.1111/j.1349-7006.2011.01953.

[37] Gibbs CP, Kukekov VG, Reith JD, et al. Stem-like cells in bone sarcomas: implications for tumorigenesis. Neoplasia. 2005;7:967–976.

[38] Yan GN, Lv YF, Guo QN. Advances in osteosarcoma stem cell research and opportunities for novel therapeutic targets. Cancer Lett. 2016 Jan 28;370(2):268–274. DOI:10.1016/j.canlet.2015.11.003.

[39] Adhikari AS, Agarwal N, Wood BM, et al. CD117 and Stro-1 identify osteosarcoma tumor-initiating cells associated with metastasis and drug resistance. Cancer Res. 2010 Jun 1;70(11):4602–4612. doi: 10.1158/0008-5472.CAN-09-3463].

[40] Fujii H, Honoki K, Tsujiuchi T, et al. Sphere-forming stem-like cell populations with drug resistance in human sarcoma cell lines. Int J Oncol. 2009 May;34(5):1381–1386. DOI: 10.3892/ijo_00000265.

[41] Martins-Neves SR, Lopes ÁO, do Carmo A, et al. Therapeutic implications of an enriched cancer stem-like cell population in a human osteosarcoma cell line. BMC Cancer. 2012 Apr 4;12:139. DOI: 10.1186/1471-2407-12-139.

[42] Gonçalves C, Martins-Neves SR, Paiva-Oliveira D, et al. Sensitizing osteosarcoma stem cells to doxorubicin-induced apoptosis through retention of doxorubicin and modulation of apoptotic-related proteins. Life Sci. 2015 Jun 1;130:47–56. DOI: 10.1016/j.lfs.2015.03.009.

[43] Mongre RK, Sodhi SS, Ghosh M, et al. The novel inhibitor BRM270 downregulates tumorigenesis by suppression of NF-κB signaling cascade in MDR-induced stem like cancer-initiating cells. Int J Oncol. 2015;46(6):2573–2585. DOI: 10.3892/ijo.2015.2961.

[44] Menendez JA, Alarcón T, Corominas-Faja B, et al. Reprogramming the epigenetic landscapes of patient-derived cancer genomes. Cell Cycle. 2014 Feb 1;13(3):358–370. DOI: 10.4161/cc.27770.

[45] Yang RS, Wu CT, Lin KH, et al. Relation between histological intensity of transforming growth factor-beta isoforms in human osteosarcoma and the rate of lung metastasis. Tohoku J Exp Med. 1998;184(2):133–142.

[46] Li F, Li S, Cheng T. TGF-β1 promotes osteosarcoma cell migration and invasion through the miR-143-versican pathway. Cell Physiol Biochem. 2014;34(6):2169–2179. DOI: 10.1159/000369660.

[47] Liu Y, Zheng QX, Du JY, et al. Effects of TGF beta1 autocrine blockage on osteosarcoma cells. Chin Med Sci J. 2004 Jun;19(2):155–156.

[48] Silva G, Aboussekhra A. p16(INK4A) inhibits the pro-metastatic potentials of osteosarcoma cells through targeting the ERK pathway and TGF-β1. Mol Carcinog. 2016 May;55(5):525–536. DOI: 10.1002/mc.22299.

[49] Tu B, Peng ZX, Fan QM et al. Osteosarcoma cells promote the production of pro-tumor cytokines in mesenchymal stem cells by inhibiting their osteogenic differentiation through the TGF-β/Smad2/3 pathway. Exp Cell Res. 2014 Jan 1;320(1):164–173. DOI: 10.1016/j.yexcr.2013.10.013.

[50] Hung SP, Yang MH, Tseng KF, Lee OK. Hypoxia-induced secretion of TGF-β1 in mesenchymal stem cell promotes breast cancer cell progression. Cell Transplant. 2013;22(10):1869–1882. DOI: 10.3727/096368912X657954.

[51] Massagué J. TGFbeta in cancer. Cell. 2008 Jul 25;134(2):215–230. DOI: 10.1016/j.cell.2008.07.001.

[52] Copson ER, White HE, Blaydes JP, et al. Influence of the MDM2 single nucleotide polymorphism SNP309 on tumor development in BRCA1 mutation carriers. BMC Cancer. 2006;6(1):80–86. DOI: 10.1186/1471-2407-6-80.

[53] Liu F, Kong X, Lv L, Gao J. TGF-β1 acts through miR-155 to down-regulate TP53INP1 in promoting epithelial-mesenchymal transition and cancer stem cell phenotypes. Cancer Lett. 2015 Apr 10;359(2):288–298. DOI: 10.1016/j.canlet.2015.01.030.

[54] Yue D, Zhang Z, Li J, et al. Transforming growth factor-beta1 promotes the migration and invasion of sphere-forming stem-like cell subpopulations in esophageal cancer. Exp Cell Res. 2015 Aug 1;336(1):141–149. DOI: 10.1016/j.yexcr.2015.06.007.

[55] Lamora A, Talbot J, Bougras G, et al. Overexpression of smad7 blocks primary tumor growth and lung metastasis development in osteosarcoma. Clin Cancer Res. 2014 Oct 1;20(19):5097–5112. DOI: 10.1158/1078-0432.CCR-13-3191.

[56] Lamora A, Mullard M, Amiaud J, et al. Anticancer activity of halofuginone in a preclinical model of osteosarcoma: inhibition of tumor growth and lung metastases. Oncotarget. 2015 Jun 10;6(16):14413–14427. DOI: 10.18632/oncotarget.3891.

[57] Kumar V, Gabrilovich DI. Hypoxia-inducible factors in regulation of immune responses in tumor microenvironment. Immunology. 2014 Dec;143(4):512–519. DOI: 10.1111/imm.12380.

[58] Feng H, Wang J, Chen W, et al. Hypoxia-induced autophagy as an additional mechanism in human osteosarcoma radioresistance. J Bone Oncol. 2016 Mar 9;5(2):67–73. DOI: 10.1016/j.jbo.2016.03.001.

[59] Lv F, Du R, Shang W, et al. HIF-1α silencing inhibits the growth of osteosarcoma cells by inducing apoptosis. Ann Clin Lab Sci. 2016 Mar;46(2):140–146.

[60] Guan G, Zhang Y, Lu Y, et al. The HIF-1α/CXCR4 pathway supports hypoxia-induced metastasis of human osteosarcoma cells. Cancer Lett. 2015 Feb 1;357(1):254–264. DOI: 10.1016/j.canlet.2014.11.034.

[61] Ren HY, Zhang YH, Li HY, et al. Prognostic role of hypoxia-inducible factor-1 alpha expression in osteosarcoma: a meta-analysis. Onco Targets Ther. 2016 Mar 14;9:1477–1487. DOI: 10.2147/OTT.S95490.

[62] Ouyang Y, Li H, Bu J, et al. Hypoxia-inducible factor-1 expression predicts osteosarcoma patients' survival: a meta-analysis. Int J Biol Markers. 2016 Jun 11. DOI: 10.5301/jbm.5000216.

[63] Covello KL, Kehler J, Yu H, et al. HIF-2alpha regulates Oct-4: effects of hypoxia on stem cell function, embryonic development, and tumor growth. Genes Dev. 2006;20:557–570. DOI: 10.1101/gad.1399906.

[64] Gordan JD, Bertout JA, Hu CJ, et al. HIF-2alpha promotes hypoxic cell proliferation by enhancing c-myc transcriptional activity. Cancer Cell. 2007;11:335–347. DOI: 10.1016/j.ccr.2007.02.006.

[65] Wang Y, Yao J, Meng H, et al. A novel long non-coding RNA, hypoxia-inducible factor-2α promoter upstream transcript, functions as an inhibitor of osteosarcoma stem cells *in vitro*. Mol Med Rep. 2015 Apr;11(4):2534–2540. DOI: 10.3892/mmr.2014.3024.

[66] Zeng W, Wan R, Zheng Y, et al. Hypoxia, stem cells and bone tumor. Cancer Lett. 2011 Dec 27;313(2):129–136. DOI: 10.1016/j.canlet.2011.09.023.

[67] Kawasoe Y, Yokouchi M, Ueno Y, et al. Hyperbaric oxygen as a chemotherapy adjuvant in the treatment of osteosarcoma. Oncol Rep. 2009 Nov;22(5):1045–1050. DOI: 10.3892/or_00000534.

[68] Hanahan D, Weinberg RA. Hallmarks of cancer: the next generation. Cell. 2011 Mar 4;144(5):646–674. DOI: 10.1016/j.cell.2011.02.013.

[69] Martinez-Outschoorn UE, Peiris-Pagés M, Pestell RG, et al. Cancer metabolism: a therapeutic perspective. Nat Rev Clin Oncol. 2016 May 4. DOI: 10.1038/nrclinonc.2016.60.

[70] Mitsuishi Y, Taguchi K, Kawatani Y, et al. Nrf2 redirects glucose and glutamine into anabolic pathways in metabolic reprogramming. Cancer Cell. 2012 Jul 10;22(1):66–79. DOI: 10.1016/j.ccr.2012.05.016.

[71] Bensaad K, Vousden KH. p53: new roles in metabolism. Trends Cell Biol. 2007 Jun;17(6):286–291. DOI: 10.1016/j.tcb.2007.04.004.

[72] Giang AH, Raymond T, Brookes P, et al. Mitochondrial dysfunction and permeability transition in osteosarcoma cells showing the Warburg effect. J Biol Chem. 2013 Nov 15;288(46):33303–33311. DOI: 10.1074/jbc.M113.507129.

[73] Wang DW, Yu SY, Cao Y, et al. A novel mechanism of mTORC1-mediated serine/glycine metabolism in osteosarcoma development. Cell Signal. 2016 Jun 10. DOI: 10.1016/j.cellsig.2016.06.008.

[74] Gupte A, Baker EK, Wan SS, et al. Systematic screening identifies dual PI3K and mTOR inhibition as a conserved therapeutic vulnerability in osteosarcoma. Clin Cancer Res. 2015 Jul 15;21(14):3216–3229. DOI: 10.1158/1078-0432.CCR-14-3026.

[75] Im HJ, Kim TS, Park SY, et al. Prediction of tumor necrosis fractions using metabolic and volumetric 18F-FDG PET/CT indices, after one course and at the completion of neoadjuvant chemotherapy, in children and young adults with osteosarcoma. Eur J Nucl Med Mol Imaging. 2012 Jan;39(1):39–49. DOI: 10.1007/s00259-011-1936-4.

[76] Byun BH, Kong CB, Park J, et al. Initial metabolic tumor volume measured by 18F-FDG PET/CT can predict the outcome of osteosarcoma of the extremities. J Nucl Med. 2013 Oct;54(10):1725–1732. DOI: 10.2967/jnumed.112.117697.

[77] Gao S, Tu DN, Li H, et al. Pharmacological or genetic inhibition of LDHA reverses tumor progression of pediatric osteosarcoma. Biomed Pharmacother. 2016 Jul;81:388–393. DOI: 10.1016/j.biopha.2016.04.029.

[78] Sottnik JL, Lori JC, Rose BJ, Thamm DH. Glycolysis inhibition by 2-deoxy-d-glucose reverts the metastatic phenotype *in vitro* and *in vivo*. Clin Exp Metastasis. 2011 Dec;28(8):865–875. DOI: 10.1007/s10585-011-9417-5.

[79] Maschek G, Savaraj N, Priebe W, et al. 2-deoxy-D-glucose increases the efficacy of adriamycin and paclitaxel in human osteosarcoma and non-small cell lung cancers *in vivo*. Cancer Res. 2004 Jan 1;64(1):31–34. DOI: 10.1158/0008-5472.CAN-03-3294.

[80] Hanahan D, Coussens LM. Accessories to the crime: functions of cells recruited to the tumor microenvironment. Cancer Cell. 2012 Mar 20;21(3):309–322. DOI: 10.1016/j.ccr.2012.02.022.

[81] Mueller MM, Fusenig NE. Friends or foes—bipolar effects of the tumor stroma in cancer. Nature Nat Rev Cancer. 2004 Nov;4(11):839–849. DOI: 10.1038/nrc1477.

[82] Martinez-Outschoorn UE, Lisanti MP, Sotgia F. Catabolic cancer-associated fibroblasts transfer energy and biomass to anabolic cancer cells, fueling tumor growth. Semin Cancer Biol. 2014 Apr;25:47–60. DOI: 10.1016/j.semcancer.2014.01.005.

[83] Chiavarina B, Whitaker-Menezes D, Migneco G, et al. HIF1-alpha functions as a tumor promoter in cancer-associated fibroblasts, and as a tumor suppressor in breast cancer cells. Cell Cycle. 2010 Sep 1;9(17):3534–3551. DOI: 10.4161/cc.9.17.12908.

[84] Rattigan YI, Patel BB, Ackerstaff E, et al. Lactate is a mediator of metabolic cooperation between stromal carcinoma associated fibroblasts and glycolytic tumor cells in the tumor microenvironment. Exp Cell Res. 2012 Feb 15;318(4):326–335. DOI: 10.1016/j.yexcr.2011.11.014.

[85] Nieman KM, Kenny HA, Penicka CV, et al. Adipocytes promote ovarian cancer metastasis and provide energy for rapid tumor growth. Nat Med. 2011 Oct 30;17(11):1498–1503. DOI: 10.1038/nm.2492.

[86] Garris CS, Pittet MJ. ER stress in dendritic cells promotes cancer. Cell. 2015 Jun 18;161(7):1492–1493. DOI: 10.1016/j.cell.2015.06.006.

[87] Cubillos-Ruiz JR, Silberman PC, Rutkowski MR, et al. ER stress sensor XBP1 controls anti-tumor immunity by disrupting dendritic cell homeostasis. Cell. 2015 Jun 18;161(7):1527–1538. DOI: 10.1016/j.cell.2015.05.025.

[88] Chang CH, Qiu J, O'Sullivan D, et al. Metabolic competition in the tumor microenvironment is a driver of cancer progression. Cell. 2015 Sep 10;162(6):1229–1241. DOI: 10.1016/j.cell.2015.08.016.

[89] Ho PC, Bihuniak JD, Macintyre AN, et al. Phosphoenolpyruvate is a metabolic checkpoint of anti-tumor T cell responses. Cell. 2015 Sep 10;162(6):1217–1228. DOI: 10.1016/j.cell.2015.08.012.

[90] Chang CH, Curtis JD, Maggi LB Jr, et al. Posttranscriptional control of T cell effector function by aerobic glycolysis. Cell. 2013 Jun 6;153(6):1239–1251. DOI: 10.1016/j.cell.2013.05.016.

[91] Bonuccelli G, Avnet S, Grisendi G. Role of mesenchymal stem cells in osteosarcoma and metabolic reprogramming of tumor cells. Oncotarget. 2014 Sep 15;5(17):7575–7588. DOI: 10.18632/oncotarget.2243.

[92] Folkman J. Tumor angiogenesis: therapeutic implications. N Engl J Med. 1971 Nov 18;285(21):1182–1186. DOI: 10.1056/NEJM197111182852108.

[93] Handa A, Tokunaga T, Tsuchida T, et al. Neuropilin-2 expression affects the increased vascularization and is a prognostic factor in osteosarcoma. Int J Oncol. 2000 Aug;17(2):291–295. DOI: 10.3892/ijo.17.2.291.

[94] Habel N, Vilalta M, Bawa O, et al. Cyr61 silencing reduces vascularization and dissemination of osteosarcoma tumors. Oncogene. 2015 Jun 11;34(24):3207–3213. DOI: 10.1038/onc.2014.232.

[95] Clark ER, Clark EL. Observations on living preformed blood vessels as seen in a transparent chamber inserted into the rabbit's ear. Am J Anat. 1932;49(3):441–477. DOI: 10.1002/aja.1000490306.

[96] Gerhardt H, Golding M, Fruttiger M, et al. VEGF guides angiogenic sprouting utilizing endothelial tip cell filopodia. J Cell Biol. 2003 Jun 23;161(6):1163–1177. DOI: 10.1083/jcb.200302047.

[97] Algire GH, Chalkley HW, Legallais FY, Park HD. Vasculae reactions of normal and malignant tissues *in vivo*. I. Vascular reactions of mice to wounds and to normal and neoplastic transplants. J Natl Cancer Inst. 1945;6(1):73–85. DOI: 10.1093/jnci/6.1.73.

[98] Mantadakis E, Kim G, Reisch J, et al. Lack of prognostic significance of intratumoral angiogenesis in nonmetastatic osteosarcoma. J Pediatr Hematol Oncol. 2001 Jun-Jul;23(5):286–289. DOI: 10.1097/00043426-200106000-00010.

[99] Mikulić D, Ilić I, Cepulić M, et al. Tumor angiogenesis and outcome in osteosarcoma. Pediatr Hematol Oncol. 2004 Oct-Nov;21(7):611–619. DOI: 10.1080/08880010490501015.

[100] Kunz P, Fellenberg J, Moskovszky L, et al. Improved survival in osteosarcoma patients with atypical low vascularization. Ann Surg Oncol. 2015 Feb;22(2):489–496. doi: 10.1245/s10434-014-4001-2.

[101] Mori S, Ueda T, Kuratsu S, et al. Suppression of pulmonary metastasis by angiogenesis inhibitor TNP-470 in murine osteosarcoma. Int J Cancer. 1995 Mar 29;61(1):148–152. DOI: 10.1002/ijc.2910610125.

[102] Ferrara N, Gerber HP, LeCouter J. The biology of VEGF and its receptors. Nat Med. 2003 Jun;9(6):669–676. DOI: 10.1038/nm0603-669.

[103] Kaya M, Wada T, Nagoya S, et al. The level of vascular endothelial growth factor as a predictor of a poor prognosis in osteosarcoma. J Bone Joint Surg Br. 2009 Jun;91(6):784–788. DOI:10.1302/0301-620X.91B6.

[104] Kaya M, Wada T, Kawaguchi S, et al. Vascular endothelial growth factor expression in untreated osteosarcoma is predictive of pulmonary metastasis and poor prognosis. Clin Cancer Res. 2000 Feb;6(2):572–577.

[105] Kaya M, Wada T, Kawaguchi S, et al. Increased pre-therapeutic serum vascular endothelial growth factor in patients with early clinical relapse of osteosarcoma. Br J Cancer. 2002 Mar 18;86(6):864–869. DOI: 10.1038/sj/bjc/6600201.

[106] Lee YH, Tokunaga T, Oshika Y, et al. Cell-retained isoforms of vascular endothelial growth factor (VEGF) are correlated with poor prognosis in osteosarcoma. Eur J Cancer. 1999 Jul;35(7):1089–1093. DOI: 10.1016/S0959-8049(99)00073-8.

[107] Yang SY, Yu H, Krygier JE, et al. High VEGF with rapid growth and early metastasis in a mouse osteosarcoma model. Sarcoma. 2007;2007:95628. DOI:10.1155/2007/95628.

[108] Yin D, Jia T, Gong W, et al. VEGF blockade decelerates the growth of a murine experimental osteosarcoma. Int J Oncol. 2008 Aug;33(2):253–259. DOI: 10.3892/ijo_00000004.

[109] Wu X, Chen Z, Zeng W, et al. Silencing of eag1 gene inhibits osteosarcoma proliferation and migration by targeting STAT3-VEGF pathway. Biomed Res Int. 2015;2015:617316. DOI: 10.1155/2015/617316.

[110] Zhao J, Zhang ZR, Zhao N, et al. VEGF silencing inhibits human osteosarcoma angiogenesis and promotes cell apoptosis via PI3K/AKT signaling pathway. Cell Biochem Biophys. 2015 Nov;73(2):519–525. DOI: 10.1007/s12013-015-0692-7.

[111] Tzeng HE, Tsai CH, Chang ZL, et al. Interleukin-6 induces vascular endothelial growth factor expression and promotes angiogenesis through apoptosis signal-regulating kinase 1 in human osteosarcoma. Biochem Pharmacol. 2013 Feb 15;85(4):531–540. DOI: 10.1016/j.bcp.2012.11.021.

[112] Wang M, Wang L, Ren T, et al. IL-17A/IL-17RA interaction promoted metastasis of osteosarcoma cells. Cancer Biol Ther. 2013 Feb;14(2):155–163. DOI: 10.4161/cbt.22955.

[113] de Nigris F, Schiano C, Infante T, Napoli C. CXCR4 inhibitors: tumor vasculature and therapeutic challenges. Recent Pat Anticancer Drug Discov. 2012 Sep;7(3):251–264. DOI: 10.2174/157489212801820039.

[114] Fan L, Wu Q, Xing X, et al. MicroRNA-145 targets vascular endothelial growth factor and inhibits invasion and metastasis of osteosarcoma cells. Acta Biochim Biophys Sin (Shanghai). 2012 May;44(5):407–414. DOI: 10.1093/abbs/gms019.

[115] Abdollahi A, Hahnfeldt P, Maercker C, et al. Endostatin's antiangiogenic signaling network. Mol Cell. 2004 Mar 12;13(5):649–663.

[116] Folkman J. Antiangiogenesis in cancer therapy—endostatin and its mechanisms of action. Exp Cell Res. 2006 Mar 10;312(5):594–607. DOI: 10.1016/j.yexcr.2005.11.015.

[117] Kaya M, Wada T, Nagoya S, Yamashita T. Prevention of postoperative progression of pulmonary metastases in osteosarcoma by antiangiogenic therapy using endostatin. J Orthop Sci. 2007 Nov;12(6):562–567. DOI 10.1007/s00776-007-1179-1.

[118] Maniotis AJ, Folberg R, Hess A, et al. Vascular channel formation by human melanoma cells *in vivo* and *in vitro*: vasculogenic mimicry. Am J Pathol. 1999 Sep;155(3):739–752. DOI: 10.1016/S0002-9440(10)65173-5.

[119] Ren K, Yao N, Wang G, et al. Vasculogenic mimicry: a new prognostic sign of human osteosarcoma. Hum Pathol. 2014 Oct;45(10):2120–2129. DOI: 10.1016/j.humpath.2014.06.013.

[120] Zhang LZ, Mei J, Qian ZK, et al. The role of VE-cadherin in osteosarcoma cells. Pathol Oncol Res. 2010 Mar;16(1):111–117. DOI: 10.1007/s12253-009-9198-1.

[121] Alfranca A, Martinez-Cruzado L, Tornin J, et al. Bone microenvironment signals in osteosarcoma development. Cell Mol Life Sci. 2015 Aug;72(16):3097–3113. DOI: 10.1007/s00018-015-1918-y.

[122] Xu WT, Bian ZY, Fan QM, et al. Human mesenchymal stem cells (hMSCs) target osteosarcoma and promote its growth and pulmonary metastasis. Cancer Lett. 2009 Aug 18;281(1):32–41. DOI:10.1016/j.canlet.2009.02.022.

[123] Tsukamoto S, Honoki K, Fujii H, et al. Mesenchymal stem cells promote tumor engraftment and metastatic colonization in rat osteosarcoma model. Int J Oncol. 2012;40(1):163–169. DOI: 10.3892/ijo.2011.1220.

[124] Tu B, Du L, Fan QM, et al. STAT3 activation by IL-6 from mesenchymal stem cells promotes the proliferation and metastasis of osteosarcoma. Cancer Lett. 2012 Dec 1;325(1):80–88. DOI: 10.1016/j.canlet.2012.06.006.

[125] Williams SA, Maecker HL, French DM, et al. USP1 deubiquitinates ID proteins to preserve a mesenchymal stem cell program in osteosarcoma. Cell. 2011 Sep 16;146(6):918–930. DOI: 10.1016/j.cell.2011.07.040.

[126] Moschoi R, Imbert V, Nebout M, et al. Protective mitochondrial transfer from bone marrow stromal cells to acute myeloid leukemic cells during chemotherapy. Blood. 2016 Jul 14;128(2):253–264. DOI: 10.1182/blood-2015-07-655860.

[127] Denbo JW, Zhu L, Srivastava D, et al. Long-term pulmonary function after metastasectomy for childhood osteosarcoma: a report from the St Jude lifetime cohort study. J Am Coll Surg. 2014 Aug;219(2):265–271. DOI: 10.1016/j.jamcollsurg.2013.12.064.

[128] Mirabello L, Troisi RJ, Savage S. Osteosarcoma incidence and survival rates from 1973 to 2004: data from the surveillance, epidemiology, and end results program. Cancer. 2009 Apr 1;115(7):1531–1543. DOI: 10.1002/cncr.24121.

[129] Robbins PD, Morelli AE. Regulation of immune responses by extracellular vesicles. Nat Rev Immunol. 2014;14(3):195–208. DOI: 10.1038/nri3622.

[130] van der Pol E, Böing AN, Harrison P, et al. Classification, functions, and clinical relevance of extracellular vesicles. Pharmacol Rev. 2012;64(3):676–705. DOI: 10.1124/pr.112.005983.

[131] Lai FW, Lichty BD, Bowdish DM. Microvesicles: ubiquitous contributors to infection and immunity. J Leukoc Biol. 2015;97(2):237–245. DOI: 10.1189/jlb.3RU0513-292RR.

[132] Li XB, Zhang ZR, Schluesener HJ, Xu SQ. Role of exosomes in immune regulation. J Cell Mol Med. 2006;10(2):364–375. DOI: 10.1038/nri3622.

[133] Anderson MR, Kashanchi F, Jacobson S. Exosomes in viral disease. Neurotherapeutics. 2016 Jun 20. DOI: 10.1007/s13311-016-0450-6.

[134] Chen WX, Cai YQ, Lv MM, et al. Exosomes from docetaxel-resistant breast cancer cells alter chemosensitivity by delivering microRNAs. Tumor Biol. 2014;35(10):9649–9659. DOI: 10.1007/s13277-014-2242-0.

[135] Torreggiani E, Roncuzzi L, Perut F, et al. Multimodal transfer of MDR by exosomes in human osteosarcoma. Int J Oncol. 2016 Jul;49(1):189–196. DOI: 10.3892/ijo.2016.3509.

[136] Jerez S, Araya H, Thaler R, et al. Proteomic analysis of exosomes and exosome-free conditioned media derived from human osteosarcoma cell lines reveal differential secretion of proteins related to biological functions and tumor progression. J Cell Biochem. 2016 Jun 30. DOI: 10.1002/jcb.25642

[137] Mu X, Agarwal R, March D, et al. Notch signaling mediates skeletal muscle atrophy in cancer cachexia caused by osteosarcoma. Sarcoma. 2016;2016:3758162. DOI:10.1155/2016/3758162.

[138] Hildenbrand R, Allgayer H, Marx A, Stroebel P. Modulators of the urokinase-type plasminogen activation system for cancer. Expert Opin Investig Drugs. 2010;19(5):641–652. DOI: 10.1517/13543781003767400.

[139] Endo-Munoz L, Cai N, Cumming A, et al. Progression of osteosarcoma from a non-metastatic to a metastatic phenotype is causally associated with activation of an autocrine and paracrine uPA Axis. PLoS One. 2015 Aug 28;10(8):e0133592. DOI: 10.1371/journal.pone.0133592.

[140] Vallabhaneni KC, Penfornis P, Dhule S, et al. Extracellular vesicles from bone marrow mesenchymal stem/stromal cells transport tumor regulatory microRNA, proteins, and metabolites. Oncotarget. 2015;6(7):4953–4967. DOI: 10.18632/oncotarget.3211.

[141] Shimbo K, Miyaki S, Ishitobi H, et al. Exosome-formed synthetic microRNA-143 is transferred to osteosarcoma cells and inhibits their migration. Biochem Biophys Res Commun. 2014 Mar 7;445(2):381–387. DOI: 10.1016/j.bbrc.2014.02.007.

[142] Lässer C. Identification and analysis of circulating exosomal microRNA in human body fluids. Methods Mol Biol. 2013;1024:109–128. DOI: 10.1007/978-1-62703-453-1_9.

[143] Lässer C, Seyed Alikhani V, Ekström K, et al. Human saliva, plasma and breast milk exosomes contain RNA: uptake by macrophages. J Transl Med. 2011 Jan 14;9:9. DOI: 10.1186/1479-5876-9-9.

[144] Miranda KC, Bond DT, McKee M, et al. Nucleic acids within urinary exosomes/microvesicles are potential biomarkers for renal disease. Kidney Int. 2010 Jul;78(2):191–199. DOI:10.1038/ki.2010.106.

[145] Wang ZQ, Liang J, Schellander K, et al. c-fos-induced osteosarcoma formation in transgenic mice: cooperativity with c-jun and the role of endogenous c-fos. Cancer Res. 1995 Dec 15;55(24):6244–6251.

[146] Entz-Werlé N, Choquet P, Neuville A, et al. Targeted apc;twist double-mutant mice: a new model of spontaneous osteosarcoma that mimics the human disease. Transl Oncol. 2010 Dec 1;3(6):344–353.

[147] Elliott NT, Yuan F. A review of three-dimensional *in vitro* tissue models for drug discovery and transport studies. J Pharm Sci. 2011 Jan;100(1):59–74. DOI: 10.1002/jps.22257.

[148] Merlino G, Khanna C. Fishing for the origins of cancer. Genes Dev. 21(11):1275–1279. DOI: 10.1101/gad.1563707.

[149] Langenau DM, Keefe MD, Storer NY, et al. Effects of RAS on the genesis of embryonal rhabdomyosarcoma. Genes Dev. 21(11):1382–1395. DOI: 10.1101/gad.1545007.

[150] Feitsma H, Kuiper RV, Korving J, et al. Zebrafish with mutations in mismatch repair genes develop neurofibromas and other tumors. Cancer Res. 68(13):5059–5066. DOI: 10.1158/0008-5472.CAN-08-0019.

[151] Etchin J, Kanki JP, Look AT. Zebrafish as a model for the study of human cancer. Methods Cell Biol. 105:309–337. DOI: 10.1016/B978-0-12-381320-6.00013-8.

[152] He S, Krens SG, Zhan H, et al. A DeltaRaf1-ER-inducible oncogenic zebrafish liver cell model identifies hepatocellular carcinoma signatures. J Pathol. 225(1):19–28. DOI: 10.1002/path.2936.

[153] Alford AI, Kozloff KM, Hankenson KD. Extracellular matrix networks in bone remodeling. Int J Biochem Cell Biol. 2015 Aug;65:20–31. DOI: 10.1016/j.biocel.2015.05.008.

[154] Alemany-Ribes M, Semino CE. Bioengineering 3D environments for cancer models. Adv Drug Deliv Rev. 2014 Dec 15;79–80:40–49. DOI: 10.1016/j.addr.2014.06.004.

[155] Zhang W, Zhu Y, Li J, et al. Cell-derived extracellular matrix: basic characteristics and current applications in orthopedic tissue engineering. Tissue Eng Part B Rev. 2016 Jun;22(3):193–207. DOI: 10.1089/ten.TEB.2015.0290.

[156] Beck EC, Barragan M, Tadros MH, et al. Approaching the compressive modulus of articular cartilage with a decellularized cartilage-based hydrogel. Acta Biomater. 2016 Apr;38:pp. 94–105. DOI: 10.1016/j.actbio.2016.04.019.

[157] Datta N, Holtorf HL, Sikavitsas VI, et al. Effect of bone extracellular matrix synthesized *in vitro* on the osteoblastic differentiation of marrow stromal cells. Biomaterials. 2005 Mar;26(9):971–977. DOI: 10.1016/j.biomaterials.2004.04.001.

[158] Benders KE, van Weeren PR, Badylak SF, et al. Extracellular matrix scaffolds for cartilage and bone regeneration. Trends Biotechnol. 2013 Mar;31(3):169–176. DOI: 10.1016/j.tibtech.2012.12.004.

[159] Mohseny AB, Xiao W, Carvalho R, et al. An osteosarcoma zebrafish model implicates Mmp-19 and Ets-1 as well as reduced host immune response in angiogenesis and migration. J Pathol. 2012 Jun;227(2):245–253. DOI: 10.1002/path.3998.

[160] Bulut G, Hong SH, Chen K, et al. Small molecule inhibitors of ezrin inhibit the invasive phenotype of osteosarcoma cells. Oncogene. 2012 Jan 19;31(3):269–281. DOI: 10.1038/onc.2011.245.

[161] Rodriguez CO Jr. Using canine osteosarcoma as a model to assess efficacy of novel therapies: can old dogs teach us new tricks?. Adv Exp Med Biol. 2014;804:237–256. DOI: 10.1007/978-3-319-04843-7_13.

[162] Gordon N, Koshkina NV, Jia SF, et al. Corruption of the Fas pathway delays the pulmonary clearance of murine osteosarcoma cells, enhances their metastatic potential, and reduces the effect of aerosol gemcitabine. Clin Cancer Res. 2007 Aug 1;13(15 Pt 1):4503–4510. DOI: 10.1158/1078-0432.CCR-07-0313.

[163] Koshkina NV, Kleinerman ES. Aerosol gemcitabine inhibits the growth of primary osteosarcoma and osteosarcoma lung metastases. Int J Cancer. 2005 Sep 1;116(3):458–463. DOI: 10.1002/ijc.21011.

[164] Rodriguez CO Jr, Crabbs TA, Wilson DW, et al. Aerosol gemcitabine: preclinical safety and *in vivo* antitumor activity in osteosarcoma-bearing dogs. J Aerosol Med Pulm Drug Deliv. 2010 Aug;23(4):197–206. DOI: 10.1089/jamp.2009.0773.

Chapter 6

Immune Environment and Osteosarcoma

Marie-Françoise Heymann and
Dominique Heymann

Additional information is available at the end of the chapter

http://dx.doi.org/10.5772/67448

Abstract

Immune niche with its huge cell diversity including more specifically tumour infiltrating lymphocytes (TILs), tumour-associated macrophages (TAMs) regulate osteosarcoma (OS) microenvironment. TAMs exert differential activities in the tumour development according to their polarisation. Indeed, in oncology, M1-polarised macrophages are considered as anti-tumour effectors, and M2-polarised macrophages are defined as protumour modulators by increasing the neoangiogenic process. TAM density is correlated with tumour cell proliferation, invasion, metastasis and poor prognosis in various epithelial and haematological cancers and in bone metastasis. Similarly, tumour infiltrating lymphocytes play a key role in tumour development by inducing a local tolerant environment favourable for the tumour growth. The present chapter will describe the main roles of the immune system in the pathogenesis of osteosarcoma and the most recent therapeutic development based on its regulation.

Keywords: osteoimmunology, osteosarcoma, macrophage, lymphocyte, microenvironment

1. Introduction

In recent years, there has been a dramatic increase in the importance given to the theory that the tissue microenvironment participates in determining the "bone niche" in the progression of bone tumours and in establishing resistance processes to conventional therapies. Originally, the concept of tumour niche has emerged based on the "seed and soil theory" proposed by Stephan Paget at the end of the nineteenth century [1, 2]. This tumour niche is defined as a specific microenvironment promoting the emergence of cancer initiating cells and providing all the factors required for their quiescence, proliferation and migration.

Therefore, the tumour microenvironment is composed of a complex, interconnected network of protagonists, including soluble factors such as cytokines, extracellular matrix components, interacting with fibroblasts, endothelial cells, immune cells and various specific cell types depending on the location of the cancer cells (e.g. osteoblasts, osteoclasts in the bone tissue or pulmonary epithelium in case of lung metastasis). This cellular diversity defines three main "niches" depending on their functional implication: an *immune niche* involved in local immune tolerance, a *vascular niche* associated with tumour cell extravasation/migration and a *metastatic niche* (e.g. bone, lung and liver) hosting the metastatic tumour cells [3, 4].

The concept of "bone niche" was initially described in the context of haematological malignancies, such as leukaemia [5] or multiple myeloma [6], and then extended to bone metastases, such as breast or prostate cancers [7]. As all tumours, the pathogenesis of osteosarcoma (OS) is closely related to the microenvironment in which the tumour grows. Even though the aetiology of OS has not been clearly established, its development has the special feature of being strongly associated with the "soil" described by Paget. In physiological and pathological bone tissue, the various cells communicate together by direct contacts involving adhesion molecules or channels, but also in an autocrine/paracrine/endocrine manner involving cytokines and growth factors [8]. Among these glycoproteins, the triad osteoprotegerin (OPG)/Receptor Activator of NF-κB (RANK)/RANK Ligand (RANKL) plays a pivotal role in OS development [9]. In case of OS, there is effectively a dysregulation in this balance between OPG/RANK/RANKL, provoking exacerbated local bone remodelling (**Figure 1**). As a result, numerous factors initially trapped in this matrix are released, which in turn stimulate sarcoma cell proliferation, leading to the establishment of a vicious cycle between bone and tumour cells [10]. These events are associated with early and late events in the metastatic process by promoting the neoangiogenesis and extravasation of tumour cells [11, 12]. But until today, the characterisation of the microenvironment of OS has not been fully documented [13, 14]. The immune niche, with its huge cell diversity including more specifically tumour infiltrating lymphocytes (TILs) and tumour-associated macrophages (TAMs), regulates the OS microenvironment [15, 16]. TAMs exert different effects on tumour development because of their polarisation. In oncology, M1-polarised macrophages are considered to be anti-tumour effectors, and M2-polarised macrophages are defined as pro-tumour modulators as they increase the neoangiogenic process [17–19]. The density of TAMs is correlated with tumour cell proliferation, invasion, metastasis and poor prognosis in various epithelial and haematological cancers and in bone metastases [20].

Osteoimmunology is a recent term proposed for describing the complex immune environment controlling the bone remodelling and related diseases [21]. Several reports have underlined the therapeutic interest to use immunotherapies or immunomodulatory-based therapies for OS. In this context, the number of new drugs activating the immune system has exploded in the last 10 years, and numerous phase I and II clinical trials are in progress in OS. The present chapter will describe the main roles of the immune system in the pathogenesis of OS and the most recent therapeutic development based on its regulation.

http://dx.doi.org/10.5772/67448

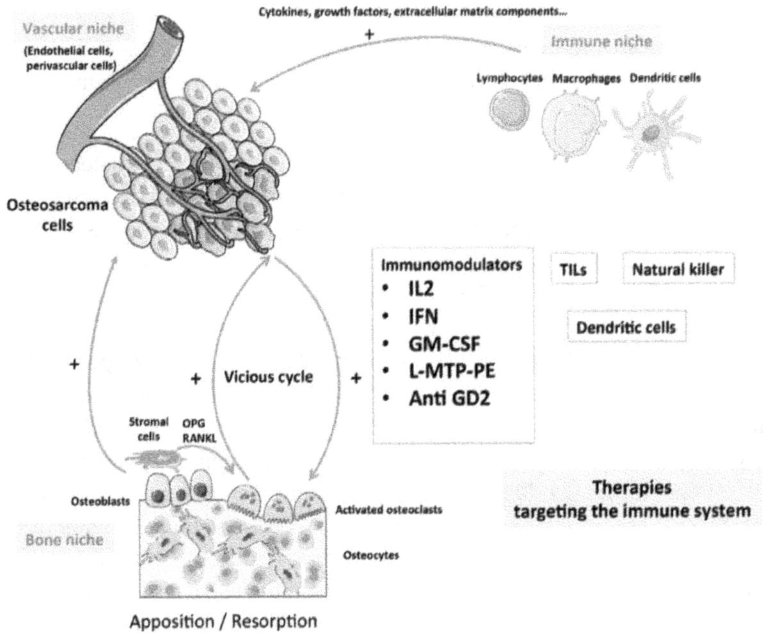

Figure 1. Osteosarcoma and its niches. In osteosarcoma, the microenvironment plays a pivotal role in the pathogenesis of tumour cells. It facilitates the transport of gas and nutriments to cancer cells and extravasation to their metastatic location (vascular niche), induces a tolerant environment (immune niche) and dysregulates bone remodelling (bone niche), in which the molecular OPG/RANKL/RANK triad plays a key role in regulation. OPG and RANKL are produced by osteoblasts and/or stromal cells, whereas RANK is expressed at the surface of osteoclasts and their precursors. The immune niche is one of the source of therapeutic targets against osteosarcoma.

2. The immune niche in osteosarcoma

As said above, the niche of OS is composed of a complex network of diverse cells, which interact together by direct contacts, or in an autocrine/paracrine/endocrine manner involving cytokines and growth factors. This chapter will focus specifically on the main cellular protagonists: lymphocytes, macrophages and the principal associated cytokines.

2.1. Tumour infiltrating lymphocytes (TILs)

Heterogeneity of tumour cells with various osteosarcoma sub-entities further complicates identification of robust biomarkers with broad clinical application [22]. Analysis of the tumour microenvironment in patients with a variety of haematological pathologies and solid tumours such as bone metastases and soft tissue sarcomas has revealed that a major subset of tumours shows evidence of a T cell–infiltrated phenotype [23, 24]. Selected T lymphocytes migrate from secondary lymphoid organs to the tumour sites and invade the tumour tissues. They are composed of various T lymphocyte subpopulations, which exhibit highly specific immunological reactivity compared to circulating and non-infiltrating lymphocytes [25]. The final immune response resulting from the activation of T lymphocytes is complex and depends on the nature of these T cells (e.g. Treg, CD4$^+$) and the presence of the other immune protagonists such as macrophages.

As other immune cells, lymphocytes seem to play an essential role in osteosarcoma growth and prognosis, but publications reporting this population in OS remain rare [16, 22, 26]. The presence of T lymphocytes in human OS tissues was previously studied by Trieb et al. by immunohistochemical techniques [26]. Phenotypic analyses have revealed that the infiltrating lymphocytes into OS were 95% CD3$^+$ and 68% CD8$^+$. At this time, human CD4$^+$ Treg was unknown and not included in the study, which did not detect any correlation of TILs with OS outcome. A few years later, Theoleyre et al. supported the presence of specific T subpopulations in OS: TILs isolated from OS samples exhibited lytic activity *in vitro*, which were apparently no efficient in patients [16]. The study of the microenvironment has a strong impact on targeted patient treatment for which little progress has been achieved since introduction of neo-adjuvant chemotherapy 30 years ago. Prognostic biomarkers for risk stratification at the time of diagnosis are missing and are a major drawback in clinical testing of novel therapeutic agents. Alternatively, analysis of the tumour microenvironment for osteosarcoma outcome-related biomarkers might be less dependent from the osteosarcoma subtype. Recently, Fritzsching et al. have reported for the first time CD8$^+$/FOXP3$^+$ ratio as strong prognostic factor at time of OS diagnosis, pointing out the functional key role of Treg in OS pathogenesis. Multivariate analysis showed that this novel parameter was independent from tumour metastasis and response to neoadjuvant chemotherapy and could be validated in an independent patient cohort with current state of diagnosis and treatment of OS [22]. It has been suggested in other solid tumours (e.g. colon cancers) that intensity of tumour microenvironment infiltration with T-cells, especially cytotoxic tumour infiltrating CD8$^+$T-cells (CD8$^+$ TILs) allows more powerful prognostic staging than traditional staging. The characterisation of this simple immune system-based biomarker has been termed the "immunoscore", and this is currently tested for some tumours in a multicenter study [27, 28].

Lymphocytes are immune cells regulated by diverse cytokines, in particular the triad OPG/RANK/RANKL, which represents a setting up a fertile soil for cancer cells as well [9]. Bone remodelling results from a balance between two opposite cellular activities: (i) osteoblasts in charge of the synthesis of new organic extracellular matrix, which will become progressively mineralized and (ii) osteoclasts specialised in the degradation of the mineralised extracellular matrix, process named bone resorption. Osteoclastogenesis and osteoclast activities are regulated by a master cytokine called NF-κB Ligand (RANKL), member of the tumour necrosis factor (TNF) superfamily (official TNF nomenclature: TNFSF11) [9]. RANKL is a soluble and/or membrane cytokine expressed by osteoblasts and stromal cells, binds to RANK a membrane receptor expressed at the surface of mature osteoclasts and their precursors. RANKL binding to RANK induces specific NF-κB–dependent signal transduction pathways and stimulates osteoclast differentiation, survival and resorption activity. RANKL binds to a soluble receptor named osteoprotegerin (OPG), which is a ubiquitous protein and acts as a decoy blocking RANKL binding to RANK [29]. OPG is then considered as a strong inhibitor of osteoclastogenesis and bone resorption. LGR4 is the last receptor of RANK recently identified. LGR4 expressed at the osteoclast/osteoclast precursor membrane is a negative regulator of RANKL-RANK activation (see review in Ref. [9]). It is widely accepted that the multiple components of the bone niche (e.g. soluble factors, extracellular matrix) strongly contribute to the bone tumour initiation and the metastatic process [30, 31]. RANKL influences the microenvironment of cancer cells by acting on the local immunity. Indeed, the major role of RANKL in the immune system has been initially identified in RANKL-knockout mice in which the development of secondary lymphoid organs was impaired especially the lymph nodes [32] but also at the "central" level where the maturation of thymic epithelial cells necessary for T cell development was affected [33]. RANKL is also involved in the modulation of the immune response by inducing T cell proliferation [34] and dendritic cells survival [29]. Indeed, activated T cells through RANKL expression stimulate dendritic cells, expressing RANK, to enhance their survival and thereby increase the T cell memory response [34]. More recently, Khan et al. demonstrated that RANKL blockade can rescue melanoma-specific T cells from thymic deletion and increases anti-tumour immune response as shown in melanoma [35]. In 2007, Mori et al. reported for the first time functional RANK expression in human OS cells strengthening the involvement of the RANK/RANKL/OPG axis in OS [36, 37]. Moreover, in animal OS models, OPG gene transfer prevents the formation of osteolytic lesions associated with OS development, in reducing the tumour incidence and the local tumour growth, leading to a fourfold increase in mice survival 28 days post-implantation [38]. This opened a new door of novel therapeutic approaches for OS.

2.2. Tumour-associated macrophages (TAMs)

The mononuclear phagocyte system is composed by heterogeneous populations participating in the body's first line of defence against pathogens and parasites [39]. This system includes cells circulating cells into the body fluids such as monocytes, and integrates resident cells such as macrophages, dendritic cells (DC) and their precursors located in the bone marrow [40]. Their production and activities are controlled by numerous cytokines and growth factors but are more specifically regulated by the two ligands of macrophage-colony stimulating factor (M-CFR, cFMS or CD115): M-CSF (or CSF-1) and interleukin (IL)-34 [41, 42].

TAMs are the predominant leukocytes infiltrating solid tumours and can represent up to 50% of the tumour mass. These cells play a pivotal role in tumour behaviour illustrated by the significant link between TAM number and density and the prognosis [18, 43, 44]. Whereas TAMs can exert anti-tumour activities, the ambiguous role of macrophages in tumour progression is reflected in the finding that TAMs can also actively contribute to each stage of cancer development and progression [45]. Macrophage subtypes are conventionally classified in M1 considered as the classical population and M2 identified as an alternative subpopulation in link to their differentiation/activation state. However, if the parallel between M1 and M2 can be drawn with the Th1 and Th2 T lymphocyte classification, Th1/Th2 cells do not regulate macrophage polarisation. On the contrary, macrophage subtypes are versatile, are non-permanent cell populations, initiate and influence T lymphocyte polarisation resulting in differential immune response (e.g. Th1 response against virus and bacteria, Th2 response against parasites) [46]. Indeed, M1 and M2 macrophages are characterised by specific profiles of cytokine secretion. M1 macrophages are characterised by the secretion of IL-12, IL-1, IL-6, TNF or ROS, considered as pro-inflammatory mediators and directly involved in the control of infections and anti-tumour activities. On the opposite, M2 macrophages constitute a heterogeneous population (M2a, b and c) inducing a Th2 immune response and secreting IL-4, IL-10 and IL-13. M2 macrophages are pro-angiogenic, pro-fibrotic and pro-tumorigenic.

The exact role of macrophages in OS is still unclear and controversial. Some studies have defined TAMs as anti-tumour effectors. Buddingh et al. thus demonstrated that higher TAM infiltration was associated with better overall survival in high-grade osteosarcoma. However, the authors did not observe any differences between metastatic and non-metastatic osteosarcomas, and TAMs exhibited both M1 and M2 characteristics [47]. On the contrary, the impact of macrophages in tumour development has been also suspected. Lewis and Pollard distinguished the anti-tumour M1-macrophages from M2-macrophages leading to tumour growth and invasion, angiogenesis, metastasis and immune-suppression [18]. OS development may thus be accompanied by a switch in the phenotype of infiltrating TAMs, from anti-metastatic M1-macrophages to pro-metastatic M2-macrophages. This hypothesis is in agreement with the *in vivo* work described by Xiao et al. who showed a switch in macrophage subpopulations in a mouse model of human osteosarcoma from M1-macrophages during the first week of tumour growth, to M2-macrophages after 2–3 weeks [48]. In addition, Pahl et al. demonstrated that human M1-like macrophages can be induced to exert direct anti-tumour activity against osteosarcoma cells, mediated by TNF-α and IL-1β [49]. In the same manner, Ségaliny et al. demonstrated that osteosarcoma cells expressed IL-34, increasing the recruitment of M2-polarised macrophages into the tumour tissue, which correlates with tumour vascularization and the metastatic process [50]. TAMs accumulate in tumour microenvironment and according to their M2 or M1 phenotype contribute to tumour growth, angiogenesis and metastasis [51]. RANK is present at the cell membrane of monocytes/macrophages and RANKL acts as chemoattractant factor for these cells [52]. M2 subtype is strongly associated with the angiogenic process and interestingly RANK is mainly expressed by M2 macrophage subtype [53]. RANK/RANKL signalling in M2 subtype modulates the production of chemokines promoting the proliferation of Treg lymphocytes in favour of an immunosuppressive environment [54]. In breast carcinoma, RANKL is mainly produced by $CD4^{+}CD25^{+}$ T lymphocytes expressing Foxp3 and corresponding to Treg lymphocytes. In this context, a vicious cycle is established between TAMs, Treg and tumour cells resulting in the tumour growth, the spreading of cancer cells and the amplification of the metastatic process [55].

2.3. Recent therapeutic developments based on the regulation of the immune system of osteosarcoma: immunomodulating drugs

The therapeutic protocol currently used for osteosarcoma was established by Rosen et al. at the end of the 1970s [56]. It comprises preoperative (neoadjuvant) chemotherapy associating mainly four drugs (doxorubicin, cisplatin, methotrexate and ifosfamide) [57], and followed by surgical removal of all detectable disease (including metastases), and postoperative (adjuvant) chemotherapy, preferably within the setting of clinical trials [58]. OS is considered resistant to applicable doses of radiation [59, 60]. Supplemental therapeutic approaches such as chemoembolisation or angioembolisation, thermal ablation, radiofrequency ablation and cryotherapy are experimental or palliative [59]. Unfortunately, patients, who are diagnosed with metastatic disease or who relapse post-therapy have an extremely poor prognosis, with little to no improvements in survival seen over the past 30 years [61]. Several reports have underlined the therapeutic value of using immunotherapies or immunomodulatory-based therapies for osteosarcoma [15, 62–64]. In this context, the number of new drugs activating the immune system has exploded in the last 10 years and numerous phase I and II clinical trials are in progress in osteosarcoma (**Figure 1**). In this chapter, the most recent therapeutic developments targeting the regulation of T lymphocytes and macrophages will be exposed.

2.3.1. T-cell therapies

Detection of specific T lymphocyte populations in the tumour microenvironment and in human tumour tissues defines an immunoscore and leads to patient stratification based on this immunophenotyping. These analyses have identified new predictive biomarkers and new therapeutic targets, which have stimulated the development of immunotherapies [65].

2.3.1.1. Disialoganglioside (GD2)

Monoclonal antibodies targeted against cell surface antigens specific to tumour cells have been proven to be effective in patients with breast cancer, lymphoma and neuroblastoma [66–68]. Usually these bispecific antibodies are engineered antibodies linking a tumour antigen recognition domain to a second domain that activates a receptor on immune effector cells, typically T cells. The expression of the glycosphingolipid GD2 is restricted to the central and peripheral nervous system, skin (melanocyte) and mesenchymal cells located in the stroma [69–71]. In addition to the healthy tissues, GD2 was detected in neuroblastomas, melanomas, sarcomas, lung and central nervous system tumours, in which a variable number of cancer cells express this antigen [72–75]. Based on this relative restricted distribution, GD2-targeting appeared very quickly as an interesting immunotherapy, especially for high-risk neuroblastomas, for which anti-GD2 antibodies improved significantly patient survival [68, 76]. In patients with stage IV neuroblastoma, anti-GD2 antibody ch14.18 has been shown to improve EFS effectively when given in the setting of minimal residual disease. The rationale for using this antibody in patients with OS lies in that 95% of osteosarcoma express GD2 [77]. Consequently, given the success of anti-GD2 mAb therapy in neuroblastoma, studies exploring the use of these mAbs in OS are underway [78]. Current trials include the GD2mAbs humanized3F8 (NCT01419834 and NCT01662804) and hu14.18K322A (NCT00743496) [61].

2.3.1.2. Nivolumab

Nivolumab is an immunomodulator, which acts by blocking the activation of the programmed cell death-1 (PD-1) receptor, induced by one of its two ligands (PD-L1) on activated T cells [79]. Numerous preclinical investigations have demonstrated that inhibition of the interaction between PD-1 and PD-L1 enhances the T-cell response, resulting in increased anti-tumour activity. PD-L1 or PD-1 blockade with monoclonal antibodies results in strong and often rapid anti-tumour effects in several mouse models. A high PD-L1 expression has been identified in OS cell lines [80], and PD-1 expression on CD4 and CD8 T-cells was found higher in OS patients than in healthy controls and in patients with metastasis at diagnosis, high tumour stage or bone fracture [81]. A phase I/II trial will be conclude in 2016 on refractory solid tumours and sarcomas including osteosarcoma. A total of 242 patients will be enrolled and treated with Nivolumab IV over 60 minutes twice a month. Courses repeat every 28 days in the absence of disease progression or unacceptable toxicity.

2.3.2. *Immune and dendritic cell vaccine*

Dendritic cells have the specific ability to initiate and modulate adaptive immune responses [82]. This specificity, associated with their role in antigen presentation, has led to their use in vaccine approaches in cancer. Matured autologous dendritic cells loaded with tumour lysates derived from tumour tissue were used as the vaccine product. In a pre-clinical model of osteosarcoma, it has been demonstrated that killer dendritic cells were able to induce an adaptive anti-tumour immune response with a decrease in tumour development after cross-presentation of the tumour cell-derived antigen [83]. A phase I clinical trial demonstrated the feasibility and good tolerance of dendritic cells pulsed with MAGE-A1, MAGE-A3 and NYESO-1 full length peptides in combination with decitabine. Anti-tumour activity was observed in some patients [84]. In 2012, 12 osteosarcoma patients were vaccinated with tumour lysate pulsed dendritic cells, but evidence of a clinical benefit was observed in only two of these patients [85]. These authors concluded that osteosarcoma patients may be relatively insensitive to DC-based vaccine treatments. A new clinical trial was initiated, enrolling 56 patients (>1 year) with confirmed sarcoma, either relapsed or without known curative therapies, and treated with autologous dendritic cells pulsed with tumour lysate. NCT02409576 is a pilot trial ("Pilot Study of Expanded, Activated Haploidentical Natural Killer Cell Infusions for Sarcomas (NKEXPSARC)") analysing the effect of donor NK cells on clinical response determined by imaging. About 20 patients (aged 6 months–80 years) will be included between 2015 and 2016. The patients will receive lymphodepleting chemotherapy with cyclophosphamide (1 day) followed by fludarabine (5 days) and each patient will receive IL-2 1 day before infusion of the NK cell (total six doses).

2.3.3. *Mifamurtide (liposomal-muramyl tripeptide phosphatidyl-ethanolamine L-MTP-PE)*

As it has been discussed above, the density of TAM is linked to a poor diagnosis. In osteosarcoma, Buddingh et al. showed that macrophages exhibit M1 and M2 phenotypes and demonstrated a link between M2 macrophages and angiogenesis. Similarly, in preclinical models of osteosarcoma, the recruitment of the M2 subtype is correlated with tumour angiogenesis and lung metastasis [47, 50].

L-MTP-PE is a synthetic analogue of muramyl dipeptide of the bacterial cell walls, which was identified as a powerful activator or monocyte/macrophage lineage. Indeed, L-MTP-PE induces the expression of pro-inflammatory mediators such TNF-α, IL-1, IL-6, lymphocyte function-associated antigen 1 (LFA-1) and intercellular adhesion molecule 1 (ICAM1) leading to an M1 macrophage response. The therapeutic interest of L-MTP-PE was widely studied in osteosarcoma [86, 87]. The largest clinical experience with combination chemotherapy and L-MTP derives from the Intergroup 0133 osteosarcoma study. No difference in survival was found for patients who received ifosfamide in addition to the standard three-drug chemotherapy (doxorubicin, cisplatin and methotrexate). But this study did suggest that L-MTP had a beneficial impact on survival, improving the 5-year overall survival rate from 70 to 78% ($p = 0.03$) [88]. However, no significant difference in survival was observed between the two groups of treatment concerning the patients with metastatic disease (40% without L-MTP versus 53% with L-MTP, $p = 0.27$). Based on these results, the European Medicines Agency granted L-MTP an indication for the treatment of non-metastatic osteosarcoma in 2009; the American Food and Drug Administration (FDA) did not. L-MTP is also approved for use in Turkey, Mexico and Israel. Recently, Biteau et al. have proved the efficacy of association of zoledronate and L-mifamurtide combination in osteosarcoma. This association induced an additional and in some cases synergistic inhibition of primary tumour progression [89].

2.3.4. Inhaled granulocyte-macrophage colony stimulating factor (GM-CSF)

GM-CSF is one of the master regulators of myeloid cell lineage by controlling their differentiation, proliferation and activities. Indeed, this growth factor exerts immunomodulatory and immunostimulatory activities by stimulating the functional activities of neutrophil granulocytes but also of macrophages and DC. More specifically, GM-CSF promotes the recruitment and cytotoxic functions of macrophages, stimulates natural killer and dendritic cells, and consequently, upmodulates the number of CD4 T lymphocytes [90]. Arndt et al. have recently performed a phase I clinical trial using inhaled GM-CSF in patients with first isolated pulmonary recurrence of OS. Unfortunately, even though the clinical studies demonstrated the safety of administered GM-CSF (e.g. aerosolized delivery), no biological benefit (e.g. local immunomodulation in lung metastases) or improved clinical outcome was demonstrated. A future larger prospective randomised trial may demonstrate improved outcomes in OS patients probably [91, 92].

3. Conclusion

The therapies focused on the immune niche partially represent the potential therapeutic targets available for OS nowadays. Blood vessels, bone cells and tumour cells are targeted as well in the current clinical trials. However, in the future, the key to success will lie in better understanding and characterisation of the disease, leading to better patient stratification and, consequently, to personalised medicine.

Acknowledgements

This work was supported by the Bone Cancer Research Trust (UK, research project number 144681).

Author details

Marie-Françoise Heymann* and Dominique Heymann

*Address all correspondence to: m.heymann@sheffield.ac.uk

Department of Oncology and Metabolism, European Associated Laboratory "Sarcoma Research Unit", INSERM, Medical School, University of Sheffield, Sheffield, UK

References

[1] Fidler IJ. The pathogenesis of cancer metastasis: the 'seed and soil' hypothesis revisited. Nat Rev Cancer 2003;3:453–8.

[2] Paget S. The distribution of secondary growths in cancer of the breast. Cancer Metastasis Rev 1989;8:98–101.

[3] Plaks V, Kong N, Werb Z. The cancer stem cell niche: how essential is the niche in regulating stemness of tumour cells? Cell Stem 2015;16:225–38.

[4] Ordóñez-Morán P, Huelsken J. Complex metastatic niches: already a target for therapy? Curr Opin Cell Biol 2014;3:29–38.

[5] Iwasaki H, Suda T. Cancer stem cells and their niche. Cancer Sci 2009;100:1166–72.

[6] Basak GW, Srivastava AS, Malhotra R, Carrier E. Multiple myeloma bone marrow niche. Curr Pharm Biotechnol 2009;10:345–6.

[7] Wan L, Pantel K, Kang Y. Tumour metastasis: moving new biological insights into the clinic. Nat Med 2013;19:1450–64.

[8] Landskron G, De la Fuente M, Thuwajit P, Hermoso MA. Chronic inflammation and cytokines in the tumour microenvironment. J Immunol Res 2014;2014:149185.

[9] Renema N, Navet B, Heymann MF, Lezot F, Heymann D. RANK-RANKL signalling in cancer. Biosci Rep. 2016;36:e00366.

[10] Grimaud E, Soubigou L, Couillaud S, Coipeau P, Moreau A, Passuti N, et al. Receptor activator of nuclear factor kappa B ligand (RANKL)/osteoprotegerin (OPG) ratio is increased in severe osteolysis. Am J Pathol 2003;163:2021–31.

[11] Ungefroren H, Sebens S, Seidl D, Lehnert H, Hass R. Interaction of tumour cells with the microenvironment. Cell Commun Signal 2011;9:18.

[12] Zhu L, McManus MM, Hughes DPM. Understanding the biology of bone sarcoma from early initiating events through late events in metastasis and disease progression. Front Oncol 2013;3:230.

[13] Alfranca A, Martinez-Cruzado L, Tornin J, Abarrategi A, Amaral T, de Alava E, et al. Bone microenvironment signals in osteosarcoma development. Cell Mol Life Sci 2015;72:3097–113.

[14] Ando K, Heymann MF, Stresing V, Mori K, Rédini F, Heymann D. Current therapeutic strategies and novel approaches in osteosarcoma. Cancers 2013;5:591–616.

[15] Endo-Munoz L, Evdokiou A, Saunders NA. The role of osteoclasts and tumour-associated macrophages in osteosarcoma metastasis. Biochim Biophys Acta 1826;2012:434–42.

[16] Theoleyre S, Mori K, Cherrier B, Passuti N, Gouin F, Rédini F, et al. Phenotypic and functional analysis of lymphocytes infiltrating osteolytic tumours: use as a possible therapeutic approach of osteosarcoma. BMC Cancer 2005;5:123.

[17] Gordon S, Martinez FO. Alternative activation of macrophages: mechanism and functions. Immunity 2010;32:593–604.

[18] Lewis CE, Pollard JW. Distinct role of macrophages in different tumour microenvironments. Cancer Res 2006;66:605–12.

[19] Qian BZ, Pollard JW. Macrophage diversity enhances tumour progression and metastasis. Cell 2010;141:39–51.

[20] Rogers TL, Holen I. Tumour 469 macrophages as potential targets of bisphosphonates. J Transl Med 2011;9:177.

[21] Criscitiello C, Viale G, Gelao L, Esposito A, De Laurentiis M, De Placido S, Santangelo M, Goldhirsch A, Curigliano G. Crosstalk between bone niche and immune system: osteoimmunology signaling as a potential target for cancer treatment. Cancer Treat Rev 2015;41(2):61–8.

[22] Fritzsching B, Fellenberg J, Moskovszky L, Sápi Z, Krenacs T, Machado I, Poeschl J, Lehner B, Szendrõi M, Bosch AL, Bernd L, Csóka M, Mechtersheimer G, Ewerbeck V, Kinscherf R, Kunz P. $CD8^{+}/FOXP3^{+}$-ratio in osteosarcoma microenvironment separates survivors from non-survivors: a multicenter validated retrospective study. Oncoimmunology. 2015;4(3):e990800.

[23] Adams S, Gray RJ, Demaria S, Goldstein L, Perez EA, Shulman LN, Martino S, Wang M, Jones VE, Saphner TJ, Wolff AC, Wood WC, Davidson NE, Sledge GW, Sparano JA, Badve SS. Prognostic value of tumour-infiltrating lymphocytes in triple-negative breast cancers from two phase III randomized adjuvant breast cancer trials: ECOG 2197 and ECOG 1199. J Clin Oncol 2014;32(27):2959–66.

[24] Sorbye SW, Kilvaer T, Valkov A, Donnem T, Smeland E, Al-Shibli K, Bremnes RM, Busund LT. Prognostic impact of lymphocytes in soft tissue sarcomas. PLoS One. 2011;6(1):e14611.

[25] Rosenberg SA. Progress in human tumour immunology and immunotherapy. Nature 2001;411:380–4.

[26] Trieb K, Lechleitner T, Lang S, Windhager R, Kotz R, Dirnhofer S. Evaluation of HLA-DR expression and T-lymphocyte infiltration in osteosarcoma.Pathol Res Pract 1998;194(10):679–84.

[27] Galon J, Pages F, Marincola FM, Angell HK, Thurin M, Lugli A, Zlobec I, Berger A, Bifulco C, Botti G, et al. Cancer classification using the Immunoscore: a world-wide task force. J Transl Med 2012;10:205.

[28] Mlecnik B, Tosolini M, Kirilovsky A, Berger A, Bindea G, Meatchi T, Bruneval P, Trajanoski Z, Fridman WH, Pages F, et al. Histopathologic-based prognostic factors of colorectal cancers are associated with the state of the local immune reaction. J Clin Oncol 2011;29:610–8.

[29] Wong BR, Josien R, Lee SY, Sauter B, Li HL, Steinman RM, Choi Y. TRANCE (tumour necrosis factor [TNF]-related activation-induced cytokine), a new TNF family member

predominantly expressed in T cells,isadendritic cells pecific survival factor. J Exp Med 1997;186:2075–80.

[30] Yasuda H, Shima N, Nakagawa N, Mochizuki SI, Yano K, Fujise N, Sato Y, Goto M, Yamaguchi K, Kuriyama M, Kanno T, Murakami A, Tsuda E, Morinaga T, Higashio K. Osteoclast differentiation factor is a ligand for osteoprotegerin/osteoclastogenesis-inhibitory factor and is identical to TRANCE/RANKL. Proc Natl Acad Sci U S A 1998;95:3597–602.

[31] Ikeda T, Kasai M, Utsuyama M, Hirokawa K. Determination of three isoforms of the receptor activator of nuclear factor-kappa B ligand and their differential expression in bone and thymus. Endocrinology 2001;142:1419–26.

[32] Mueller CG, Hess E. Emerging functions of RANKL in lymphoid tissues. Front Immunol 2012;3:261.

[33] Akiyama T, Shimo Y, Yanai H, Qin J, Ohshima D, Maruyama Y, Asaumi Y, Kitazawa J, Takayanagi H, Penninger JM, Matsumoto M, Nitta T, Takahama Y, Inoue J. The tumour necrosis factor family receptors RANK and CD40 cooperatively establish the thymic medullary microenvironment and self-tolerance. Immunity 2008;29:423–37.

[34] Anderson DM, Maraskovsky E, Billingsley WL, Dougall WC, Tometsko ME, Roux ER, Teepe MC, DuBose RF, Cosman D, Galibert L. A homologue of the TNF Receptor and its ligand enhance T cell growth and dendritic cell function. Nature 1997;390:175–9.

[35] Khan IS, Mouchess ML, Zhu ML,Conley B, Fasano KJ, Hou Y, Fong L, Su MA. Enhancement of an anti-tumour immune response by transient blockade of central T cell tolerance. J Exp Med 2014;211:761–8.

[36] Mori K, Rédini F, Gouin F, Cherrier B, Heymann D. Osteosarcoma: current status of immunotherapy and future trends. Oncol Rep 2006;15(3):693–700.

[37] Mori K, Le Goff B, Berreur M, Riet A, Moreau A, Blanchard F, Chevalier C, Guisle-Marsollier I, Léger J, Guicheux J, Masson M, Gouin F, Rédini F, Heymann D. Human osteosarcoma cells express functional receptor activator of nuclear factor-kappa B. J Pathol 2007;11:555–62.

[38] Lamoureux F, Richard P, Wittrant Y, Battaglia S, Pilet P, Trichet V, Blanchard F, Gouin F, Pitard B, Heymann D, Redini F. Therapeutic relevance of osteoprotegerin gene therapy in osteosarcoma: blockade of the vicious cycle between tumour cell proliferation and bone resorption. Cancer Res 2007;67(15):7308–18.

[39] van Furth R, Cohn ZA. The origin and kinetics of mononuclear phagocytes. J Exp Med 1968;128:415–35.

[40] Taylor PR, Gordon S. Monocytes heterogeneity and innate immunity. Immunity 2003; 19:2–4.

[41] Lin H, Lee E, Hestir K, Leo C, Huang M, Bosch E, et al. Discovery of a cytokine and its receptor by functional screening of the extracellular proteome. Science 2008;320:807–11.

[42] Heymann D. Interleukin-34: an enigmatic cytokine. IBMS BoneKey 2010;7:406–13.

[43] Bingle L, Brown NJ, Lewis CE. The role of tumour-associated macrophages in tumour progression: implications for new anticancer therapies. J Pathol 2002;196(3):254–65.

[44] Zhang QW, Liu L, Gong CY, Shi HS, Zeng YH, Wang XZ, Zhao YW, Wei YQ. Prognostic significance of tumor-associated macrophages in solid tumor: a meta-analysis of the literature. PLoS One 2012;7(12):e50946.

[45] Laoui D, Van Overmeire E, De Baetselier P, Van Ginderachter JA, Raes G. Functional relationship between tumor-associated macrophages and macrophage colony-stimulating factor as contributors to cancer progression. Front Immunol 2014;5:489.

[46] Mills CD, Kincaid K, Alt JM, Heilman MJ, Hill AM. M-1/M-2 macrophages and the Th1/Th2 paradigm. J Immunol 2000;164:6166–73.

[47] Buddingh EP, Kuijjer ML, Duim RA, Bürger H, Agelopoulos K, Myklebost O, et al. Tumour-infiltrating macrophages are associated with metastasis suppression in high-grade osteosarcoma: a rationale for treatment with macrophage activating agents. Clin Cancer Res 2011;17:2110–9.

[48] Xiao Q, Zhang X, Wu Y, Yang Y. Inhibition of macrophage polarization prohibits growth of human osteosarcoma. Tumour Biol 2014;35:7611–6.

[49] Pahl JHW, Kwappenberg KM, Varypataki EM, Santos SJ, Kuijjer ML, Mohamed S, et al. Macrophages inhibit human osteosarcoma cell growth after activation with the bacterial cell wall derivative liposomal muramyl tripeptide in combination with interferon-γ. J Exp Clin Cancer Res 2014;33:27.

[50] Ségaliny AI, Mohamadi A, Dizier B, Lokajczyk A, Brion R, Lanel R, et al. Interleukin-34 promotes tumour progression and metastatic process in osteosarcoma through induction of angiogenesis and macrophage recruitment. Int J Cancer 2015;137:73–85.

[51] Cook J, Hagemann T. Tumour-associated macrophages and cancer. Curr Opin Pharmacol 2013;13:595–601.

[52] Breuil V, Schmid-Antomarchi H, Schmid-Alliana A, Rezzonico R, Euller-Ziegler L, Rossi B. The receptor activator of nuclear factor (NF)-kappa B lignad (RANKL) is a new chemotactic for human monocytes. FASEB J 2003;17:2163–5.

[53] Kambayashi Y, Fujimura T, Furudate S, Asano M, Kakizaki A, Aiba S. The possible interaction between receptor activator of nuclear factor kappa-B ligand expressed by extramammary paget cells and its ligand on dermal macrophages. J Invest Dermatol 2015;135:2547–50.

[54] Fujimura T, Kambayashi Y, Furudate S, Asano M, Kakizaki A, Aiba S. Receptor activator of NF-[kappa] B ligand promotes the production of CCL17 from RANK+ M2 macrophages. J Invest Dermatol 2015;135:2884–7.

[55] Tan W, Zhang W, Strasner A, Grivennikov S, Cheng JQ, Hoffman RM, Karin M. Tumour-infiltrating regulatory T cells stimulate mammary cancer metastasis through RANKL-RANK signalling. Nature 2011;470:548–53.

[56] Rosen G, Tan C, Sanmaneechai A, Beattie EJ Jr, Marcove R, Murphy ML. The rationale for multiple drug chemotherapy in the treatment of osteogenic sarcoma. Cancer 1975;35:936–45.

[57] Bacci G, Longhi A, Fagioli F, Briccoli A, Versari M, Picci P. Adjuvant and neoadjuvant chemotherapy for osteosarcoma of the extremities: 27 year experience at Rizzoli Institute, Eur J Cancer 2005;41:2836–45.

[58] Chou AJ, Geller DS, Gorlick R. Therapy for osteosarcoma: where do we go from here? Paediatr Drugs 2008;10:315–27.

[59] Errani C, Longhi A, Rossi G, et al. Palliative therapy for osteosarcoma. Expert Rev Anticancer Ther 2011;11:217–27.

[60] Schwarz R, Bruland O, Cassoni A, Schomberg P, Bielack S. The role of radiotherapy in oseosarcoma. Cancer Treat Res 2009;152:147–64.

[61] Roberts SS, Chou AJ, Cheung NK. Immunotherapy of Childhood Sarcomas. Front Oncol 2015;5:181.

[62] DeRenzo C, Gottschalk S. Genetically modified T-cell therapy for osteosarcoma. Adv Exp Med Biol 2014;804:323–40.

[63] Li Z. Potential of human γδ T cells for immunotherapy of osteosarcoma. Mol Biol Rep 2013;40:427–37.

[64] Tarek N, Lee DA. Natural killer cells for osteosarcoma. Adv Exp Med Biol 2014;804:341–53.

[65] Gajewski TF, Schreiber H, Fu YX. Innate and adaptive immune cells in the tumor microenvironment. Nat Immunol 2013;14(10):1014–22.

[66] Coiffier B, Lepage E, Brière J, et al. CHOP chemotherapy plus rituximab compared with CHOP alone in elderly patients with diffuse large-B-cell lymphoma. N Engl J Med 2002;346(4):235–42.

[67] Piccart-Gebhart MJ, Procter M, Leyland-Jones B, et al. Trastuzumab after adjuvant chemotherapy in HER2-positive breast cancer. N Engl J Med 2005;353(16):1659–72.

[68] Yu AL, Gilman AL, Ozkaynak MF, et al. Anti-GD2 antibody with GM-CSF, interleukin-2, and isotretinoin for neuroblastoma. N Engl J Med 2010;363(14):1324–34.

[69] Hersey P, Jamal O, Henderson C, Zardawi I, D'Alessandro G. Expression of the gangliosides GM3, GD3 and GD2 in tissue sections of normal skin, naevi, primary and metastatic melanoma. Int J Cancer 1988;41(3):336–43.

[70] Martinez C, Hofmann TJ, Marino R, Dominici M, Horwitz EM. Human bone marrow mesenchymal stromal cells express the neural ganglioside GD2: a novel surface marker for the identification of MSCs. Blood 2007;109(10):4245–8.

[71] Svennerholm L, Boström K, Fredman P, et al. Gangliosides and allied glycosphingolipids in human peripheral nerve and spinal cord. Biochim Biophys Acta 1994;1214(2):115–23.

[72] Cheung N, Kushner B, Yeh S, Larson S. 3F8 monoclonal antibody treatment of patients with stage 4 neuroblastoma: a phase II study. Int J Oncol 1998;12(6):1299.

[73] Cheung N, Lazarus H, Miraldi FD, et al. Ganglioside GD2 specific monoclonal antibody 3F8: a phase I study in patients with neuroblastoma and malignant melanoma. J Clin Oncol 1987;5(9):1430–40.

[74] Heiner JP, Miraldi F, Kallick S, et al. Localization of GD2-specific monoclonal antibody 3F8 in human osteosarcoma. Cancer Res 1987;47(20):5377–81.

[75] Cheung NKV, Canete A, Cheung IY, Ye JN, Liu C. Disialoganglioside GD2 anti-idiotypic monoclonal antibodies. Int J Cancer 1993;54(3):499–505.

[76] Cheung N-KV, Cheung IY, Kushner BH, et al. Murine anti-GD2 monoclonal antibody 3F8 combined with granulocyte-macrophage colony-stimulating factor and 13-cis-retinoic acid in highrisk patients with stage 4 neuroblastoma in first remission. J Clin Oncol 2012;30(26):3264–70.

[77] Roth M, Linkowski M, Tarim J, et al. Ganglioside GD2 as a therapeutic target for antibodymediated therapy in patients with osteosarcoma. Cancer 2014;120(4):548–54.

[78] Gorlick R, Janeway K, Lessnick S, Randall RL, Marina N. COG Bone Tumor Committee. Children's Oncology Group's 2013 blueprint for research: bone tumors. Pediatr Blood Cancer 2013;60(6):1009–15.

[79] Hamanishi J, Mandai M, Matsumura N, Abiko K, Baba T, Konishi I. PD-1/PD-L1 blockade in cancer treatment: perspectives and issues. Int J Clin Oncol. 2016;21(3):462–73.

[80] Shen JK, Cote GM, Choy E, et al. Targeting programmed cell death ligand 1 in osteosarcoma: an auto-commentary on therapeutic potential. Oncoimmunology 2014;3(8):e954467.

[81] Zheng W, Xiao H, Liu H, Zhou Y. Expression of programmed death 1 is correlated with progression of osteosarcoma. APMIS 2015;123(2):102–7.

[82] Constantino J, Gomes C, Falcão A, Cruz MT, Neves BM. Antitumor dendritic cell-based vaccines: lessons from 20years of clinical trials and future perspectives. Transl Res 2016;168:74–95.

[83] Chauvin C, Philippeau JM, Hémont C, Hubert FX, Wittrant Y, Lamoureux F, Trinité B, Heymann D, Rédini F, Josien R. Killer dendritic cells link innate and adaptive immunity against established osteosarcoma in rats. Cancer Res 2008;68:9433–40

[84] Krishnadas DK, Shusterman S, Bai F, Diller L, Sullivan JE, Cheerva AC, George RE, Lucas KG. A phase I trial combining decitabine/dendritic cell vaccine targeting MAGE-A1, MAGE-A3 and NY-ESO-1 for children with relapsed or therapy-refractory neuroblastoma and sarcoma. Cancer Immunol Immunother 2015;64:1251–60.

[85] Himoudi N, Wallace R, Parsley KL, Gilmour K, Barrie AU, Howe K, Dong R, Sebire NJ, Michalski A, Thrasher AJ, Anderson J. Lack of T-cell responses following autologous

tumour lysate pulsed dendritic cell vaccination, in patients with relapsed osteosarcoma. Clin Transl Oncol 2012;14:271–9.

[86] Kleinerman ES, Jia SF, Gri NJ, Seibel NL, Benjamin RS, Ja EN. Phase II study of liposomal muramyl tripeptide in osteosarcoma: the cytokine cascade and monocyte activation following administration. J Clin Oncol 1992;10(8):1310–6.

[87] Ando K, Mori K, Corradini N, Redini F, Heymann D. Mifamurtide for the treatment of nonmetastatic osteosarcoma. Expert Opin Pharmacother 2011;12(2):285–92.

[88] Meyers PA, Schwartz CL, Krailo MD, Healey JH, Bernstein ML, Betcher D, et al. Osteosarcoma: the addition of muramyl tripeptide to chemotherapy improves overall survival—a report from the children's oncology group. J Clin Oncol 2008;26(4):633–8

[89] Biteau K, Guiho R, Chatelais M, Taurelle J, Chesneau J, Corradini N, Heymann D, Redini F. L-MTP-PE and zoledronic acid combination in osteosarcoma: preclinical evidence of positive therapeutic combination for clinical transfer. Am J Cancer Res 2016;6(3):677–89.

[90] Lamplot JD, Denduluri S, Qin J, Li R, Liu X, Zhang H, Chen X, Wang N, Pratt A, Shui W, Luo X, Nan G, Deng ZL, Luo J, Haydon RC, He TC, Luu HH. The current and future therapies for human osteosarcoma. Curr Cancer Ther Rev 2013;9(1):55–77.

[91] Arndt CA, Koshkina NV, Inwards CY, Hawkins DS, Krailo MD, Villaluna D, Anderson PM, Goorin AM, Blakely ML, Bernstein M, Bell SA, Ray K, Grendahl DC, Marina N, Kleinerman ES. Inhaled granulocyte-macrophage colony stimulating factor for first pulmonary recurrence of osteosarcoma: effects on disease-free survival and immunomodulation. A report from the Children's Oncology Group. Clin Cancer Res. 2010;16(15):4024–30.

[92] Heymann MF, Brown HK, Heymann D. Drugs in early clinical development for the treatment of osteosarcoma. Expert Opin Investig Drugs 2016;25(11):1265–80.

Chapter 7

Immune Checkpoint Blockade: Subjugation of the Masses

Danielle M. Lussier, Nicole T. Appel,
John L. Johnson and Joseph N. Blattman

Additional information is available at the end of the chapter

http://dx.doi.org/10.5772/67687

Abstract

Osteosarcoma remains the most common form of bone cancer in adolescents. Standard of care treatment for osteosarcoma includes chemotherapy combined with limb-salvage surgery or amputation. Survival rates for compliant patients are 60–80% for those with localized tumors and 15–30% if the tumor metastasizes or reoccurs. Given the successes of monoclonal antibody blockades in other cancers, clinical trials for applying immunotherapies to osteosarcoma are underway. Antibody blockades reinvigorate T cells to eliminate cancer cells thereby leading to decreased tumor burden and long-term regression. Single monoclonal antibody therapy has shown modest efficacy compared to standard of care. However, treating with only a single antibody can ultimately result in immune evasion by heterogeneous tumors via selection of cells expressing other inhibitory ligands. Hence, combination immunotherapies have yielded the most promising results for eliminating tumors or preventing reoccurrence in other cancer types and will likely be the most efficacious strategy for treating osteosarcoma. Here, we review current immunotherapies for other cancers and their potential application to osteosarcoma.

Keywords: osteosarcoma, monoclonal antibody blockade, PD-1, PD-L1, CTLA-4, LAG-3, TIM-3, combination antibody blockade, tumor escape

1. Introduction

Multiple tumor types have been shown to co-opt the use of immune inhibitory receptors to evade immune detection and killing [1–5], including metastatic osteosarcoma. Several immune inhibitory receptors have been identified and shown to decrease tumor-specific T-cell killing and induce an exhausted T-cell state [6]. The use of blocking monoclonal antibodies in experimental settings can prevent tolerance, reinvigorate T-cell function at the tumor site increasing T-cell killing, cytokine production, and proliferation, or induce new systemic T-cell responses [7]. The prevention of T-cell exhaustion or reinvigoration at the tumor site has led to improved clinical results in using these monoclonal antibodies to reduce tumor burden in human patients [8, 9]. However, outcomes after blocking monoclonal antibody therapy vary by tumor type/stage (i.e., primary versus metastatic), amount of tumor infiltrating lymphocyte (TIL) infiltration, and amount and combinational inhibitory receptor expression. Early studies investigating the role of the immune system in preventing metastatic tumor development, while allowing primary tumor growth, shed light on the importance of T-cell-tumor mingling in order to effectively suppress tumor growth through immune-mediated killing [10]. Suppressive tumor microenvironments that inhibit TIL infiltration leading to immune-privileged sites would not benefit from increased tumor-reactive T-cell responses via blocking monoclonal antibodies. Additionally, tumor-reactive T cells require inhibition via inhibitory receptors to benefit from blocking monoclonal antibody treatments [11]. Ultimately, with new advances in immunotherapies to alleviate microenvironment suppression, combinational treatments to increase T-cell function, increased immune effector access to tumors, and prevention of T-cell exhaustion may have increased curative potential.

2. Successes of single checkpoint mAb blockade strategies in the treatment of progressive tumors

2.1. PD-1 blockade

The efficacy of programmed death receptor-1 (PD-1) blockade in initial clinical trials of several tumor types has been reviewed extensively by Pardoll, Momtaz and Postow, and Sharma and Allison [9, 12, 13]. Nivolumab, pembrolizumab, and pidilizumab are α-PD-1 blocking antibodies developed by various pharmaceutical companies. Investigators are trying to identify biomarkers to classify cancer patients that will benefit most from PD-1 blockade. Programmed death ligand 1 (PD-L1) expression on tumors correlates with poor prognosis; however, high expression of PD-L1/PD-1 in tumors correlates with responses to blockade therapy [14]. However, patients with PD-L1 negative tumor expression still benefit from PD-1 blockade in some cases [15]. Briefly, overall response rate from patients with different progressive solid tumors treated with nivolumab was 31%, and duration of response was approximately 2 years, with median overall survival of 16.8 months [14, 16]. This is in comparison to malignant melanoma patients treated with pembrolizumab with an overall response rate of 38%, although treatment dose varied [17]. Additionally, chemotherapy-resistant hematologic malignancies treated with pidilizumab saw clinical benefit in 33% of patients [18]. Clinical success of the PD-1 monoclonal antibody blockade in treating multiple progressive tumors has inspired the field of tumor immunology, by leading to some of the best clinical efficacies and long-term durable regression. Currently, clinical trials for treating recurrent or refractory osteosarcoma with nivolumab, with and without ipilimumab, are in phase I/II [19].

2.2. CTLA-4 blockade

Successes of cytotoxic lymphocyte associated antigen-4 (CTLA-4) monoclonal antibody blockade have been reviewed extensively in Ref. [13]. Briefly, patients with advanced stage melanoma when treated with ipilimumab had long-term durable responses with over 20% surviving longer than 4 years [20, 21]. However, other tumor types, such as prostate cancer, saw no improvement in survival in patients treated with ipilimumab at multiple stages of disease progression [22].

2.3. LAG-3 blockade

Lymphocyte activating gene protein 3 (LAG-3) inhibitors have begun phase I/II trials in human patients. Both renal cell carcinoma and metastatic breast cancer patients saw objective responses when treated with LAG-3 inhibitors and durable disease stabilization [23, 24]. Ongoing trials are beginning with a monoclonal antibody to LAG-3; however, no results have been reported.

2.4. TIM-3 blockade

Preclinical tumor models suggest that blocking T-cell immunoglobulin mucin domain molecule 3 (TIM-3) activation in combination with PD-1 may improve survival, as the majority of TILs are both TIM-3 and PD-1 positive, and these TILs have the most profound exhaustion at the tumor site [25]. In a mouse model of solid-tumor CT26 colon carcinoma, mice treated with dual TIM-3 and PD-1 blocking mAb had significantly decreased tumor growth; however, TIM-3 mAb treatment alone provided no benefits. The combinational approach appeared to have some synergistic effects [25].

3. Resistance to blockade treatment

3.1. Resistance to blockade treatment in tumor settings

Tumor heterogeneity provides the fuel for the evolution of therapeutic resistance [26]. A more diverse tumor has a greater likelihood of possessing a pre-existing resistance mutation than a less heterogeneous one, and a more mutable tumor has a greater likelihood of generating a *de novo* mutation during therapy. Even before immunotherapy, cells in the tumor will have undergone extensive selection for the capacity to evade the immune system during the course of progression. This means that cell-level capacities that enable resistance to immunotherapy pre-exist in some tumors. In immunotherapy, cells that preferentially survive treatment are likely to be those with the ability to create an immunosuppressive environment around the tumor and/or reduce immunogenicity through loss of antigens or downregulation of MHC I.

Taube et al. introduced the adaptive immune resistance hypothesis to explain selection of PD-L1 positive tumor cells by endogenous immune response pressure [27]. Initially proposed by Robert Schreiber, the now widely accepted hypothesis of tumor immune editing describes how immune responses can both eliminate and promote tumor formation. This fine line between elimination and immune driven escape explains the ability of the adaptive immune resistance hypothesis to select for PD-L1 positive tumor cells, suppressing immune-mediated killing. Overwhelming evidence exists for the use of PD-1/PD-L1 blockade in reinvigorating immune-mediated tumor killing. However, little is known regarding immune-mediated tumor escape after monoclonal antibody blockade TIL reinvigoration. Responses in only a fraction of patients and incomplete tumor control from PD-1 blockade may be due to the upregulation of compensatory regulatory pathways or the selection of nonimmunogenic tumors. As stated earlier, clinical trials are in the early stages for recurring and refractory osteosarcoma treatments with monoclonal antibody blockade both as a singular drug and in combination with another monoclonal antibody blockade therapy. Therefore, little data are currently available regarding how combination immunotherapies affect human patients. Nonetheless, scientific research highly suggests increased expression of other regulatory pathways when only one immunotherapy is administered [28].

Knowing the mechanism of immune escape from blockade therapy will guide the clinician in choosing more effective treatments to combat escape and lead to durable responses or complete remission. It may also be possible to measure existing immune evasion strategies in a tumor before therapy begins in order to limit the use of immunotherapies for which the tumor may already be preadapted (e.g., where there are pre-existing resistance mutations). However, to prevent escape from occurring, it may be necessary to administer combinational treatments concurrently and early in treatment history, similar to treatment to persistent viral infections.

3.2. Viral resistance to therapy, what can we learn

T-cell exhaustion was first observed in a mouse model of chronic lymphocytic choriomeningitis virus (LCMV), in which exhausted T cells were unable to proliferate rapidly, produce antitumor cytokines, or perform cytotoxic functions [29]. PD-1 blockade in mice infected with chronic LCMV could reinvigorate T cells and rescue function. However, due to only a subset of exhausted CD8 T cells regaining function after blockade, PD-1/PD-L1 blockade is not fully effective at restoring function to all exhausted T cells [30], leaving open the potential for additional T-cell exhaustion, and ultimately viral escape. T-cell exhaustion has been observed in many chronic virally infected humans with HIV, hepatitis B virus, or hepatitis C virus, and immune checkpoint blockade can restore T-cell function *in vitro*. However, HIV escape from adaptive immune responses has led to persistent viremia with no immune control. Even in the presence of combinational antiretroviral therapy, HIV still increases inflammation, leads to increased apoptosis, and induces oxidative stress in the host. However, physicians treat with combination antiretroviral therapy at the beginning of a treatment regimen to reduce chance of viral resistance and escape.

There may be limitations to the application of viral antiresistance strategies to cancer immunotherapy including the differences in population sizes, with tumors having several orders of magnitude more cells than are typically virally infected in HIV [31, 32]. This larger population size means that there is a greater likelihood of pre-existing resistance in cancer relative to viral infections and that it may be easier for tumor cell populations to evolve resistance.

Nonetheless, just as cancer immunologists learned from virologists about T-cell exhaustion in chronic viral settings, we may be able to apply the same strategies of early combinational treatments to try to prevent overall escape.

4. Potential escape through upregulation of other inhibitory receptors

Blockade of other inhibitory receptors in combination with PD-1 blockade is of clinical interest as responding TILs often co-express multiple inhibitory receptors, which may be an appropriate marker for potential escape through additional T-cell suppression [33].

Multiple studies have now shown increased expression of co-inhibitory receptors on infiltrating CD4 and CD8 T cells after blockade therapy including α-CTLA-4 alone, α-PD-1 alone, α-PD-L1 alone, or combinational therapies. Curran et al. observed a twofold increase in the percentage of CTLA-4+ expressing cells after treatment with anti-PD-1 mAb in their B16-BL6 melanoma mouse model [34]. Additionally, treatment with CTLA-4 mAb led to an approximate 10% increase in PD-1+ CD8+ TILs [34]. In a metastatic mouse model of osteosarcoma, treatment with anti-PD-L1 led to a twofold increase in CTLA-4 expression and selection of a PD-L1 negative tumor [28]. Sznol and Chen, in personal communications with J. Weber, confirmed this effect in human patients treated with α-PD-1 blockade noting an increase in CTLA-4 expression on TILs [35]. In an implantable mouse model of metastatic osteosarcoma, the authors of this review discovered resistance to α-PD-L1 blockade following treatment due to increases in co-inhibitory receptor expression on TILs, which dual CTLA-4/PD-1 blockade treatment could prevent [28]. These studies confirm changes in co-inhibitory receptor expression on TILs following blockade therapy and confer additional mechanisms for tumor cells to evade immune killing in response to blockade treatment. Conversely, the other co-inhibitory receptors LAG-3 and TIM-3 appear to decrease in an methylcholanthrene (MCA) induced sarcoma model following anti-PD-1 alone, anti-CTLA-4 alone, or anti-PD-1 and anti-CTLA-4 in combination [36]. The most likely explanation for increased co-inhibitory receptors following blockade is due to compensatory mechanisms preventing pathology against persistent antigen exposure.

Tumor resistance to blockade treatment generated through additional upregulation and ligation of co-inhibitory receptors may direct physicians to treat with combinational immunotherapies to target multiple inhibitory receptors. Whereas tumor resistance to blockade treatment generated through decreased immunogenicity may warrant chemotherapy or radiation in combination with blockade to increase the expression of immunogenic antigens.

5. Successes of combinational blockade strategies

5.1. Immunotherapy combinational blockades

CTLA-4 and PD-1 combinational blockade has shown promise in clinical trials against advanced melanoma with 50% of patients in the highest dose cohort achieving objective responses and a large reduction in tumor burden [37]. The inhibitory pathways of PD-1 and CTLA-4 appear to be nonredundant with distinct mechanisms in the maintenance of peripheral tolerance, as well as biased effects on distinct subsets of T cells, making the combination of the two of particular interest.

The combination of anti-PD-L1 or anti-PD-1 and anti-CTLA-4 mAb improved tumor control, increased IL-2 production and proliferation of CD8+ TILs, and increased the ratio of intratumoral CD8+ T cells to Tregs in the B16 melanoma mouse model [34, 38]. In the GL261 glioma model, the combination of CTLA-4 and PD-L1 mAb blockade provided long-term survival and significantly reduced the proportion of Tregs in the brain [39]. Moreover, the combination potentiated the eradication of tumors in the CT26 colon carcinoma and 4T1 breast cancer model compared to the modest effects of single-agent treatment.

In a metastatic osteosarcoma model, combining PD-L1 and CTLA-4 blockade allowed for over 50% rate in mice, while neither PD-L1 nor CTLA-4 blockade alone eliminated tumor burden. Furthermore, tumor did not come back even when mice were challenged [28].

Clinical success of α-CTLA-4 and α-PD-1 monoclonal antibodies has inspired investigators to identify other potential inhibitory receptors that modulate T-cell responses in nonredundant mechanisms. Other co-inhibitory receptors of clinical interest include LAG-3 and TIM-3 [40, 41]. Blockade of both LAG-3 and PD-1 in the Sa1N fibrosarcoma model and MC38 colon adenocarcinoma model exhibited complete tumor control with effects that appear to be synergistic compared to single-agent therapy. No effect was seen against established B16 melanoma tumors again suggesting the presence of other regulatory or resistance mechanisms [40]. The blockade of both TIM3 and PD-1 in methylcholanthrene-induced fibrosarcomas suppressed growth of established tumors and even completely cleared tumors in a small fraction of mice [41]. However, the mechanism of action of anti-TIM3 blockade alone or in combination with other immunomodulatory mAbs has not been well characterized [42]. Additionally, upregulation of PD-L1 homologs B7-H3 and B7-H4 or the induction of expression of these homologs on macrophages within the tumor microenvironment presents additional opportunities for tumors to mediate effector T-cell inhibition through PD-1, when PD-L1 mAb blockade is used [43–45].

Although the mechanisms underlying resistance to PD-1/PD-L1 blockade have not yet been clearly elucidated, the success of combinational immunotherapies suggests that tumors use multiple and nonoverlapping mechanisms of resistance in order to maintain an immunosuppressive environment or to escape T-cell recognition altogether. Combinational treatment with monoclonal inhibitory blockade antibodies may be necessary for optimal anti-tumor responses and prevention of additional escape mechanisms through other T-cell inhibitory receptor suppression. Therefore, the type of blockade-driven tumor resistance may alter the choice of combinational therapies.

6. Decreased immunogenicity leading to escape

Another possible mechanism of acquired resistance to PD-1/PD-L1 blockade includes the selection of nonimmunogenic tumors [46]. Loss of antigens or downregulation of MHC I allow the

http://dx.doi.org/10.5772/67687

tumor to escape from T-cell recognition, possibly following blockade reinvigoration. There is currently no evidence that we are aware of for selection of tumors with decreased immunogenicity after monoclonal antibody blockade therapy, although selection of PD-L1+ tumors during initial tumor immune responses suggests that similar mechanisms may exist following TIL reinvigoration with checkpoint inhibitor blockade. The use of radiation to overcome this type of resistance has shown promise by causing immunogenic cell death. After radiation, tumors upregulate MHC I, Fas (CD95), ICAM-1, and NKG2D ligands to become optimized targets for CTLs and lead to the release of more tumor antigens and activation of a broader T-cell repertoire [47]. Significant tumor regression in metastatic melanoma patients was seen with combinational anti-CTLA-4 blockade and radiation [48]. Another study showed the combination of radiation and PD-L1 blockade was more effective than either single agent treatment in TUBO breast cancer and MC38 colon adenocarcinoma tumor models, reduced myeloid derived suppressor cells (MDSCs), and led to eradication of tumor and protection against further rechallenge [49]. Hypofractionated radiotherapy appears to be more effective than single high-dose radiotherapy, and the combination of hypofractionated radiation with anti-PD-1 mAb increased tumor antigen–specific CD8 T cells, improved survival, increased tumor control, and elicited the abscopal effect in 4T1 and B16 tumor models [50]. Additionally, fractioned radiation required concurrent administration of PD-1 or PD-L1 to elicit a synergistic effect in CD26 colon carcinoma, 4434 melanoma, and 4T1 breast cancer models, and no synergistic effect was seen if blockade was administered sequentially after completion of radiation [51]. Combination of PD-1 blockade with targeted therapies such as BRAF inhibitors in melanoma—which has been shown to decrease IL-10 production and enhance expression of tumor-specific antigens—may also prove promising, and clinical trials of the combination are underway [52–54]. Chemotherapy can also cause immunogenic cell death and lead to maturation and recruitment of antigen presenting cells (APCs), upregulation of antigens, increased MHC I expression, and increased CD8+ TIL infiltration [55]. α-PD-1/PD-L1 mAb treatment can select for nonimmunogenic tumors via antigen loss, MHC downregulation, selection of less immunogenic antigens, etc. Combinational therapies that increase TIL repertoire, antigen diversity, and tumor-specific antigens can combat this type of resistance after PD-1/PD-L1 blockade.

Another opportunity in designing combinatorial treatments from an evolutionarily informed perspective is that of shaping selection pressures so as to make resistant cells least fit by using antagonistic drug interactions [56]. This approach uses two therapeutic agents with antagonistic effects, making the fitness of cells with resistance to one therapy or the other less fit than cells that lack resistance entirely. This strategy could potentially be leveraged in immunotherapy by employing immunotherapeutic approaches that have some antagonistic effects.

7. Conclusion

Therapeutic resistance is one of the most difficult challenges in cancer treatment. At its root, this therapeutic resistance is driven by heterogeneity of cancer cells and their capacity to evolve quickly in response to treatments. From an evolutionary perspective, immunotherapy offers a unique approach that can harness the power of the adaptive immune systems to generate and respond to novelty rapidly and with a precision that may not be possible with other treatment approaches.

There are several potential mechanisms of resistance to PD-1/PD-L1 blockade that lead to upregulation of co-expression of inhibitory receptors and/or selection of less immunogenic tumors. Understanding these mechanisms will provide the opportunity to develop the right combination of therapies or to develop new therapies in order to elicit a potent anti-tumor T-cell response.

Author details

Danielle M. Lussier, Nicole T. Appel, John L. Johnson and Joseph N. Blattman*

*Address all correspondence to: joseph.blattman@asu.edu

Center for Immunotherapy, Vaccines, and Virotherapy, Biodesign Institute, Arizona State University, Tempe, AZ, USA

References

[1] Boorjian SA, Sheinin Y, Crispen PL, Farmer SA, Lohse CM, Kuntz SM, Leibovich BC, Kwon ED, Frank I. T-cell coregulatory molecule expression in urothelial cell carcinoma: clinicopathologic correlations and association with survival. Clinical Cancer Research: An Official Journal of the American Association for Cancer Research 2008; 14:4800-8.

[2] Lyford-Pike S, Peng S, Young GD, Taube JM, Westra WH, Akpeng B, Bruno TC, Richmon JD, Wang H, Bishop JA, et al. Evidence for a role of the PD-1: PD-L1 pathway in immune resistance of HPV-associated head and neck squamous cell carcinoma. Cancer Research 2013; 73:1733-41.

[3] Muenst S, Hoeller S, Dirnhofer S, Tzankov A. Increased programmed death-1+ tumor-infiltrating lymphocytes in classical Hodgkin lymphoma substantiate reduced overall survival. Human Pathology 2009; 40:1715-22.

[4] Nomi T, Sho M, Akahori T, Hamada K, Kubo A, Kanehiro H, Nakamura S, Enomoto K, Yagita H, Azuma M, et al. Clinical significance and therapeutic potential of the programmed death-1 ligand/programmed death-1 pathway in human pancreatic cancer. Clinical Cancer Research: An Official Journal of the American Association for Cancer Research 2007; 13:2151-7.

[5] Thompson RH, Dong H, Lohse CM, Leibovich BC, Blute ML, Cheville JC, Kwon ED. PD-1 is expressed by tumor-infiltrating immune cells and is associated with poor outcome for patients with renal cell carcinoma. Clinical Cancer Research: An Official Journal of the American Association for Cancer Research 2007; 13:1757-61.

[6] Seliger B, Quandt D. The expression, function, and clinical relevance of B7 family members in cancer. Cancer Immunology, Immunotherapy: CII 2012; 61:1327-41.

[7] Lussier DM, O'Neill L, Nieves LM, McAfee MS, Holechek SA, Collins AW, Dickman P, Jacobsen J, Hingorani P, Blattman JN. Enhanced T-cell immunity to osteosarcoma through antibody blockade of PD-1/PD-L1 interactions. Journal of Immunotherapy (Hagerstown, Md: 1997) 2015; 38:96-106.

[8] Brahmer JR, Tykodi SS, Chow LQ, Hwu WJ, Topalian SL, Hwu P, Drake CG, Camacho LH, Kauh J, Odunsi K, et al. Safety and activity of anti-PD-L1 antibody in patients with advanced cancer. The New England Journal of Medicine 2012; 366:2455-65.

[9] Pardoll DM. The blockade of immune checkpoints in cancer immunotherapy. Nature Reviews Cancer 2012; 12:252-64.

[10] Joyce JA, Fearon DT. T cell exclusion, immune privilege, and the tumor microenvironment. Science (New York, NY) 2015; 348:74-80.

[11] Tumeh PC, Harview CL, Yearley JH, Shintaku IP, Taylor EJ, Robert L, Chmielowski B, Spasic M, Henry G, Ciobanu V, et al. PD-1 blockade induces responses by inhibiting adaptive immune resistance. Nature 2014; 515:568-71.

[12] Momtaz P, Postow MA. Immunologic checkpoints in cancer therapy: focus on the programmed death-1 (PD-1) receptor pathway. Pharmacogenomics and Personalized Medicine 2014; 7:357-65.

[13] Sharma P, Allison JP. The future of immune checkpoint therapy. Science (New York, NY) 2015; 348:56-61.

[14] Topalian SL, Hodi FS, Brahmer JR, Gettinger SN, Smith DC, McDermott DF, Powderly JD, Carvajal RD, Sosman JA, Atkins MB, et al. Safety, activity, and immune correlates of anti-PD-1 antibody in cancer. The New England Journal of Medicine 2012; 366:2443-54.

[15] Weber JS, Kudchadkar RR, Yu B, Gallenstein D, Horak CE, Inzunza HD, Zhao X, Martinez AJ, Wang W, Gibney G, et al. Safety, efficacy, and biomarkers of nivolumab with vaccine in ipilimumab-refractory or -naive melanoma. Journal of Clinical Oncology: Official Journal of the American Society of Clinical Oncology 2013; 31:4311-8.

[16] Topalian SL, Sznol M, McDermott DF, Kluger HM, Carvajal RD, Sharfman WH, Brahmer JR, Lawrence DP, Atkins MB, Powderly JD, et al. Survival, durable tumor remission, and long-term safety in patients with advanced melanoma receiving nivolumab. Journal of Clinical Oncology: Official Journal of the American Society of Clinical Oncology 2014; 32:1020-30.

[17] Hamid O, Robert C, Daud A, Hodi FS, Hwu WJ, Kefford R, Wolchok JD, Hersey P, Joseph RW, Weber JS, et al. Safety and tumor responses with lambrolizumab (anti-PD-1) in melanoma. The New England Journal of Medicine 2013; 369:134-44.

[18] Armand P, Nagler A, Weller EA, Devine SM, Avigan DE, Chen YB, Kaminski MS, Holland HK, Winter JN, Mason JR, et al. Disabling immune tolerance by programmed death-1 blockade with pidilizumab after autologous hematopoietic stem-cell transplantation for diffuse large B-cell lymphoma: results of an international phase II trial. Journal of Clinical Oncology: Official Journal of the American Society of Clinical Oncology 2013; 31:4199-206.

[19] COG Phase I Consortium; National Cancer Institute. Nivolumab with or without ipilimumab in treating younger patients with recurrent or refractory solid tumors or sarcomas. In: ClinicalTrails.gov [Internet]. Bethesda (MD): National Library of Medicine (US). Available from: http://clinicaltrials.gov/show/NCT02304458. NLM Identifier: NCT02304458. [Accessed 2016-12-02].

[20] Hodi FS, O'Day SJ, McDermott DF, Weber RW, Sosman JA, Haanen JB, Gonzalez R, Robert C, Schadendorf D, Hassel JC, et al. Improved survival with ipilimumab in patients with metastatic melanoma. The New England Journal of Medicine 2010; 363:711-23.

[21] Robert C, Thomas L, Bondarenko I, O'Day S, Weber J, Garbe C, Lebbe C, Baurain JF, Testori A, Grob JJ, et al. Ipilimumab plus dacarbazine for previously untreated metastatic melanoma. The New England Journal of Medicine 2011; 364:2517-26.

[22] van den Eertwegh AJ, Versluis J, van den Berg HP, Santegoets SJ, van Moorselaar RJ, van der Sluis TM, Gall HE, Harding TC, Jooss K, Lowy I, et al. Combined immunotherapy with granulocyte-macrophage colony-stimulating factor-transduced allogeneic prostate cancer cells and ipilimumab in patients with metastatic castration-resistant prostate cancer: a phase 1 dose-escalation trial. The Lancet Oncology 2012; 13:509-17.

[23] Brignone C, Escudier B, Grygar C, Marcu M, Triebel F. A phase I pharmacokinetic and biological correlative study of IMP321, a novel MHC class II agonist, in patients with advanced renal cell carcinoma. Clinical Cancer Research: An Official Journal of the American Association for Cancer Research 2009; 15:6225-31.

[24] Brignone C, Gutierrez M, Mefti F, Brain E, Jarcau R, Cvitkovic F, Bousetta N, Medioni J, Gligorov J, Grygar C, et al. First-line chemoimmunotherapy in metastatic breast carcinoma: combination of paclitaxel and IMP321 (LAG-3Ig) enhances immune responses and antitumor activity. Journal of Translational Medicine 2010; 8:71.

[25] Sakuishi K, Apetoh L, Sullivan JM, Blazar BR, Kuchroo VK, Anderson AC. Targeting Tim-3 and PD-1 pathways to reverse T cell exhaustion and restore anti-tumor immunity. The Journal of Experimental Medicine 2010; 207:2187-94.

[26] Greaves M and Maley CC. Clonal evolution in cancer. Nature 2012; 481(7381):306-13

[27] Taube JM, Anders RA, Young GD, Xu H, Sharma R, McMiller TL, Chen S, Klein AP, Pardoll DM, Topalian SL, et al. Colocalization of inflammatory response with B7-h1 expression in human melanocytic lesions supports an adaptive resistance mechanism of immune escape. Science Translational Medicine 2012; 4:127ra37.

[28] Lussier, et al. Combination immunotherapy with α-CLTA-4 and α-PD-L1 antibody blockade prevents immune escape and leads to complete control of metastatic osteosarcoma. Journal for ImmunoTherapy of Cancer 2015; 3:1.

[29] Zajac AJ, Blattman JN, Murali-Krishna K, Sourdive DJ, Suresh M, Altman JD, Ahmed R. Viral immune evasion due to persistence of activated T cells without effector function. The Journal of Experimental Medicine 1998; 188:2205-13.

[30] Blackburn SD, Shin H, Freeman GJ, Wherry EJ. Selective expansion of a subset of exhausted CD8 T cells by alphaPD-L1 blockade. Proceedings of the National Academy of Sciences of the United States of America 2008; 105:15016-21.

[31] Del Monte U. Does the cell number 109 still really fit one gram of tumor tissue?. Cell Cycle 2009; 8(3):505-6.

[32] Coffin J and Swanstrom R. HIV pathogenesis: dynamics and genetics of viral populations and infected cells. Cold Springs Harbor Perspectives in Medicine 2013; 3:1.

[33] Nirschl CJ, Drake CG. Molecular pathways: coexpression of immune checkpoint molecules: signaling pathways and implications for cancer immunotherapy. Clinical Cancer Research: An Official Journal of the American Association for Cancer Research 2013; 19:4917-24.

[34] Curran MA, Montalvo W, Yagita H, Allison JP. PD-1 and CTLA-4 combination blockade expands infiltrating T cells and reduces regulatory T and myeloid cells within B16 melanoma tumors. Proceedings of the National Academy of Sciences of the United States of America 2010; 107:4275-80.

[35] Sznol M, Chen L. Antagonist antibodies to PD-1 and B7-H1 (PD-L1) in the treatment of advanced human cancer. Clinical Cancer Research: An Official Journal of the American Association for Cancer Research 2013; 19:1021-34.

[36] Gubin MM, Zhang X, Schuster H, Caron E, Ward JP, Noguchi T, Ivanova Y, Hundal J, Arthur CD, Krebber WJ, et al. Checkpoint blockade cancer immunotherapy targets tumour-specific mutant antigens. Nature 2014; 515:577-81.

[37] Wolchok JD, Kluger H, Callahan MK, Postow MA, Rizvi NA, Lesokhin AM, Segal NH, Ariyan CE, Gordon RA, Reed K, et al. Nivolumab plus ipilimumab in advanced melanoma. The New England Journal of Medicine 2013; 369:122-33.

[38] Spranger S, Koblish HK, Horton B, Scherle PA, Newton R, Gajewski TF. Mechanism of tumor rejection with doublets of CTLA-4, PD-1/PD-L1, or IDO blockade involves restored IL-2 production and proliferation of CD8(+) T cells directly within the tumor microenvironment. Journal for Immunotherapy of Cancer 2014; 2:3.

[39] Wainwright DA, Chang AL, Dey M, Balyasnikova IV, Kim CK, Tobias A, Cheng Y, Kim JW, Qiao J, Zhang L, et al. Durable therapeutic efficacy utilizing combinatorial blockade against IDO, CTLA-4, and PD-L1 in mice with brain tumors. Clinical Cancer Research: An Official Journal of the American Association for Cancer Research 2014; 20:5290-301.

[40] Woo SR, Turnis ME, Goldberg MV, Bankoti J, Selby M, Nirschl CJ, Bettini ML, Gravano DM, Vogel P, Liu CL, et al. Immune inhibitory molecules LAG-3 and PD-1 synergistically regulate T-cell function to promote tumoral immune escape. Cancer Research 2012; 72:917-27.

[41] Ngiow SF, von Scheidt B, Akiba H, Yagita H, Teng MW, Smyth MJ. Anti-TIM3 antibody promotes T cell IFN-gamma-mediated antitumor immunity and suppresses established tumors. Cancer Research 2011; 71:3540-51.

[42] Ngiow SF, Teng MW, Smyth MJ. Prospects for TIM3-targeted antitumor immunotherapy. Cancer Research 2011; 71:6567-71.

[43] Miyatake T, Tringler B, Liu W, Liu SH, Papkoff J, Enomoto T, Torkko KC, Dehn DL, Swisher A, Shroyer KR. B7-H4 (DD-O110) is overexpressed in high risk uterine endometrioid adenocarcinomas and inversely correlated with tumor T-cell infiltration. Gynecologic Oncology 2007; 106:119-27.

[44] Chen C, Shen Y, Qu QX, Chen XQ, Zhang XG, Huang JA. Induced expression of B7-H3 on the lung cancer cells and macrophages suppresses T-cell mediating anti-tumor immune response. Experimental Cell Research 2013; 319:96-102.

[45] Sun Y, Wang Y, Zhao J, Gu M, Giscombe R, Lefvert AK, Wang X. B7-H3 and B7-H4 expression in non-small-cell lung cancer. Lung Cancer (Amsterdam, Netherlands) 2006; 53:143-51.

[46] Matsushita H, Vesely MD, Koboldt DC, Rickert CG, Uppaluri R, Magrini VJ, Arthur CD, White JM, Chen YS, Shea LK, et al. Cancer exome analysis reveals a T-cell-dependent mechanism of cancer immunoediting. Nature 2012; 482:400-4.

[47] Pilones KA, Vanpouille-Box C, Demaria S. Combination of radiotherapy and immune checkpoint inhibitors. Seminars in Radiation Oncology 2015; 25:28-33.

[48] Twyman-Saint Victor C, Rech AJ, Maity A, Rengan R, Pauken KE, Stelekati E, Benci JL, Xu B, Dada H, Odorizzi PM, et al. Radiation and dual checkpoint blockade activate non-redundant immune mechanisms in cancer. Nature 2015; 520:373-7.

[49] Deng L, Liang H, Burnette B, Beckett M, Darga T, Weichselbaum RR, Fu YX. Irradiation and anti-PD-L1 treatment synergistically promote antitumor immunity in mice. The Journal of Clinical Investigation 2014; 124:687-95.

[50] Sharabi A, Nirschl C, Ceccato T, Nirschl T, Francica B, Alme A, Velarde E, DeWeese T, Drake C. Role of radiation therapy in inducing antigen specific antitumor immune responses when combined with anti-PD1 checkpoint blockade: mechanism and clinical implications. International Journal of Radiation Oncology 2014; 90.

[51] Dovedi SJ, Adlard AL, Lipowska-Bhalla G, McKenna C, Jones S, Cheadle EJ, Stratford IJ, Poon E, Morrow M, Stewart R, et al. Acquired resistance to fractionated radiotherapy can be overcome by concurrent PD-L1 blockade. Cancer Research 2014; 74:5458-68.

[52] Azijli K, Stelloo E, Peters GJ, VDE AJ. New developments in the treatment of metastatic melanoma: immune checkpoint inhibitors and targeted therapies. Anticancer Research 2014; 34:1493-505.

[53] Cooper ZA, Juneja VR, Sage PT, Frederick DT, Piris A, Mitra D, Lo JA, Hodi FS, Freeman GJ, Bosenberg MW, et al. Response to BRAF inhibition in melanoma is enhanced when combined with immune checkpoint blockade. Cancer Immunology Research 2014; 2:643-54.

[54] Frederick DT, Piris A, Cogdill AP, Cooper ZA, Lezcano C, Ferrone CR, Mitra D, Boni A, Newton LP, Liu C, et al. BRAF inhibition is associated with enhanced melanoma antigen

expression and a more favorable tumor microenvironment in patients with metastatic melanoma. Clinical Cancer Research: An Official Journal of the American Association for Cancer Research 2013; 19:1225-31.

[55] Frey B, Rubner Y, Kulzer L, Werthmoller N, Weiss EM, Fietkau R, Gaipl US. Antitumor immune responses induced by ionizing irradiation and further immune stimulation. Cancer Immunology, Immunotherapy: CII 2014; 63:29-36.

[56] Yeh PJ et al. Drug interactions and the evolution of antibiotic resistance. Nature Reviews Microbiology 2009; 7(6):460-6.

Section 3

Clinical Implications of Basic Sciences

Chapter 8

Osteosarcomagenesis: Biology, Development, Metastasis, and Mechanisms of Pain

Branden A. Smeester, Branden S. Moriarity and Alvin J. Beitz

Additional information is available at the end of the chapter

http://dx.doi.org/10.5772/67070

Abstract

Osteosarcoma is the most common primary cancer of the bone and third most common cancer in children and adolescents with approximately 900 new cases annually in the United States. A major facet of osteosarcoma is its high level of genomic instability, in particular chromosomal instability, which is the result of increased or decreased chromosome number in a cell. Furthermore, pain is the most common symptomatic feature of osteosarcoma that lacks effective therapy. Pain in osteosarcoma is relatively more complicated than many other painful conditions requiring a more thorough understanding of its etiology, pathobiology, and neurobiology to allow the development of better therapies for reducing pain in osteosarcoma patients. Studies are underway to define the diverse modalities of presentation, growth, development, metastases, and nociception in osteosarcoma. New data from human studies in combination with data from studies incorporating transgenic mouse models of osteosarcoma are providing valuable insights into the mechanisms underlying the development of both the tumor and the tumor-induced pain. These new data will undoubtedly lead to improved prognoses, as well as the development of novel therapeutics that will significantly decrease bone cancer pain.

Keywords: osteosarcoma, genetics, pain, bone tumors, pathobiology

1. Introduction

Osteosarcoma is the most common malignant bone tumor found in children and adolescents and is associated with many complications including metastases and intractable cancer pain [1, 2]. Typically, the prevalence of osteosarcoma shows a strong relationship with skeletal growth. The main incidence peak occurs in the second decade of life and generally is associated with a highly defined phenotype. Osteosarcoma also occurs in elderly adults in the sixth and seventh decades of life and is often preceded by certain genetic predispositions [3]. Osteosarcomas predominately form in the metaphyses of the long bones in the major growth centers such as the distal femur, proximal tibia, and proximal humerus. Osteosarcomas are quite aggressive locally but often produce early, lethal systemic metastases [4]. According to the National Cancer Institute, as many as 20% of patients will have radiographically detectable metastases at diagnosis, and ultimately nearly 90% of patients have radiographically undetectable metastatic lesions, particularly to the lungs [5, 6]. However, chest CTs have been estimated to miss nearly 25% of metastatic nodules found during thoracotomy, and up to 14% of metastases are not nodular in shape, which complicates the metastatic picture in many patients [7]. With no known precursor to osteosarcoma, treatment options are extremely limited. Adjuvant chemotherapy and surgical resection are standard therapies, but treatment efficacy still remains poor for over one-third of osteosarcoma patients [5, 8]. Although our understanding of the mechanisms underlying tumor development, tumor progression, and metastasis is improving [6, 9–12], the complex nature of the bone tumor microenvironment presents unique challenges to identifying novel drug targets and treatment strategies.

The most common presenting symptom of osteosarcoma is pain, particularly with activity. Osteosarcoma pain can start in adolescence, leading to hospitalization, reduced survival, and poor quality of life. Pain in osteosarcoma is unique because of unpredictable and recurrent episodes of acute pain due to vaso-occlusive crises (VOC), in addition to chronic pain experienced by a majority of adult patients on a daily basis [13]. As detection and survival among cancer patients have improved, pain has become an increasing challenge, because traditional therapies are often only partially effective [14]. In this regard, the treatment of osteosarcoma pain is complicated because long-term treatment choices remain limited and generally involve opioids, which impose liabilities of their own including constipation, mast cell activation, addiction, and respiratory depression [15]. Moreover, significantly larger doses of opioids are required to treat pain in osteosarcoma as compared to other acute and chronic pain conditions. Pain can be lifelong in osteosarcoma and may therefore influence cognitive function and lead to depression and anxiety, which can in turn promote the perception of pain [13]. In general, the treatment of chronic pain remains unsatisfactory, perhaps due to the diverse pathobiology in different diseases. Therefore, it is critical to understand the mechanisms specific to the genesis of osteosarcoma-related pain to develop targeted therapies.

2. Normal bone development

The bone is a readily adaptive, mineralized tissue that performs diverse functions including enabling locomotion, storing nutrients such as phosphate and calcium, and protecting soft tissues among many others. Despite its static appearance, osteoclasts and osteoblasts, two major cell types abundant throughout bone tissue are constantly remodeling bone.

Osteoblasts are the resident bone-producing cells of the body. Osteoblasts are derived from a lineage of cells arising from a mesenchymal origin [16], while osteoclasts arise from a hematopoietic lineage [17]. The remodeling of the bone is a tightly coupled process. From a physiological perspective, distinct differentiation and maturation pathways of these two cell types allows for uninterrupted maintenance of bone homeostasis [18]. The differentiation process of osteoblasts is often divided in specific stages: mesenchymal progenitors, preosteoblasts, and osteoblasts. Similarly, this process also occurs in osteoclastogenesis where cells of myeloid origin differentiate into one of four cell types, one being osteoclasts [17]. While differentiation stages are useful for cellular identification, the maturation process is not well understood. Often, the identities of cells during each stage are characterized by expression of various molecular markers highly associated with osteoblast development. Markers of cells from mesenchymal origin are not well defined and are still a matter of intense debate. Similarly, preosteoblast markers are also difficult to identify. These cells are highly heterogeneous in their expression patterns, as this stage can encompass various cell types during maturation into osteoblasts, bone-lining cells, or osteocytes. However, two common transcription factors, Runt-Related Transcription Factor 2 (*RUNX2*) and later OSTERIX (also known as *SP7*), are expressed during maturation and are highly associated with maturation of the preosteoblast lineage [19], while hematopoietic transcription factor (*PU.1*), microphthalmia-associated transcription factor (*MITF*), and *c-FOS* are associated with osteoclast precursors [17].

3. Tumorigenesis

There is currently no known origin to osteosarcoma; however, much research has pointed to osteoblasts as the progenitor cell type. The single most shared feature of all osteosarcomas histologically is the presence of osteoid matrix, secreted by malignant cells in the growing tumor. In addition, the presence and quantity of this matrix do not define the disease, as osteosarcomas may be composed of many tissue types including chondroblastic, fibroblastic, and osteoblastic [20]. Osteosarcoma has been shown to be associated with loss of key tumor suppressor genes such as tumor protein P53 (*TP53*) and retinoblastoma 1 (*RB1*) [21], and alterations in *p53* are associated with reduced event-free survival [22]. Moreover, sporadic osteosarcomas are highly associated with mutations in the *RB* gene. Additionally, germ line mutations in the *p53* gene predispose patients with Li-Fraumeni syndrome (LFS) to osteosarcoma [23] with an incidence of up to 12% [24].

4. Chromosomal abnormalities

Despite its well-defined phenotypic characteristics, genetically speaking, osteosarcoma is chaotic and disordered. It is often associated with massive chromosomal rearrangements, cytogenetic aberrations, and numerous mutations [25]. Numerous cytogenetic and molecular studies of osteosarcoma have been conducted in recent years yielding interesting results but often with conflicting findings [26]. Many of these studies have limited prognostic and diagnostic value and fail to understand the driving events necessary for osteosarcoma development. However, the overall infrequency of this disease makes elucidating these factors all the more challenging. It has been apparent since early studies that osteosarcomas have a significant propensity toward aneuploidy with over 96% of high-grade cases being hyperploid [26]. Furthermore, cytogenetic analyses have provided evidence for enormous variation in karyotypic alterations. A major facet of osteosarcoma is its high level of genomic instability, in particular chromosomal instability (CIN). CIN can contribute to tumor initiation and progression through altering the expression of proto-oncogenes or tumor suppressor genes. The rate of gain or loss of entire chromosomes or sections is significant in the pathogenesis of osteosarcoma resulting in numerous aberrations and wide variability between cells and tumors [27].

5. Oncogene/tumor suppressor gene dysfunction

The search for specific drivers of osteosarcoma development has stemmed from the early cytogenetic and molecular findings. Initial genetic studies sought to identify important genes involved in cancers although not necessarily specific to osteosarcoma. These early studies have implicated a number of important tumor suppressors, oncogenes, and growth factors that are implicated in other sarcomas and carcinomas as well [26]. As stated earlier, perhaps the best two characterized examples of this are the tumor suppressor gene *TP53* and the retinoblastoma *RB1* gene. The location of *TP53* on chromosome 17p13 is an area frequently altered in osteosarcomas and is readily apparent in cytogenetic analyses. Alterations in the *TP53* gene have significant effects on the downstream signaling targets, many of which are normally involved in cell cycle control and apoptosis. Gene rearrangements, point mutations, epigenetic modification [28, 29], and/or allelic loss can presumably lead to inactivation of normal *TP53* function, and these aberrations have been associated with the development of osteosarcoma. In a recent study that characterized the genomic landscape of osteosarcoma via whole genome sequencing (WGS), the majority of *TP53* inactivation in osteosarcoma was found to be due to translocations [30]. Furthermore, this study highlights the fact that *TP53* mutation is highly prevalent in osteosarcoma, with >90% of all tumors containing a mutation in at least one allele, and upward of 80% containing mutations in both alleles. In addition to the *TP53* gene, associations between osteosarcoma and *RB1* are well recognized as well, especially in patients with hereditary retinoblastoma, in which osteosarcoma incidence is 1000 times higher than in the general population. The loss of heterozygosity and/or sporadic alterations in the *RB1* gene is apparent in >60% of osteosarcoma cases, and these genetic changes have significant prognostic value [31]. As only these prototypical cancer genes and a few others have been definitively implicated in osteosarcoma, there is a pressing need to identify more genes and pathways governing its development and metastasis to better treat osteosarcoma patients and their associated pain.

6. Axonal guidance genes in osteosarcoma

Recently, a new pathway has been identified using the Sleeping Beauty mutagenesis system in mice implicating axon guidance genes such as semaphorin-4D (*SEMA4D*) in osteosarcoma [25]. During normal bone homeostasis, osteoclasts express high levels of *Sema4d*, whereas osteoblasts do not. Instead, osteoblasts express its cognate receptor and co-receptor, Plexin B1 (*Plxnb1*) and Erb-B2 receptor tyrosine kinase 2 (*Erbb2*), respectively. Thus, it is possible that misexpression of *SEMA4D* and MET proto-oncogene, receptor tyrosine kinase (*MET*) in osteoblasts might give rise to a subset of osteosarcomas. Similarly, the tumorigenic properties induced by overexpression of *SEMA4D* in human osteosarcoma cells are dependent on MET and ERBB2 levels, which has been reported [32]. Previous studies in osteosarcoma showed that high levels of *ERBB2* are associated with a good outcome and that overexpression of *MET* can directly transform osteoblasts into osteosarcomas [33, 34]. The fact that *SEMA4D* is a cell surface receptor makes it an attractive candidate for novel therapies. This will be addressed later in the chapter.

7. Metastasis

Approximately 20–30% of osteosarcoma patients have overt metastases at diagnosis, and about 40% of patients will develop lung metastases during the course of treatment [35–37]. Analysis of clinical outcomes of patients without overt metastasis at diagnosis prior to the advent of chemotherapy demonstrated >90% of patients developed lung metastasis 6–36 months after surgical resection, indicating the majority of seemingly nonmetastatic patients actually have micrometastatic disease at diagnosis [30]. While it is largely believed that the implementation of chemotherapy eradicates these developing micrometastases in many cases, these data highlight the fact that metastasis is the most important factor associated with poor outcome in osteosarcoma [38]. Recent work from Moriarity and colleagues identified many genes that promote osteosarcoma development and metastasis through a forward genetic screen in mice using the *SB* transposon-based mutagenesis system. Both classes of genes (oncogenes and tumor suppressors) may be critical for development of detectable metastases present at diagnosis and/or the ability of latent micrometastases to develop to a detectable level. Subsets of genes identified via the SB screen were only present in the metastatic lesions, while others were found both in primary tumors and metastases. Among those genes were phosphatase and tensin homolog (*Pten*), glycogen synthase kinase 3 beta (*Gsk3b*), synaptosome-associated protein 23 kDa (*Snap23*), mitogen-activated protein kinase kinase kinase kinase 3 (*Map4k3*), Rho GTPase-activating protein 35 (*Arhgap35* (*Grlf1*)), Rho/Rac guanine nucleotide exchange factor 18 (*Arhgef18*), Axin 1 (*Axin1*), Raf-1 proto-oncogene, serine/threonine kinase (*Raf1*), and ubiquitin-associated protein 2 like (*Ubap2l*). Interestingly, all of these genes have been previously implicated in metastasis of other cancers, which supports the conclusion that these genes are likely involved in osteosarcoma metastasis [25]. Additionally, bone metastases are also highly painful. The ability of osteosarcoma to successfully metastasize relies in part on its ability to exploit many mechanisms of normal bone remodeling [39]. Two such examples of this are the Wnt family of proteins and bone morphogenetic proteins (BMPs), both of which are critical in bone development and are implicated in cancer pain [40, 41]. The evolving physiologic and pathological roles of the Wnt/β-catenin signaling pathway may offer attractive therapeutic targets for novel antagonists and inhibitors for patients with primary and metastatic osteosarcoma. Likewise, BMPs are responsible for numerous osteoinductive cellular processes including bone growth, differentiation, and matrix maintenance [40]. In vitro examination in numerous osteosarcoma cell lines revealed highly abundant expression of BMPs in virtually all lines tested [42–44]. Moreover, BMP expression has been found to correlate with metastasis in osteosarcoma [45], while overexpression of BMP-9 reduces invasion and migration properties of osteosarcoma cells [46]. Conversely, analysis of 47 human osteosarcomas found no correlations between BMP expression and prognostic outcomes [47]. Furthermore, BMPs have also been shown to induce bone formation in human osteosarcoma cells [48]. As mentioned earlier, osteosarcomas can present with mixed cell lineages and differentiation patterns [20]. These studies and others suggest that perhaps BMPs may be expressed at differing levels depending on the cellular state, and their presence may offer an attractive therapeutic option for the treatment of osteosarcoma. While the significance of BMP signaling in osteosarcomagenesis is not yet fully understood, current research suggests BMPs may play an important role.

8. Characteristics of pain in osteosarcoma

Cancer-induced bone pain is a complex pain state involving a combination of background, spontaneous, and incident (movement-evoked) pain [14, 49]. Regional pain alone or in conjunction with a palpable mass are the two main reasons that osteosarcoma patients consult a doctor. Patients with osteosarcoma of the jaws typically present with pain, swelling, ulceration, or neurological deficit [50], but again pain is a major symptom causing these patients to seek medical attention. Currently only about half of patients with cancer-induced bone pain experience temporary relief from conventional therapies [51], which stresses the need for the development of more effective treatments. **Table 1** summarizes some of the types of pain experienced by bone cancer patients and animal models of bone cancer pain.

Characteristics of pain	Pain phenotyping method	
	Subjects with OSA	Mice with bone tumor
Mechanical allodynia	Patients with cancer pain were evaluated for mechanical allodynia [52]	Paw withdrawal responses to von Frey monofilaments in bone cancer mice or rats [1, 53–55]
Heat hyperalgesia	Patients with cancer pain were evaluated for heat hyperalgesia [52]	Paw withdrawal latency and frequency in response to static heat stimuli in mice or rats [53, 54, 56]
Movement-evoked pain	The use of a pain verbal rating scale during movement [57]	Count the number of spontaneous flinches of the hind limb in bone tumor mice [55]

Note: most human cancer pain studies have employed visual analogue scales (VAS), numerical rating scales, or verbal reporting to quantify pain, and thus it is often difficult to compare nociceptive behavioral testing results from cancer pain studies using animal models with human cancer pain studies because of the differences in pain assessment.

Table 1. Characteristics of pain in osteosarcoma.

http://dx.doi.org/10.5772/67070

9. Peripheral and central mechanisms of pain in osteosarcoma

While our knowledge of the mechanisms of bone cancer pain is ever expanding, part of our failure to adequately manage osteosarcoma and other forms of bone cancer pain is an inadequate understanding of the etiology and mechanisms involved. Cancer-induced bone pain is a mixed-mechanism pain state exhibiting elements of inflammatory, neuropathic, and ischemic pain, but with distinctive effects on the tissues and nerves in the periphery, as well as unique biochemical changes within the spinal cord [14, 58].

9.1. Peripheral mechanisms

As summarized by Falk and colleagues, the biology of cancer-induced bone pain involves a complex interplay among the tumor cells, peripheral nerves, and cells of the bone [14]. The tumor cells trigger a number of nociceptive and immune responses that ultimately recruit inflammatory cells including macrophages, neutrophils, and T cells to the bone resulting in release of a plethora of endogenous chemicals acting on bone cells, cancer cells, and importantly on primary afferent nerve fibers [59, 60]. Thus, tumor and tumor-associated cells in the cancer microenvironment may release various peripheral mediators. These include adenosine triphosphate (ATP), formaldehyde, protons, proteases, endothelin, bradykinin, tumor necrosis factor (TNF), and nerve growth factor (NGF) that result in the activation and/or sensitization of peripheral and central neurons [61, 62]. The complexity of this neuroimmune and inflammatory effect on cancer pain has been recently reviewed [63]. Ultimately this cascade of events leads to the activation and sensitization of nociceptors, the degradation of the bone, and subsequent increased tumor growth [14]. Furthermore, studies have shown that cancer cells in the bone induce a highly disorganized sprouting of sensory and sympathetic fibers, leading to the formation of small neuromas. These disorganized bundles of nerve fibers are thought to contribute to episodes of breakthrough pain or even movement-induced pain [64, 65]. In addition to changes in nerve fibers, bone tumors in mice have also been shown to be associated with changes in both blood vessels and lymphatics, which may facilitate metastasis and which, interestingly, can be altered by acupuncture treatment [66].

9.2. Central mechanisms

Both the spinal cord dorsal horn and dorsal root ganglia undergo unique changes induced by bone tumors suggesting that the peripheral alterations drive central alterations. Some of the bone tumor-induced changes observed in the spinal glial and neurons are distinct, but many are reflective of changes seen with other chronic pain states. Thus, tumors are associated with increased expression of dynorphin with accompanying spinal astrocyte hypertrophy and upregulation of galanin and AF3 [14, 66]. Clearly, the recent identification of a vast number of mediators and receptors that contribute to bone cancer-related pain, as well as more detailed knowledge of the peripheral and central mechanisms underlying the development of bone tumor nociception, will provide novel therapeutic targets for treating patients with osteosarcoma pain. Subsets of these targets are discussed in more detail below.

10. Treatment of osteosarcoma

From the discussion above, it is clear that due to the complex nature of osteosarcoma pathobiology and the neurobiological mechanisms that underlie the development of bone cancer pain, it may be necessary to target multiple receptors, mediators, and genes to adequately treat osteosarcomas and osteosarcoma-associated pain. Below we review some of the established and novel targets for the treatment of osteosarcoma and its associated pain.

10.1. Immunomodulation

10.1.1. Semaphorins

VX15/2503 (Vaccinex, Inc.) is a highly novel, immunomodulatory monoclonal antibody that specifically targets *SEMA4D* (CD100), a receptor and soluble protein from the semaphorin family known to be involved in immune modulation [67] and regulation of normal bone formation [68]. Initial interest in this monoclonal antibody was rooted in results indicating that immune cell-dependent interactions were in fact responsible for its antitumor activity [67]. Early preclinical studies have determined that high concentrations of *SEMA4D* are expressed at the invasive border of many human cancers and that this border restricts the antitumor cell infiltrate from effectively combating the growing tumor. Treatment with anti-*SEMA4D* restores the inhibited immune response leading to reduced tumor burden and delayed growth in animal models. Furthermore, anti-*SEMA4D* blockade results in phase I clinical trials of 42 adult patients with advanced solid tumors have been well tolerated with many exhibiting stable disease over various treatment regimens. Antibody therapy targeting *SEMA4D* has also been shown to reduce tumor growth in a xenograft model of soft tissue sarcoma (STS) when combined with antibody therapy for vascular endothelial growth factor (VEGF) [69].

10.2. Intracellular signaling pathway inhibitors

10.2.1. Hedgehog (Hh)

While encompassing diverse functions such as tissue homeostasis and embryonic development, Hedgehog (Hh) signaling is highly complex and not completely understood [70]. Signaling through its receptor Patched-1 (PTCH), Smoothened is activated and promotes subsequent downstream signaling pathway of the Hedgehog (Hh) pathway [71]. This activation has been implicated in many cancers including osteosarcoma where aberrant activation increases cell proliferation but can be reduced through inhibition of the signaling [72]. Hedgehog inhibitors have been successfully tested in clinical trials of other cancers such as chondrosarcoma [73, 74], carcinoma [75], and medulloblastoma [76] providing solid evidence for consideration as a novel therapeutic in osteosarcoma.

10.2.2. Mammalian target of rapamycin (mTOR)

The mammalian target of rapamycin (mTOR) is a protein kinase that regulates cell survival and proliferation [77]. Due to its diverse functions, mTOR is implicated in many cancers making it an attractive target in treating tumors, including osteosarcoma. In one recent study, activated mTOR was visualized in osteosarcoma and the staining positively correlated to metastasis and necrosis [78]. Targeted inhibition of the signaling pathway of mTOR has been shown to reduce metastatic behavior in a mouse model of osteosarcoma [79] as well as human xenograft models [80]. Current and future clinical trials using mTOR inhibitors may prove therapeutically fruitful in the treatment of osteosarcoma [81].

10.3. Tyrosine kinase receptors

10.3.1. Human epidermal growth factor receptor 2 (HER2)

HER2 is a member of the human epidermal growth factor receptor family. Located on chromosome 17, activation and overexpression have been implicated in a number of cancers including osteosarcoma. *HER2* is overexpressed in ~40% of osteosarcomas and has been found to occur more frequently in metastatic patients [82]. Expression was also found to correlate with decreased tumor necrosis and event-free survival [83]. Chimeric antigen receptor (CAR)-modified T cells have been shown to kill *HER2*-positive osteosarcoma cells in xenograft and metastatic mouse models [84].

10.3.2. Vascular endothelial growth factor (VEGF)

VEGF expression has been shown to involve in osteosarcoma [85], correlated with overall survival [86] and implicated in metastatic development [82]. A recent paper by Zhou and colleagues found anti-VEGF strategies to be antiangiogenic in osteosarcoma [69]. Interestingly, *SEMA4D* blockade enhanced the anticancer activity of anti-VEGF treatment that provides a viable adjunct to *VEGF* therapy alone. While discussed above, development of a highly novel monoclonal antibody to *SEMA4D* is underway and may provide further insight into targeting *VEGF*-resistant tumors as well as associated malignancies.

11. Treatment of osteosarcoma pain

With a growing population of patients receiving inadequate treatment for intractable bone cancer pain, new targets need to be considered to better address this largely unmet clinical need for improving their quality of life. In general, while there are a variety of methods that are used to treat bone cancer pain, including bisphosphonates, radiation therapy, chemotherapy, hormone therapy, and surgery, the clinical treatment of bone cancer pain still focuses on the three-step program. This program was established by the World Health Organization and includes NSAIDs and narcotics as therapeutic treatment options. However, as we learn more about the mechanisms responsible for cancer pain and the genetic basis for the development of osteosarcomas, there are several areas that offer hope for the development of novel treatments for bone cancer pain. It is important to point out that bone cancer pain can be treated by both systemic and local administration of drugs as well as alternative medical approaches. The obvious advantage of peripheral targets is the reduced potential for CNS side effects, such as the sedation and nausea that often accompany opiate analgesics.

11.1. Cytokines

Pain is a complex trait, and thus, the influence of genetics on pain sensitivity and the efficacy of analgesics are an ongoing challenge. A recent study found that polymorphisms in the Interleukin 1 Beta (IL-1β) family have a significant influence on cytokine serum levels and maximum pain intensity in cancer patients, as well as affecting cancer proliferation [87]. IL-1β has been shown to be expressed in astrocytes and microglia and in nociceptive dorsal root ganglion neurons [88] and thus may represent a target for the treatment of cancer pain.

11.2. TRPV1 receptors

TRP channels were first identified in Drosophila [89], and TRPV1 denotes the transient receptor potential channel family number 1 and was the first mammalian TRP channel to be cloned [90]. Capsaicin and other TRPV1 agonists selectively stimulate nociceptive neurons, and thus while it induces pain, it is possible to treat pain by boosting analgesic pathways [91]. In this regard the use of the TRPV1 agonist, resiniferatoxin (RTX), to block cancer pain has recently been reviewed [92]. In human cancer patients, RTX was given by intrathecal injection into the lumbar cistern, and all patients experienced substantial analgesia without significant side effects. In addition, a recent study has shown that cancer cells undergo numerous metabolic changes that include increased glutamine catabolism and overexpression of the enzyme glutaminase, which mediates glutaminolysis. This produces large pools of intracellular glutamate [93]. This is coupled to an upregulation of the plasma membrane antiporter, system x_c^-. System x_c^- is an amino acid antiporter that typically mediates the exchange of extracellular l-cystine and intracellular L-glutamate across the cellular plasma membrane. The exchange-mediated export of L-glutamate is particularly important within the nervous system, since it represents a non-vesicular route of release through which glutamate can participate in either neuronal signaling or in excitotoxic pathology. With respect to osteosarcomas, the excess glutamate is released directly from the cancer cells and can act on peripheral glutamate receptors located on nerve fibers. It is known that glutamate receptors can modulate peripheral TRPV1 receptors [78]. Thus, the released glutamate converges on peripheral afferent nerve terminals to transmit nociceptive signals through TRPV1. Activation of TRPV1 receptors can ultimately initiate central sensitization in response to tumor-released glutamate [93]. Thus, using RTX to block peripheral TRPV1 channels would block this excess glutamate effect on TRPV1 and reduce both tumor-induced peripheral and central sensitization.

11.3. Opioid receptors

Three members of the opioid receptor family were cloned in the early 1990s, including the delta-opioid receptor (DOR1), the mu-opioid receptor (MOR1), and the kappa-opioid receptor (KOR1) [94]. These three receptors and their corresponding peptide systems are significantly implicated in antinociceptive processes. Opiates have long been the mainstay of treatment for chronic bone cancer pain. However, there is increasing pressure to ensure that prescribing opioid analgesics is minimized to reduce not only the risk of dependence and illicit diversion but also the potential harms associated with tolerance, side effects, and complications, since opioid doses required for bone cancer patients are associated with adverse side effects further diminishing their quality of life [95]. This has often led to opiate underdosing [96]. It is important to note that while opioids are routinely used to treat tumor-induced bone pain, Parreca's lab has shown that sustained morphine use increases pain, osteolysis, bone loss, and spontaneous fracture, as well as markers of neuronal damage in DRG cells and the expression of pro-inflammatory cytokines in a rodent model of bone cancer [97]. More recent studies indicate that morphine contributes to chemoresistance via expanding the population of cancer stem cells, promotes tumor angiogenesis, and promotes tumor growth, thereby revealing a novel role of morphine and providing some new guidelines for the clinical use of morphine [98, 99]. It is also worth noting that treatment guidelines tend to consider morphine and morphine-like opioids comparable and interchangeable in the treatment of chronic cancer pain, but individual responses can vary. A recent clinical trial found that while there were no significant analgesic differences among morphine, oxycodone, transdermal fentanyl, or buprenorphine, the dose escalation was greater with fentanyl and switches, and discontinuations were more frequent with morphine [100]. Interestingly, this study identified groups of patients that were nonresponders to opiate treatment ranging from 11.5% (morphine) to 14.4% (buprenorphine). Thus, subsets of patients that do not respond to opiates are found in the general population, and like nonresponders for acupuncture analgesia (discussed below), these patients should be considered for alternative treatments. Finally, cannabis may be used both to treat chronic cancer pain and importantly to significantly reduce opiate usage. Thus, a 2011 clinical trial that examined the administration of vaporized plant cannabis in chronic cancer pain patients on a daily regimen of morphine or oxycodone reported that inhaled cannabis augments the analgesic effect of opioids [101].

11.4. Complementary/alternative therapies

Controlling cancer pain is an important part of the palliative care of cancer patients. Although conventional medicine has well-established guidelines to systemically control cancer-related pain, over half of cancer patients still suffer from pain as indicated above. Pharmacological therapeutic approaches are not always sufficient and may produce serious side effects. Thus these limitations have led to the use of complementary and alternative medicine approaches. While acupuncture has been around for thousands of years, it is only recently that it has been evolving as a promising approach to relieve chronic cancer pain [102, 103]. A recent study has shown that acupuncture and related therapies are effective in reducing pain and fatigue and in improving quality of life when compared with conventional intervention alone among cancer patients [104]. On the other hand, a subgroup analysis of five randomized controlled trials (RCTs) that evaluated acupuncture's effect on cancer pain did not include cancer-induced bone pain, because none of the studies made any reference to bone pain [105]. At this point in time, there is not convincing evidence that acupuncture significantly reduces cancer pain in the human literature. That being said there are several studies using animal models of cancer bone pain that suggest that acupuncture can reduce bone tumor-induced pain including osteosarcoma-induced pain [1, 106, 107]. The animal data suggest that electroacupuncture can alleviate bone cancer pain, at least in part by suppressing IL-1β expression and by altering nerve innervation and the vasculature of osteosarcoma. However, the acupuncture treatment schedule can effect tumor growth, and therefore the sequence of acupuncture treatment must be determined carefully [66]. Clearly, more clinical research is required to address whether acupuncture can reproducibly reduce pain in human osteosarcoma patients without unwanted tumor-related consequences.

12. Conclusion

Despite advances in our knowledge of osteosarcoma biology, development, metastasis, and its associated pain, the current treatment options have not changed over the last four decades and continue to rely on tumor resection and nonspecific combination chemotherapy, which results in a dismal 5-year survival rate of 0–29% for patients with clinically detectable metastases [38, 108]. Additionally, severe lack of knowledge regarding osteosarcoma metastasis hinders advancement of clinical treatment in pediatric patients. With limited human samples available, animal models hold promise for further understanding of the biology, pathways, and treatment options for osteosarcoma patients. While each model has its specific limitations, the collective insight into the genetics has proven extremely fruitful. With the advent of novel genetic engineering approaches, future studies will be instrumental in better modeling of the disease and uncovering new and valuable information. While conventional chemotherapy and surgical resection remain the mainstays of osteosarcoma treatment, when these approaches are used in combination with the above novel therapies, this will lead to prolonged if not remissive prognoses as well as significantly decreased pain for osteosarcoma patients in the future.

Acknowledgments

Author B.A.S. is supported by NIH/NIAMS T32 AR050938 "Musculoskeletal Training Grant." Author B.S.M. is supported by funding from the American Association for Cancer Research (AACR), Children's Cancer Research Fund (CCRF), Karen Wyckoff Rein in Sarcoma Foundation (KWRIS), and the Randy Shaver Foundation. Author A.J.B. is supported by NIH R01DA030316, USDA/NIFA grant MIN-63-071, and U of M Academic Health Center Seed Grant number15.05.

Author details

Branden A. Smeester[1, 2, 3], Branden S. Moriarity[1, 2, 3] and Alvin J. Beitz[4*]

*Address all correspondence to: beitz001@umn.edu

1 Department of Pediatrics, University of Minnesota, Minneapolis, Minnesota, USA

2 Center for Genome Engineering, University of Minnesota, Minneapolis, Minnesota, USA

3 Masonic Cancer Center, University of Minnesota, Minneapolis, Minnesota, USA

4 Department of Veterinary and Biomedical Sciences, University of Minnesota, Minneapolis, Minnesota, USA

References

[1] Smeester BA, Al-Gizawiy M, Beitz AJ. Effects of different electroacupuncture scheduling regimens on murine bone tumor-induced hyperalgesia: sex differences and role of inflammation. Evid Based Complement Alternat Med. 2012;2012:671386.

[2] Smeester BA, Lunzer MM, Akgun E, Beitz AJ, Portoghese PS. Targeting putative mu opioid/metabotropic glutamate receptor-5 heteromers produces potent antinociception in a chronic murine bone cancer model. Eur J Pharmacol. 2014;743:48–52.

[3] Franchi A. Epidemiology and classification of bone tumors. Clin Cases Miner Bone Metab. 2012;9(2):92–95.

[4] Raymond AK, Jaffe N. Osteosarcoma multidisciplinary approach to the management from the pathologist's perspective. Cancer Treat Res. 2009;152:63–84.

[5] Tsubaki M, Satou T, Itoh T, Imano M, Ogaki M, Yanae M, et al. Reduction of metastasis, cell invasion, and adhesion in mouse osteosarcoma by YM529/ONO-5920-induced blockade of the Ras/MEK/ERK and Ras/PI3K/Akt pathway. Toxicol Appl Pharmacol. 2012;259(3):402–410.

[6] Al-Salihi MA, Ulmer SC, Doan T, Nelson CD, Crotty T, Prescott SM, et al. Cyclooxygenase-2 transactivates the epidermal growth factor receptor through specific E-prostanoid receptors and tumor necrosis factor-alpha converting enzyme. Cell Signal. 2007;19(9):1956–1963.

[7] Ciccarese F, Bazzocchi A, Ciminari R, Righi A, Rocca M, Rimondi E, et al. The many faces of pulmonary metastases of osteosarcoma: retrospective study on 283 lesions submitted to surgery. Eur J Radiol. 2015;84(12):2679–2685.

[8] Gelderblom H, Jinks RC, Sydes M, Bramwell VH, van Glabbeke M, Grimer RJ, et al. Survival after recurrent osteosarcoma: data from 3 European Osteosarcoma Intergroup (EOI) randomized controlled trials. Eur J Cancer. 2011;47(6):895–902.

[9] Copeland NG, Jenkins NA. Harnessing transposons for cancer gene discovery. Nat Rev Cancer. 2010;10(10):696–706.

[10] Kim S, Lewis C, Nadel JA. Epidermal growth factor receptor reactivation induced by E-prostanoid-3 receptor- and tumor necrosis factor-alpha-converting enzyme-dependent feedback exaggerates interleukin-8 production in airway cancer (NCI-H292) cells. Exp Cell Res. 2011;317(18):2650–2660.

[11] Sueyoshi T, Jono H, Shinriki S, Ota K, Ota T, Tasaki M, et al. Therapeutic approaches targeting midkine suppress tumor growth and lung metastasis in osteosarcoma. Cancer Lett. 2012;316(1):23–30.

[12] Tarkkanen M, Karhu R, Kallioniemi A, Elomaa I, Kivioja AH, Nevalainen J, et al. Gains and losses of DNA sequences in osteosarcomas by comparative genomic hybridization. Cancer Res. 1995;55(6):1334–1338.

[13] Ballas SK, Gupta K, Adams-Graves P. Sickle cell pain: a critical reappraisal. Blood. 2012;120(18):3647–3656.

[14] Falk S, Dickenson AH. Pain and nociception: mechanisms of cancer-induced bone pain. J Clin Oncol. 2014;32(16):1647–1654.

[15] Kohli DR, Li Y, Khasabov SG, Gupta P, Kehl LJ, Ericson ME, et al. Pain-related behaviors and neurochemical alterations in mice expressing sickle hemoglobin: modulation by cannabinoids. Blood. 2010;116(3):456–465.

[16] Long F. Building strong bones: molecular regulation of the osteoblast lineage. Nat Rev Mol Cell Biol. 2012;13(1):27–38.

[17] Yavropoulou MP, Yovos JG. Osteoclastogenesis—current knowledge and future perspectives. J Musculoskelet Neuronal Interact. 2008;8(3):204–216.

[18] Sims NA, Martin TJ. Coupling the activities of bone formation and resorption: a multitude of signals within the basic multicellular unit. BoneKEy Rep. 2014;3:481.

[19] Fakhry M, Hamade E, Badran B, Buchet R, Magne D. Molecular mechanisms of mesenchymal stem cell differentiation towards osteoblasts. World J Stem Cells. 2013;5(4):136–148.

[20] Quist T, Jin H, Zhu JF, Smith-Fry K, Capecchi MR, Jones KB. The impact of osteoblastic differentiation on osteosarcomagenesis in the mouse. Oncogene. 2015;34(32):4278–4284.

[21] Walkley CR, Qudsi R, Sankaran VG, Perry JA, Gostissa M, Roth SI, et al. Conditional mouse osteosarcoma, dependent on p53 loss and potentiated by loss of Rb, mimics the human disease. Genes Dev. 2008;22(12):1662–1676.

[22] Tsuchiya T, Sekine K, Hinohara S, Namiki T, Nobori T, Kaneko Y. Analysis of the p16INK4, p14ARF, p15, TP53, and MDM2 genes and their prognostic implications in osteosarcoma and Ewing sarcoma. Cancer Genet Cytogenet. 2000;120(2):91–98.

[23] Porter DE, Holden ST, Steel CM, Cohen BB, Wallace MR, Reid R. A significant proportion of patients with osteosarcoma may belong to Li-Fraumeni cancer families. J Bone Joint Surg Br. 1992;74(6):883–886.

[24] Siddiqui R, Onel K, Facio F, Nafa K, Diaz LR, Kauff N, et al. The TP53 mutational spectrum and frequency of CHEK2*1100delC in Li-Fraumeni-like kindreds. Fam Cancer. 2005;4(2):177–181.

[25] Moriarity BS, Otto GM, Rahrmann EP, Rathe SK, Wolf NK, Weg MT, et al. A sleeping beauty forward genetic screen identifies new genes and pathways driving osteosarcoma development and metastasis. Nat Genet. 2015;47(6):615–624.

[26] Ragland BD, Bell WC, Lopez RR, Siegal GP. Cytogenetics and molecular biology of osteosarcoma. Lab Invest. 2002;82(4):365–373.

[27] Martin JW, Squire JA, Zielenska M. The genetics of osteosarcoma. Sarcoma. 2012;2012.

[28] Mu X, Brynien D, Weiss KR. The HDAC inhibitor Vorinostat diminishes the *in vitro* metastatic behavior of osteosarcoma cells. Biomed Res Int. 2015;2015:290368.

[29] Mu X, Sultankulov B, Agarwal R, Mahjoub A, Schott T, Greco N, et al. Chick embryo extract demethylates tumor suppressor genes in osteosarcoma cells. Clin Orthop Relat Res. 2014;472(3):865–873.

[30] Chen X, Bahrami A, Pappo A, Easton J, Dalton J, Hedlund E, et al. Recurrent somatic structural variations contribute to tumorigenesis in pediatric osteosarcoma. Cell Rep. 2014;7(1):104–112.

[31] Sadikovic B, Yoshimoto M, Al-Romaih K, Maire G, Zielenska M, Squire JA. *In vitro* analysis of integrated global high-resolution DNA methylation profiling with genomic imbalance and gene expression in osteosarcoma. PLoS One. 2008;3(7):e2834.

[32] Swiercz JM, Worzfeld T, Offermanns S. ErbB-2 and met reciprocally regulate cellular signaling via plexin-B1. J Biol Chem. 2008;283(4):1893–1901.

[33] Akatsuka T, Wada T, Kokai Y, Kawaguchi S, Isu K, Yamashiro K, et al. ErbB2 expression is correlated with increased survival of patients with osteosarcoma. Cancer. 2002;94(5):1397–1404.

[34] Patane S, Avnet S, Coltella N, Costa B, Sponza S, Olivero M, et al. MET overexpression turns human primary osteoblasts into osteosarcomas. Cancer Res. 2006;66(9):4750–4757.

[35] Kager L, Zoubek A, Potschger U, Kastner U, Flege S, Kempf-Bielack B, et al. Primary metastatic osteosarcoma: presentation and outcome of patients treated on neoadjuvant Cooperative Osteosarcoma Study Group protocols. J Clin Oncol. 2003;21(10):2011–2018.

[36] Kansara M, Thomas DM. Molecular pathogenesis of osteosarcoma. DNA Cell Biol. 2007;26(1):1–18.

[37] Meyers PA, Heller G, Healey JH, Huvos A, Applewhite A, Sun M, et al. Osteogenic sarcoma with clinically detectable metastasis at initial presentation. J Clin Oncol. 1993;11(3):449–453.

[38] Allison DC, Carney SC, Ahlmann ER, Hendifar A, Chawla S, Fedenko A, et al. A meta-analysis of osteosarcoma outcomes in the modern medical era. Sarcoma. 2012;2012:704872.

[39] Sottnik JL, Hall CL, Zhang J, Keller ET. Wnt and Wnt inhibitors in bone metastasis. BoneKEy Rep. 2012;1:101.

[40] Nguyen A, Scott MA, Dry SM, James AW. Roles of bone morphogenetic protein signaling in osteosarcoma. Int Orthop. 2014;38(11):2313–2322.

[41] Zhang YK, Huang ZJ, Liu S, Liu YP, Song AA, Song XJ. WNT signaling underlies the pathogenesis of neuropathic pain in rodents. J Clin Invest. 2013;123(5):2268–2286.

[42] Anderson HC, Hsu HH, Raval P, Hunt TR, Schwappach JR, Morris DC, et al. The mechanism of bone induction and bone healing by human osteosarcoma cell extracts. Clin Orthop Relat Res. 1995;313:129–134.

[43] Hara A, Ikeda T, Nomura S, Yagita H, Okumura K, Yamauchi Y. *In vivo* implantation of human osteosarcoma cells in nude mice induces bones with human-derived osteoblasts and mouse-derived osteocytes. Lab Invest. 1996;75(5):707–717.

[44] Ogose A, Motoyama T, Hotta T, Watanabe H, Takahashi HE. Bone formation *in vitro* and in nude mice by human osteosarcoma cells. Virchows Arch. 1995;426(2):117–125.

[45] Arihiro K, Inai K. Expression of CD31, Met/hepatocyte growth factor receptor and bone morphogenetic protein in bone metastasis of osteosarcoma. Pathol Int. 2001;51(2):100–106.

[46] Lv Z, Yang D, Li J, Hu M, Luo M, Zhan X, et al. Bone morphogenetic protein 9 overexpression reduces osteosarcoma cell migration and invasion. Mol Cells. 2013;36(2):119–126.

[47] Sulzbacher I, Birner P, Trieb K, Pichlbauer E, Lang S. The expression of bone morphogenetic proteins in osteosarcoma and its relevance as a prognostic parameter. J Clin Pathol. 2002;55(5):381–385.

[48] Wang L, Park P, La Marca F, Than K, Rahman S, Lin CY. Bone formation induced by BMP-2 in human osteosarcoma cells. Int J Oncol. 2013;43(4):1095–1102.

[49] Portenoy RK, Hagen NA. Breakthrough pain: definition, prevalence and characteristics. Pain. 1990;41(3):273–281.

[50] Bennett JH, Thomas G, Evans AW, Speight PM. Osteosarcoma of the jaws: a 30-year retrospective review. Oral Surg Oral Med Oral Pathol Oral Radiol Endod. 2000;90(3):323–332.

[51] Meuser T, Pietruck C, Radbruch L, Stute P, Lehmann KA, Grond S. Symptoms during cancer pain treatment following WHO-guidelines: a longitudinal follow-up study of symptom prevalence, severity and etiology. Pain. 2001;93(3):247–257.

[52] Chazan S, Ekstein MP, Marouani N, Weinbroum AA. Ketamine for acute and subacute pain in opioid-tolerant patients. J Opioid Manag. 2008;4(3):173–180.

[53] De Felice M, Lambert D, Holen I, Escott KJ, Andrew D. Effects of Src-kinase inhibition in cancer-induced bone pain. Mol Pain. 2016;12.

[54] Meng FF, Xu Y, Dan QQ, Wei L, Deng YJ, Liu J, et al. Intrathecal injection of lentivirus-mediated glial cell line-derived neurotrophic factor RNA interference relieves bone cancer-induced pain in rats. Cancer Sci. 2015;106(4):430–437.

[55] Ren BX, Gu XP, Zheng YG, Liu CL, Wang D, Sun YE, et al. Intrathecal injection of metabotropic glutamate receptor subtype 3 and 5 agonist/antagonist attenuates bone cancer pain by inhibition of spinal astrocyte activation in a mouse model. Anesthesiology. 2012;116(1):122–132.

[56] Pevida M, Gonzalez-Rodriguez S, Lastra A, Garcia-Suarez O, Hidalgo A, Menendez L, et al. Involvement of spinal chemokine CCL2 in the hyperalgesia evoked by bone cancer in mice: a role for astroglia and microglia. Cell Mol Neurobiol. 2014;34(1):143–156.

[57] Bennett MI, Johnson MI, Brown SR, Radford H, Brown JM, Searle RD. Feasibility study of transcutaneous electrical nerve stimulation (TENS) for cancer bone pain. J Pain. 2010;11(4):351–359.

[58] Zhu XC, Zhang JL, Ge CT, Yu YY, Wang P, Yuan TF, et al. Advances in cancer pain from bone metastasis. Drug Des Devel Ther. 2015;9:4239–4245.

[59] Mantyh PW, Clohisy DR, Koltzenburg M, Hunt SP. Molecular mechanisms of cancer pain. Nat Rev Cancer. 2002;2(3):201–209.

[60] Ueno A, Oh-ishi S. Critical roles for bradykinin and prostanoids in acute inflammatory reactions: a search using experimental animal models. Curr Drug Targets Inflamm Allergy. 2002;1(4):363–376.

[61] Lam DK. Emerging factors in the progression of cancer-related pain. Pain Manag. 2016;6:487–496.

[62] Shor S, Fadl-Alla BA, Pondenis HC, Zhang X, Wycislo KL, Lezmi S, et al. Expression of nociceptive ligands in canine osteosarcoma. J Vet Intern Med. 2015;29(1):268–275.

[63] Brown MR, Ramirez JD. Neuroimmune mechanisms in cancer pain. Curr Opin Support Palliat Care. 2015;9(2):103–111.

[64] Jimenez-Andrade JM, Ghilardi JR, Castaneda-Corral G, Kuskowski MA, Mantyh PW. Preventive or late administration of anti-NGF therapy attenuates tumor-induced nerve sprouting, neuroma formation, and cancer pain. Pain. 2011;152(11):2564–2574.

[65] Mantyh WG, Jimenez-Andrade JM, Stake JI, Bloom AP, Kaczmarska MJ, Taylor RN, et al. Blockade of nerve sprouting and neuroma formation markedly attenuates the development of late stage cancer pain. Neuroscience. 2010;171(2):588–598.

[66] Smeester BA, Al-Gizawiy M, O'Brien EE, Ericson ME, Triemstra JL, Beitz AJ. The effect of electroacupuncture on osteosarcoma tumor growth and metastasis: analysis of different treatment regimens. Evid Based Complement Alternat Med. 2013;2013:387169.

[67] Evans EE, Jonason AS, Jr., Bussler H, Torno S, Veeraraghavan J, Reilly C, et al. Antibody blockade of semaphorin 4D promotes immune infiltration into tumor and enhances response to other immunomodulatory therapies. Cancer Immunol Res. 2015;3(6):689–701.

[68] Negishi-Koga T, Shinohara M, Komatsu N, Bito H, Kodama T, Friedel RH, et al. Suppression of bone formation by osteoclastic expression of semaphorin 4D. Nat Med. 2011;17(11):1473–1480.

[69] Zhou H, Binmadi NO, Yang YH, Proia P, Basile JR. Semaphorin 4D cooperates with VEGF to promote angiogenesis and tumor progression. Angiogenesis. 2012;15(3):391–407.

[70] Briscoe J, Therond PP. The mechanisms of Hedgehog signalling and its roles in development and disease. Nat Rev Mol Cell Biol. 2013;14(7):416–429.

[71] Lum L, Beachy PA. The Hedgehog response network: sensors, switches, and routers. Science. 2004;304(5678):1755–1759.

[72] Paget C, Duret H, Ngiow SF, Kansara M, Thomas DM, Smyth MJ. Studying the role of the immune system on the antitumor activity of a Hedgehog inhibitor against murine osteosarcoma. Oncoimmunology. 2012;1(8):1313–1322.

[73] Campbell VT, Nadesan P, Ali SA, Wang CY, Whetstone H, Poon R, et al. Hedgehog pathway inhibition in chondrosarcoma using the smoothened inhibitor IPI-926 directly inhibits sarcoma cell growth. Mol Cancer Ther. 2014;13(5):1259–1269.

[74] Tiet TD, Hopyan S, Nadesan P, Gokgoz N, Poon R, Lin AC, et al. Constitutive hedgehog signaling in chondrosarcoma up-regulates tumor cell proliferation. Am J Pathol. 2006;168(1):321–330.

[75] Von Hoff DD, LoRusso PM, Rudin CM, Reddy JC, Yauch RL, Tibes R, et al. Inhibition of the hedgehog pathway in advanced basal-cell carcinoma. N Engl J Med. 2009;361(12):1164–1172.

[76] Rudin CM, Hann CL, Laterra J, Yauch RL, Callahan CA, Fu L, et al. Treatment of medulloblastoma with hedgehog pathway inhibitor GDC-0449. N Engl J Med. 2009;361(12):1173–1178.

[77] Zarogoulidis P, Lampaki S, Turner JF, Huang H, Kakolyris S, Syrigos K, et al. mTOR pathway: a current, up-to-date mini-review (review). Oncol Lett. 2014;8(6):2367–2370.

[78] Zhou Q, Deng Z, Zhu Y, Long H, Zhang S, Zhao J. mTOR/p70S6K signal transduction pathway contributes to osteosarcoma progression and patients' prognosis. Med Oncol. 2010;27(4):1239–1245.

[79] Wan X, Mendoza A, Khanna C, Helman LJ. Rapamycin inhibits ezrin-mediated metastatic behavior in a murine model of osteosarcoma. Cancer Res. 2005;65(6):2406–2411.

[80] Houghton PJ, Morton CL, Kolb EA, Gorlick R, Lock R, Carol H, et al. Initial testing (stage 1) of the mTOR inhibitor rapamycin by the pediatric preclinical testing program. Pediatr Blood Cancer. 2008;50(4):799–805.

[81] Mu X, Isaac C, Schott T, Huard J, Weiss K. Rapamycin inhibits ALDH activity, resistance to oxidative stress, and metastatic potential in murine osteosarcoma cells. Sarcoma. 2013;2013:480713.

[82] Ando K, Heymann MF, Stresing V, Mori K, Redini F, Heymann D. Current therapeutic strategies and novel approaches in osteosarcoma. Cancers (Basel). 2013;5(2):591–616.

[83] Gorlick R, Huvos AG, Heller G, Aledo A, Beardsley GP, Healey JH, et al. Expression of HER2/erbB-2 correlates with survival in osteosarcoma. J Clin Oncol. 1999;17(9):2781–2788.

[84] Ahmed N, Salsman VS, Yvon E, Louis CU, Perlaky L, Wels WS, et al. Immunotherapy for osteosarcoma: genetic modification of T cells overcomes low levels of tumor antigen expression. Mol Ther. 2009;17(10):1779–1787.

[85] Hassan SE, Bekarev M, Kim MY, Lin J, Piperdi S, Gorlick R, et al. Cell surface receptor expression patterns in osteosarcoma. Cancer. 2012;118(3):740–749.

[86] Abdeen A, Chou AJ, Healey JH, Khanna C, Osborne TS, Hewitt SM, et al. Correlation between clinical outcome and growth factor pathway expression in osteogenic sarcoma. Cancer. 2009;115(22):5243–5250.

[87] Oliveira A, Dinis-Oliveira RJ, Nogueira A, Goncalves F, Silva P, Vieira C, et al. Interleukin-1beta genotype and circulating levels in cancer patients: metastatic status and pain perception. Clin Biochem. 2014;47(13–14):1209–1213.

[88] Copray JC, Mantingh I, Brouwer N, Biber K, Kust BM, Liem RS, et al. Expression of interleukin-1 beta in rat dorsal root ganglia. J Neuroimmunol. 2001;118(2):203–211.

[89] Montell C. The history of TRP channels, a commentary and reflection. Pflugers Arch. 2011;461(5):499–506.

[90] Caterina MJ, Schumacher MA, Tominaga M, Rosen TA, Levine JD, Julius D. The capsaicin receptor: a heat-activated ion channel in the pain pathway. Nature. 1997;389(6653):816–824.

[91] Fattori V, Hohmann MS, Rossaneis AC, Pinho-Ribeiro FA, Verri WA. Capsaicin: current understanding of its mechanisms and therapy of pain and other pre-clinical and clinical uses. Molecules. 2016;21(7).

[92] Iadarola MJ, Gonnella GL. Resiniferatoxin for pain treatment: an interventional approach to personalized pain medicine. Open Pain J. 2013;6:95–107.

[93] Fazzari J, Linher-Melville K, Singh G. Tumour-derived glutamate: linking aberrant cancer cell metabolism to peripheral sensory pain pathways. Curr Neuropharmacol. 2016;14.

[94] Przewlocki R, Przewlocka B. Opioids in chronic pain. Eur J Pharmacol. 2001;429(1–3):79–91.

[95] Remeniuk B, Sukhtankar D, Okun A, Navratilova E, Xie JY, King T, et al. Behavioral and neurochemical analysis of ongoing bone cancer pain in rats. Pain. 2015;156(10):1864–1873.

[96] Varilla V, Schneiderman H, Keefe S. No ceiling dose: effective pain control with extraordinary opiate dosing in cancer. Conn Med. 2015;79(9):521–524.

[97] King T, Vardanyan A, Majuta L, Melemedjian O, Nagle R, Cress AE, et al. Morphine treatment accelerates sarcoma-induced bone pain, bone loss, and spontaneous fracture in a murine model of bone cancer. Pain. 2007;132(1–2):154–168.

[98] Bimonte S, Barbieri A, Rea D, Palma G, Luciano A, Cuomo A, et al. Morphine promotes tumor angiogenesis and increases breast cancer progression. Biomed Res Int. 2015;2015:161508.

[99] Niu DG, Peng F, Zhang W, Guan Z, Zhao HD, Li JL, et al. Morphine promotes cancer stem cell properties, contributing to chemoresistance in breast cancer. Oncotarget. 2015;6(6):3963–3976.

[100] Corli O, Floriani I, Roberto A, Montanari M, Galli F, Greco MT, et al. Are strong opioids equally effective and safe in the treatment of chronic cancer pain? A multicenter randomized phase IV 'real life' trial on the variability of response to opioids. Ann Oncol. 2016;27(6):1107–1115.

[101] Johnson JR, Burnell-Nugent M, Lossignol D, Ganae-Motan ED, Potts R, Fallon MT. Multicenter, double-blind, randomized, placebo-controlled, parallel-group study of the efficacy, safety, and tolerability of THC:CBD extract and THC extract in patients with intractable cancer-related pain. J Pain Symptom Manage. 2010;39(2):167–179.

[102] Dhanani NM, Caruso TJ, Carinci AJ. Complementary and alternative medicine for pain: an evidence-based review. Curr Pain Headache Rep. 2011;15(1):39–46.

[103] Stone JA, Johnstone PA. Mechanisms of action for acupuncture in the oncology setting. Curr Treat Options Oncol. 2010;11(3–4):118–127.

[104] Lau CH, Wu X, Chung VC, Liu X, Hui EP, Cramer H, et al. Acupuncture and related therapies for symptom management in palliative cancer care: systematic review and meta-analysis. Medicine (Baltimore). 2016;95(9):e2901.

[105] Paley CA, Johnson MI, Tashani OA, Bagnall AM. Acupuncture for cancer pain in adults. Cochrane Database Syst Rev 2015;10:CD007753.

[106] Ryu HK, Baek YH, Park YC, Seo BK. Current studies of acupuncture in cancer-induced bone pain animal models. Evid Based Complement Alternat Med. 2014;2014:191347.

[107] Zhang RX, Li A, Liu B, Wang L, Ren K, Qiao JT, et al. Electroacupuncture attenuates bone cancer pain and inhibits spinal interleukin-1 beta expression in a rat model. Anesth Analg. 2007;105(5):1482–1488, table of contents.

[108] Jaffe N, Puri A, Gelderblom H. Osteosarcoma: evolution of treatment paradigms. Sarcoma. 2013;2013:203531.

Chapter 9

The Biological Role and Clinical Implication of MicroRNAs in Osteosarcoma

Yutaka Nezu, Kosuke Matsuo, Akira Kawai,
Tomoyuki Saito and Takahiro Ochiya

Additional information is available at the end of the chapter

http://dx.doi.org/10.5772/67450

Abstract

The main causes of death in osteosarcoma (OS) patients are the development of distant metastasis and resistance to chemotherapy. Clarification of the pathophysiological molecular mechanisms that contribute to the malignant phenotype in OS and identification of a molecular target, such as a diagnostic marker, prognostic predictor, or chemosensitivity sensor, are strongly desired to develop therapeutics for OS patients. Accumulating evidence has demonstrated that microRNAs (miRNAs), small endogenous single-stranded noncoding RNAs, play critical roles not only in biological but also pathological processes such as cancer. miRNAs can function as oncogenes or tumor-suppressive genes depending on the mRNA they target. They are strongly associated with OS invasion, metastasis, and chemoresistance as well as OS cancer stemness. Furthermore, miRNAs are associated with commonly altered genes, such as TP53 and RB1. Additionally, recent global microRNA expression analyses have identified specific miRNAs correlated with the clinical stage and the response to chemotherapy. In this chapter, we summarize the current understanding of the pathological roles of miRNAs as well as their potential utility as OS biomarkers.

Keywords: microRNA, metastasis, chemoresistance, cancer stem cells, therapy

1. Introduction

Osteosarcoma (OS) is the most common primary malignant bone tumor. Before the 1970s, treatment generally included only surgical resection. However, because approximately 80% of patients have developed pulmonary metastases by the initial diagnosis, the 5-year survival rate was 10–15% [1, 2]. Due to the development of multidrug chemotherapy, surgical wide resection, and reconstruction with tumor prosthesis, the prognosis has gradually improved over the past 30 years [3]. Despite advances in multimodality treatment, the prognosis is still poor in patients with metastasis and/or acquisition of anticancer drug resistance. Because the critical molecular mechanisms contributing to the development of distant metastases and acquisition of chemoresistance in OS remain largely unknown, elucidation of the detailed pathophysiological molecular mechanisms is strongly desired to develop the novel tools for OS diagnosis, prognostic prediction, and treatment against OS.

microRNAs (miRNAs) are endogenous single-stranded, noncoding RNAs with approximately 22 nucleotides in length that regulate gene expression by cleavage or translational repression at the post-transcriptional level by base pairing with the 3′ untranslated region (UTR) of their target mRNAs. To date, 2588 mature miRNAs have been identified, and they regulate the expression of more than a half of all human genes [4, 5]. Emerging evidence has demonstrated that miRNAs not only regulate biological processes such as development, differentiation, apoptosis, and proliferation but also modulate pathological conditions [6]. Genetic or epigenetic alterations, dysregulation of transcription factors, and abnormal microRNA biogenesis can alter the dysregulation of microRNA expression [7]. As a result, the misexpressed microRNAs contribute to many types of human diseases, including cancer [6–8]. miRNAs can function as either oncogenes or tumor suppressors depending on their individual target mRNAs, and abnormal miRNA expression has been observed in various solid and hematopoietic tumors in relation to the initiation and progression of tumors including growth, metastasis, and drug resistance. Furthermore, miRNA expression profiling of human tumors has identified signatures associated with diagnosis, staging, progression, prognosis, and response to treatment.

After the first study examining the association between the microRNAs and OS pathogenesis in 2009 [9], numerous studies have reported miRNA expression profiles from clinical OS samples and cell lines, and the association between miRNAs and malignant phenotypes. The altered gene expression previously reported in OS patients is closely association with altered miRNA expression. There is growing evidence that miRNAs play critical roles in various pathological processes, such as tumorigenesis, invasion, metastasis, chemoresistance, and cancer stem cell maintenance in OS [10, 11]. Therefore, altered miRNA expressions could be a useful diagnostic and prognostic tool for OS patients [10, 11].

Here, we summarize the pathological roles of miRNAs in OS and their potential value as diagnostic and prognostic biomarkers for OS patients.

2. Biological machinery and miRNA function

miRNAs are small, noncoding, single-stranded RNAs 18–25 nucleotides long that regulate gene expression at the post-transcriptional level. miRNAs are mainly transcribed by RNA polymerase II to generate primary-miRNAs (pri-miRNAs), which are usually 3–4 kb long and characterized by hairpin structures. In the nucleus, these pri-miRNAs are cleaved into 70–100 nucleotide precursor-miRNAs (pre-miRNAs) by Drosha and DGCR8 (DiGeorge Syndrome Critical Region Gene-8). Pre-miRNAs are transferred to the cytoplasm by Exportin-5 and cleaved to form a miRNA duplex by Dicer and TRBP (transactivating response RNA-binding protein). The two miRNA strands of the duplex are processed into two different mature miRNAs (-3p or -5p). Mature miRNAs are incorporated into the RNA-induced silencing complex (RISC), which contains Argonaute 2 (Ago2) and GW182. As a part of this complex, mature miRNAs suppress gene expression by binding to the 3′UTR of target mRNAs, which are recognized by 6–8 nucleotides at the miRNA 5′-terminus called seed sequence, leading to mRNA degradation or translation inhibition depending on the complementarity between the miRNA seed sequence and the 3′UTR of the mRNA (**Figure 1**) [7, 12].

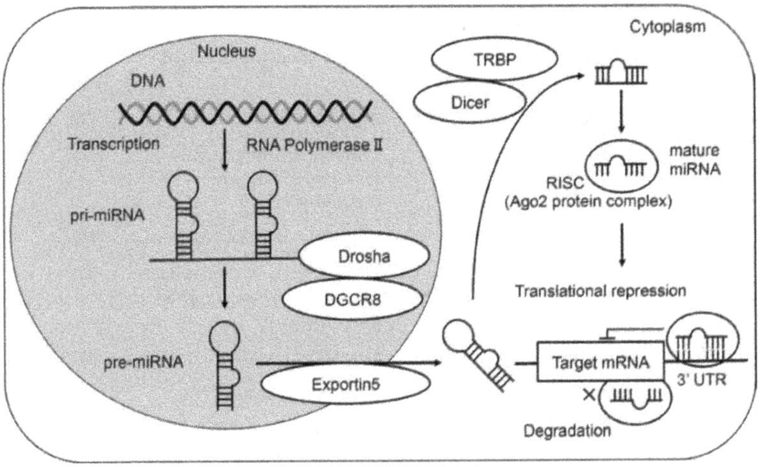

Figure 1. MicroRNA biological machinery. miRNAs are mainly transcribed by RNA polymerase-II to generate pri-miRNAs. In the nucleus, pri-miRNAs are cleaved into 70–100 nucleotide pre-miRNAs by Drosha and DGCR8. Pre-miRNAs are transferred to the cytoplasm by Exportin-5 and cleaved to form a miRNA duplex by Dicer and TRBP. The two miRNA strands of the duplex are processed into two different mature miRNAs (-3p or -5p). Mature miRNAs are incorporated into the RISC, which contains Ago2. As a part of this complex, mature miRNAs suppress gene expression by binding to the 3′UTR of target mRNAs, which are recognized by 6–8 nucleotides at the miRNA 5′-terminus called seed sequence, leading to mRNA degradation or translation inhibition.

3. miRNAs in cancer

The relationship between cancer and miRNAs was first reported in 2002. Calin et al. demonstrated that miR-15 and miR-16 at chromosome 13q14 were deleted or downregulated in the majority of chronic lymphocytic leukemia (CLL) cases and that these miRs induced apoptosis by direct suppression of Bcl-2 (B cell lymphoma 2) in CLL cells [13, 14]. Genetic or epigenetic changes, dysregulation of transcription factors, and abnormal microRNA biogenesis can alter microRNA expression [7]. Accumulating evidence suggests that dysregulated miRNAs induce cancer initiation and progression [6], and aberrant miRNAs can function as oncogenes or tumor suppressor genes depending on their target genes.

4. Dysregulation of microRNAs in OS

The relationship between OS and miRNA expression has been reported in over 400 publications to date. Aberrantly expressed miRNAs have been shown to play essential roles in the biological processes of OS pathogenesis through the regulation of numerous protein-coding genes and signaling pathways (**Tables 1** and **2**).

miRNA	Target gene	Function	Reference
miR-34a	Surviving	Proliferation, apoptosis, chemoresistance to CDDP	[21]
	mTOR, MET, MDM4	Proliferation, apoptosis	[17]
	Eag1	Proliferation, tumor growth *in vivo*	[16]
	CD44	Migration, invasion	[22]
	c-Met	Proliferation, migration, invasion, tumor growth and metastasis *in vivo*	[15]
miR-143	Bcl-2	Migration, invasion, apoptosis	[20]
	ATG2B, Bcl-2, LC-1,2	Proliferation, chemoresistance to DOX, autophagy, tumor growth *in vivo*	[23]
	VCAN	Migration, invasion	[24]
	MMP13	Invasion, metastasis	[18]
	Bcl-2	Proliferation, apoptosis, tumorigenicity	[19]
miR-144	ROCK1, ROCK2	Proliferation, invasion, tumorigenesis and metastasis *in vivo*	[25]
	ROCK1	Proliferation, migration, invasion	[26]
	Ezrin	Invasion, metastasis	[27]
	TAGLN	Proliferation, invasion	[28]
miR-145	FLI-1	Proliferation, migration, apoptosis, tumor growth *in vivo*	[29]
	ROCK1	Proliferation, migration, invasion	[30]
	ROCK1	Proliferation, invasion	[31]
	VEGF	Invasion, angiogenesis	[32]
miR-451	LRH-1	Proliferation, cell cycle	[33]
	CXCL16	Proliferation, invasion	[34]
	PGE2, CCND1	Proliferation, cell cycle, apoptosis	[35]

Table 1. Tumor suppressive microRNAs and targets in osteosarcoma.

miRNA	Target gene	Function	Reference
miR-20a	ERG2	Proliferation, cell cycle	[37]
	Fas	Metastasis	[36]
miR-21	PTEN	Proliferation, invasion, apoptosis	[39]
	SPRY2	Migration, invasion	[41]
	Bcl-2	Chemoresistance to CDDP	[38]
	RECK	Invasion, migration	[40]
miR-135b	FOXO1	Proliferation, invasion	[42]
	Myocardin	Proliferation, migration, invasion	[43]
miR-155	HBP1	Proliferation, cell cycle, tumor growth *in vivo*	[44]
	–	Proliferation, migration, invasion	[45]
	–	Autophagy, chemoresistance to DOX and CDDP	[46]
miR-214	PTEN	Proliferation, migration, invasion	[47]
	PTEN	Proliferation, apoptosis, tumorigenicity	[48]
	LZTS1	Proliferation, invasion, tumor growth *in vivo*	[49]

Table 2. Ongogenic microRNA and targets in osteosarcoma.

miR-34a: The overexpression of miR-34a inhibited the proliferation, migration, and invasion of OS cell lines (SOSP-9607 and Saos-2) *in vitro* and decreased tumor growth and pulmonary metastasis of SOSP-9607 cells *in vivo* by directly targeting c-Met [15]. Based on a bioinformatics analysis, they demonstrated that miR-34a had multiple putative targets associated with proliferation and metastasis, including members of the Wnt and Notch signaling pathways. Wu et al. demonstrated that miR-34a was significantly downregulated in clinical OS tissues and cell lines. Overexpression of miR-34a inhibited the proliferation of OS cells (MG-63 and Saos-2) *in vitro* and tumor growth *in vivo* by decreasing the expression of Ether à go-go 1 (Eag1) [16]. Furthermore, Tian et al. demonstrated that miR-34a inhibited proliferation and induced apoptosis in MG-63 cells through the p53 signaling pathway [17].

miR-143: Osaki et al. compared HOS and 143B OS cells (highly metastatic variant of HOS transformed by v-Ki-ras) using a miRNA microarray analysis [18]. miR-143 was significantly downregulated in 143B cells, and transfection of miR-143 decreased cell invasiveness by directly targeting matrix metalloproteinase 13 (MMP13). Furthermore, the systemic administration of miR-143/atelocollagen complexes significantly suppressed the lung metastasis of 143B *in vivo*. Zhang et al. demonstrated that the restoring miR-143 expression reduced OS cell (MG-63 and U-2OS) viability, promoted apoptosis *in vitro*, and suppressed tumorigenicity *in vivo* [19], and they identified Bcl-2, an important antiapoptotic protein, as a direct target of miR-143. Li et al. also showed that miR-143 promoted apoptosis in OS cells (MG-63 and U-2OS) through caspase-3 activation by targeting Bcl-2 [20]. Moreover, miR-143 overexpression significantly suppressed cell migration and invasion.

miR-20a: Huang et al. found the higher miR-20a expression in metastatic Saos-2 cells compared with original Saos-2 cells [36]. The metastatic cells expressed low levels of Fas, which is inversely correlated to lung metastasis, and miR-20a directly regulated the expression levels of Fas. The inhibition of miR-20a expression decreased the occurrence of metastasis *in vivo*. Ectopic expression of miR-20a promotes the proliferation and cell cycle progression of Saos-2 cells by directly suppressing early growth response 2 (EGR2), a key regulator of proliferation and the cell cycle [37].

miR-21: miR-21 was significantly overexpressed in OS tissues compared with matched normal bone tissues [38], and miR-21 knockdown reduced migration and invasion in MG-63 cells by directly regulating RECK (reversion-inducing-cysteine-rich protein with kazal motifs), a tumor suppressor gene. Lv et al. demonstrated that PTEN might be a potential target of miR-21 [39]. The miR-21 expression level was significantly higher in MG-63 cells than in a human fetal osteoblastic cell line, hFOB1. 19, and miR-21 overexpression increased proliferative and invasive abilities and reduced apoptosis in MG-63 cells. The authors suggested that miR-21 activates the PI3K/Akt pathway by suppressing PTEN expression. In addition, miR-21 regulates the MAPK signaling pathway by targeting SPRY2 (protein sprout homolog 2), an antagonist of MEK1/2, as an oncogenic miRNA that increases cell proliferation, cell cycle progression, and inhibits apoptosis [40].

5. miRNAs associated with dysregulated genes in OS

OS exhibits a broad range of genetic and molecular alterations, such as the gains, losses, or rearrangements of chromosomal regions that result in inactivation of tumor suppressor genes and the misregulation of major signaling pathways [50].

5.1. TP53-associated miRNAs

TP53, located in 17q13.1, is a tumor suppressor gene that is mutated in more than 20% of human OS patients, which drives OS initiation and progression of OS [51]. Recent studies have demonstrated an association between TP53 and miRNAs. He et al. demonstrated that miR-34s (miR-34a, b, and c), which was decreased OS tissues and regulated by p53, affected the expression of CDK6, E2F3, Cyclin E2, and Bcl-2, and induced G1 arrest and apoptosis partially in a p53-dependent manner [9]. Novello et al. demonstrated that miR-34a demethylation by p53 was important for etoposide sensitivity [52]. They demonstrated that U2-OS cells either with the wild-type p53 or a dominant-negative form of p53 both of which were expressing increased levels of unmethylated miR-34awere more sensitive to etoposide than p53-deficient OS cells (MG-63 and Saos-2).

5.2. RB1-associated miRNAs

RB1 on 13q14 is one of the most commonly inactivated genes in sporadic OS [53]. Poos et al. performed the miRNA expression analysis of OS cell lines based on their proliferative activity to generate a coregulatory network between miRNA and transcription factor. As a result, they found that downregulation of miR-9-5p, miR-138, and miR-214 was correlated to a strong proliferative phenotype in OS cells through their effect on NFKB and RB1 signaling pathways and focal adhesion molecules [54].

5.3. RUNX2-associated miRNA

The chromosomal region 6p 12–21 is commonly amplified and DNA gains occur in 40–50% of tumors. This region contains RUNX2 which promotes terminal osteoblast differentiation and is elevated in conventional OS [53]. van der Deen et al. demonstrated that miR-34c which is elevated by p53 and targets RUNX2, is absent in OS tissue [55]. This p53-miR-34c-RUNX2 pathway controls osteoblast growth and its alteration may impact on OS pathogenesis.

These data indicate that miRNAs play critical roles in OS pathogenesis by regulation of and interaction with commonly aberrant genes.

6. Cancer stem cell-associated miRNAs

It is widely considered that cancer stem cell (CSC) populations possibly drive the refractory nature of cancer, especially multidrug resistance and distant metastasis. OS stem cells have been isolated and identified by using cell sorting methods based on specific cell surface markers such as CD133, Hoechst dye side population assay, and sphere colony formation assays. Several groups have demonstrated that miRNAs are involved in the maintenance and stimulation of CSC population in various cancers, including OS [56]. miR-29b-1 expression was decreased in 3AB-OS cells, a CSC line selected from MG-63 cells, and its overexpression causes cell proliferation, self-renewal, and chemoresistance. This is accompanied by the downregulation of stem cell markers (Oct3/4, Sox2, Nanog, CD133, and N-Myc), cell cycle-related markers (CCND2, E2F1, E2F2), and antiapoptotic markers (Bcl-2 and IAP-2) [57]. Xu et al. demonstrated a relationship between miR-382 and CSCs in OS [58]. miR-382 expression was significantly lower in highly metastatic OS cell lines and relapsed OS clinical samples. Likewise, the overexpression of miR-382 decreased the CSC population defined by CD133 and ALDH1 expression and osteosphere capacity. *In vivo* experiments showed that miR-382 overexpression inhibited CSC-induced tumor formation. However, the association between miRNAs and CSCs is still under investigation, thus further research will be required to develop the novel therapeutic strategies targeting CSCs in OS.

7. Chemoresistance-associated miRNAs

Advances in chemotherapy have contributed to the dramatic improvement to OS patient outcomes. Most OS patients receive multidrug chemotherapy that consists of doxorubicin (DOX), cisplatin (CDDP), methotrexate (MTX), and ifosfamide (IFO), but certain population of OS patients exhibit chemoresistance. The molecular mechanisms driving poor response to chemotherapy remain largely unclear, and there are no biomarkers to discriminate between good and poor responders before chemotherapy.

DOX: miR-301a expression promoted HMGCR expression by targeting AMP-activated protein kinase alpha 1 and enhanced the resistance of OS cells (U2OS, MG-63) to DOX [59]. Chang et al. have demonstrated that miR-101 overexpression dramatically reduces DOX-induced autophagosome formation by suppressing autophagy 4 (Atg4) in U2-OS cells, thereby enhancing the sensitization of tumor cells to DOX [60]. miR-184 expression was induced by DOX, and overexpression or silencing of miR-184 reduced or enhanced DOX-induced apoptosis by targeting Bcl-2-like protein 1 (BCL2L1) [61].

CDDP: Overexpression of miR-224, which is downregulated in OS cell lines and tissues, contributed to the increased sensitivity of MG-63 cells to CDDP by targeting Rac1 [62]. miR-33a was upregulated in chemoresistant OS tissues and promoted resistance to CDDP in OS cell (MG-63, Saos-2) by downregulating TWIST [63]. Downregulation of miR-497 induced CDDP resistance through the PI3K/Akt pathway by directly targeting VEGFA in human OS [64], and miR-138 functions as a tumor suppressor by enhancing sensitivity to CDDP in OS via direct downregulation of EZH2 [65].

MTX: Decreased miR-126 reduced the sensitivity to MTX and promoted apoptosis in OS cells (MG-63 and U-2OS) [66]. According to high-throughput miRNA expression analysis, Song et al. demonstrated that miR-140 expression was associated with chemosensitivity in OS tumor xenografts [67]. The authors showed that miR-140 overexpression induced MTX resistance by targeting HDAC4 possibly through p53-dependent manner. Furthermore, they proved that miR-215 caused G2 arrest by suppressing DTL expression, and that led to chemoresistance against MTX [68].

IFO: Five miRNAs (miR-92a, miR-99b, miR-132, miR-193-5p, and miR-442a), which inhibit the TGF-β and Wnt pathways by *in silico* analysis, discriminate good from poor IFO responders against IFO [69].

These reports suggest that miRNAs associated with an anticancer drug might be potential chemosensitivity biomarkers and promising therapeutic targets for OS patients.

8. Detection of miRNA in blood samples

There are few biomarkers for the diagnosis and prognosis prediction of OS patients other than alkaline phosphatase (ALP). Meta-analysis has demonstrated that high ALP level is significantly associated with a poor overall survival and event-free survival rate and the presence of metastasis at diagnosis [70]. However, predictors of poor outcome are mainly clinical parameters, such as proximal extremity or axial skeleton involvement, large size/volume, detectable metastases at diagnosis, and poor response to preoperative chemotherapy [53]. Recently, growing evidence indicates the clinical usefulness of miRNAs as biomarkers, and numerous candidate miRNAs in blood samples have been reported in OS patients (**Table 3**).

miRNA	Blood sample	Reference
Upregulated miRNAs		
miR-221	Serum	[71]
miR-191	Serum	[73]
miR-199a-5p	Serum	[78]
miR-27a	Serum	[72]
miR-195-5p, 199a-3p, 320a, 374a-5p	Plasma	[77]
miR-155	Serum	[44]
miR-9	Serum	[83]
miR-196a, 196b	Serum	[76]
miR-21	Serum	[74]
	Plasma	[75]
Downregulated miRNAs		
miR-223	Serum	[79]
miR-106a-5p, 16-5p, 20a-5p, 425-5p, 451a, 25-3p, 139-5p	Serum	[84]
miR-195	Serum	[80]
miR-133b, 206	Serum	[82]
miR-34b	Plasma	[81]
miR-199a-3p, 143	Plasma	[75]

Table 3. Dysregulated miRNAs in blood samples of OS patients.

Upregulated miRNAs in OS: The expression level of miR-221 [71], miR-27a [72], miR-191 [73], and miR-21 [74, 75] in blood samples was increased in OS patients compared with healthy controls, and compared to preoperation and postoperation state, the expression levels of miR-199a-5p [76] and four miRNAs (miR-195-5p, miR-199a-3p, miR-320a, and miR-374a-5p; [77]) were decreased in postoperative compared to preoperative blood samples. It has been suggested that upregulations of these miRNAs were significant predictors for poor overall and disease-free survival. The expression levels of these miRNA were related to clinical stage [71–74], tumor size [73], distant metastasis [71–73, 75], and chemoresistance [50], the upregulations of these miRNAs were significant predictors for poor overall and disease-free survival.

In addition, the combination of dysregulated miRNAs was more accurate than the individual expression level of each miRNA. The coexpression of miR-196a/miR-196b [78] and the combination of four miRNAs (miR-195-5p, miR-199a-3p, miR-320a, and miR-374-5p) [77] were superior predictors to any of the miRNAs alone.

Downregulated miRNAs in OS: In contrast, the expression level of miR-223 [79], miR-195 [80], and miR-34b [81] in blood samples was significantly decreased in OS patients compared to healthy controls. These miRNAs levels were associated with clinical stage [79, 80] and distant metastasis [79–81], and the decreased expression of these miRNAs was associated with shorter overall survival and disease-free survival. In addition, the coexpression of miR-133b/miR-206 was a prognostic factor for overall survival and disease-free survival [82].

These data indicate the potential of miRNAs in blood samples as diagnostic markers, prognotic predictors, and chemosensitivity sensors.

9. Conclusion

Dysregulated miRNAs contribute to the initiation and progression of human OS in several pathobiological aspects. The detection of aberrant miRNAs could be a versatile tool for diagnosis, prognosis and chemosensitivity judgment, and inhibition of oncogenic miRNAs and/or restoration of tumor-suppressing miRNAs could be a novel strategy for treatment of OS.

Author details

Yutaka Nezu[1,2], Kosuke Matsuo[2], Akira Kawai[3], Tomoyuki Saito[2] and Takahiro Ochiya[1,*]

*Address all correspondence to: tochiya@ncc.go.jp

1 Division of Molecular and Cellular Medicine, National Cancer Center Research Institute, Tokyo, Japan

2 Department of Orthopaedic Surgery, Yokohama City University Graduate School of Medicine, Yokohama, Japan

3 Division of Musculoskeletal Oncology, National Cancer Center Hospital, Tokyo, Japan

References

[1] Bacci G, Ferrari S, Longhi A, Perin S, Forni C, Fabbri N, et al. Pattern of relapse in patients with osteosarcoma of the extremities treated with neoadjuvant chemotherapy. Eur J Cancer. 2001;**37**:32–38.

[2] Bacci G, Lari S. Adjuvant and neoadjuvant chemotherapy in osteosarcoma. Chir Organi Mov. 2001;**86**:253–268.

[3] Bielack SS, Kempf-Bielack B, Delling G, Exner GU, Flege S, Helmke K, et al. Prognostic factors in high-grade osteosarcoma of the extremities or trunk: an analysis of 1,702 patients treated on neoadjuvant cooperative osteosarcoma study group protocols. J Clin Oncol. 2002;**20**:776–790.

[4] Lopez-Serra P, Esteller M. DNA methylation-associated silencing of tumor-suppressor microRNAs in cancer. Oncogene. 2012;**31**:1609–1622. Doi: 10.1038/onc.2011.354.

[5] Friedman RC, Farh KK, Burge CB, Bartel DP. Most mammalian mRNAs are conserved targets of microRNAs. Genome Res. 2009;**19**:92–105. Doi: 10.1101/gr.082701.108.

[6] Calin GA, Croce CM. MicroRNA signatures in human cancers. Nat Rev Cancer. 2006;**6**:857–866. Doi: 10.1038/nrc1997.

[7] Iorio MV, Croce CM. MicroRNA dysregulation in cancer: diagnostics, monitoring and therapeutics. A comprehensive review. EMBO Mol Med. 2012;**4**:143–159. Doi: 10.1002/emmm.201100209.

[8] Esquela-Kerscher A, Slack FJ. Oncomirs—microRNAs with a role in cancer. Nat Rev Cancer. 2006;**6**:259–269. Doi: 10.1038/nrc1840.

[9] He C, Xiong J, Xu X, Lu W, Liu L, Xiao D, et al. Functional elucidation of MiR-34 in osteosarcoma cells and primary tumor samples. Biochem Biophys Res Commun. 2009;**388**:35–40. Doi: 10.1016/j.bbrc.2009.07.101.

[10] Kobayashi E, Hornicek FJ, Duan Z. MicroRNA involvement in osteosarcoma. Sarcoma. 2012;**2012**:359739. Doi: 10.1155/2012/359739.

[11] Kushlinskii NE, Fridman MV, Braga EA. Molecular mechanisms and microRNAs in osteosarcoma pathogenesis. Biochemistry (Mosc). 2016;**81**:315–328. Doi: 10.1134/S0006297916040027.

[12] Takahashi RU, Miyazaki H, Ochiya T. The roles of MicroRNAs in breast cancer. Cancers (Basel). 2015;**9**:598–616. Doi: 10.3390/cancers7020598.

[13] Calin GA, Dumitru CD, Shimizu M, Bichi R, Zupo S, Noch E, et al. Frequent deletions and down-regulation of micro-RNA genes miR15 and miR16 at 13q14 in chronic lymphocytic leukemia. Proc Natl Acad Sci U S A. 2002;**99**:15524–15529. Doi: 10.1073/pnas.242606799.

[14] Volinia S, Calin GA, Liu C, Ambs S, Cimmino A, Petrocca F, et al. A microRNA expression signature of human solid tumors defines cancer gene targets. Proc Natl Acad Sci USA. 2006;**103**:2257–2261. Doi: 10.1073/pnas.0510565103.

[15] Yan K, Gao J, Yang T, Ma Q, Qiu X, Fan Q, et al. MicroRNA-34a inhibits the proliferation and metastasis of osteosarcoma cells both in vitro and in vivo. PLoS One. 2012;**7**:e33778. Doi: 10.1371/journal.pone.0033778.

[16] Wu X, Zhong D, Gao Q, Zhai W, Ding Z, Wu J. MicroRNA-34a inhibits human osteosarcoma proliferation by downregulating ether à go-go 1 expression. Int J Med Sci. 2013;**10**:676–682. Doi: 10.7150/ijms.5528.

[17] Tian Y, Zhang YZ, Chen W. MicroRNA-199a-3p and microRNA-34a regulate apoptosis in human osteosarcoma cells. Biosci Rep. 2014;**34**:e00132. Doi: 10.1042/BSR20140084.

[18] Osaki M, Takeshita F, Sugimoto Y, Kosaka N, Yamamoto Y, Yoshioka Y, et al. MicroRNA-143 regulates human osteosarcoma metastasis by regulating matrix metalloprotease-13 expression. Mol Ther. 2011;**19**:1123–1130. Doi: 10.1038/mt.2011.53.

[19] Zhang H, Cai X, Wang Y, Tang H, Tong D, Ji F. microRNA-143, down-regulated in osteosarcoma, promotes apoptosis and suppresses tumorigenicity by targeting Bcl-2. Oncol Rep. 2010;**24**:223–230.

[20] Li W, Wu H, Li Y, Pan H, Meng T, Wang X. MicroRNA-143 promotes apoptosis of osteosarcoma cells by caspase-3 activation via targeting Bcl-2. Biomed Pharmacother. 2016;**80**:8–15. Doi: 10.1016/j.biopha.2016.03.001.

[21] Chen X, Chen XG, Hu X, Song T, Ou X, Zhang C, et al. MiR-34a and miR-203 inhibit surviving expression to control cell proliferation and survival in human osteosarcoma cells. J Cancer. 2016;**7**:1057–1065. Doi: 10.7150/jca.15061.

[22] Zhao H, Ma B, Wang Y, Han T, Zheng L, Sun C, et al. miR-34a inhibits the metastasis of osteosarcoma cells by repressing the expression of CD44. Oncol Rep. 2013;**29**:1027–1036. Doi: 10.3892/or.2013.2234.

[23] Zhou J, Wu S, Chen Y, Zhao J, Zhang K, Wang J, et al. microRNA-143 is associated with the survival of ALDH1+CD133+ osteosarcoma cells and the chemoresistance of osteosarcoma. Exp Biol Med (Maywood). 2015;**240**:867–875. Doi: 10.1177/1535370214563893.

[24] Li F, Li S, Cheng T. TGF-β1 promotes osteosarcoma cell migration and invasion through the miR-143-versican pathway. Cell Physiol Biochem. 2014;**34**:2169–2179. Doi: 10.1159/000369660.

[25] Wang W, Zhou X, Wei M. MicroRNA-144 suppresses osteosarcoma growth and metastasis by targeting ROCK1 and ROCK2. Oncotarget. 2015;**6**:10297–10308. Doi: 10.18632/oncotarget.3305

[26] Huang J, Shi Y, Li H, Yang M, Liu G. MicroRNA-144 acts as a tumor suppressor by targeting Rho-associated coiled-coil containing protein kinase 1 in osteosarcoma cells. Mol Med Rep. 2015;**12**:4554–4559. Doi: 10.3892/mmr.2015.3937.

[27] Cui SQ, Wang H. MicroRNA-144 inhibits the proliferation, apoptosis, invasion, and migration of osteosarcoma cell line F5M2. Tumor Biol. 2015;**36**:6949–6958. Doi: 10.1007/s13277-015-3396-0.

[28] Zhao M, Huang J, Gui K, Xiong M, Cai G, Xu J, et al. The downregulation of miR-144 is associated with the growth and invasion of osteosarcoma cells through the regulation of TAGLN expression. Int J Mol Med. 2014;**34**:1565–1572. Doi: 10.3892/ijmm.2014.1963.

[29] Wu P, Liang J, Yu F, Zhou Z, Tang J, Li K. miR-145 promotes osteosarcoma growth by reducing expression of the transcription factor friend leukemia virus integration 1. Oncotarget. 2016;**7**:42241–42251. Doi: 10.18632/oncotarget.9948.

[30] Li E, Zhang J, Yuan T, Ma B. MiR-145 inhibits osteosarcoma cells proliferation and invasion by targeting ROCK1. Tumor Biol. 2014;**35**:7645–7650. Doi: 10.1007/s13277-014-2031-9.

[31] Lei P, Xie J, Wang L, Yang X, Dai Z, Hu Y. microRNA-145 inhibits osteosarcoma cell proliferation and invasion by targeting ROCK1. Mol Med Rep. 2014;**10**:155–160. Doi: 10.3892/mmr.2014.2195.

[32] Fan L, Wu Q, Xing X, Wei Y, Shao Z. MicroRNA-145 targets vascular endothelial growth factor and inhibits invasion and metastasis of osteosarcoma cells. Acta Biochim Biophys Sin (Singhai). 2012;**44**:407–414. Doi: 10.1093/abbs/gms019.

[33] Li Z, Wu S, Lv S, Wang H, Wang Y, Guo Q. Suppression of liver receptor homolog-1 by microRNA-451 represses the proliferation of osteosarcoma cells. Biochem Biophys Res Commun. 2015;**461**:450–455. Doi: 10.1016/j.bbrc.2015.04.013.

[34] Zhang F, Huang W, Sheng M, Liu T. MiR-451 inhibits cell growth and invasion by targeting CXCL16 and is associated with prognosis of osteosarcoma patients. Tumour Biol. 2015;**36**:2041–2048. Doi: 10.1007/s13277-014-2811-2.

[35] Xu H, Mei Q, Shi L, Lu J, Zhao J, Fu Q. Tumor-suppressing effects of miR451 in human osteosarcoma. Cell Biochem Biophys. 2014;**69**:163–168. Doi: 10.1007/s12013-013-9783-5.

[36] Huang G, Nishimoto K, Zhou Z, Hughes D, Kleinerman ES. miR-20a encoded by the miR-17-92 cluster increases the metastatic potential of osteosarcoma cells by regulating fast expression. Cancer Res. 2012;**72**:908–916. Doi: 10.1158/0008-5472.CAN-11-1460.

[37] Zhuo W, Ge W, Meng G, Jia S, Zhou X, Liu J. MicroRNA-20a promotes the proliferation and cell cycle of human osteosarcoma cells by suppressing early growth response 2 expression. Mol Med Rep. 2015;**12**:4989–4994. Doi: 10.3892/mmr.2015.4098.

[38] Ziyan W, Shuhua Y, Xiufang W, Xiaoyun L. MicroRNA-21 is involved in osteosarcoma cell invasion and migration. Med Oncol. 2011:**28**;1469–1474. Doi: 10.1007/s12032-010-9563-7.

[39] Lv C, Hao Y, Tu G. MicroRNA-21 promotes proliferation, invasion and suppresses apoptosis in human osteosarcoma line MG63 through PTEN/Akt pathway. Tumour Biol. 2016;**37**:9333–9342. Doi: 10.1007/s13277-016-4807-6.

[40] Silva G, Aboussekhra A. p16 ^{INK4A} inhibits the pro-metastatic potentials of osteosarcoma cells through targeting the ERK pathway and TGF-β1. Mol Carcinog. 2016;**55**:525–536. Doi: 10.1002/mc.22299.

[41] Ziyan W, Yang L. MicroRNA-21 regulates the sensitivity to cisplatin in a human osteosarcoma cell line. Ir J Med Sci. 2016;**185:**85–91. Doi: 10.1007/s11845-014-1225-x.

[42] Pei H, Jin Z, Chen S, Sun X, Yu J, Guo W. MiR-135b promotes proliferation and invasion of osteosarcoma cells via targeting FOXO1. Mol Cell Biochem. 2015;**400**:245–252. Doi: 10.1007/s11010-014-2281-2.

[43] Xu WG, Shang YL, Cong XR, Bian X, Yuan Z. MicroRNA-135b promotes proliferation, invasion and migration of osteosarcoma cells by degrading myocardin. Int J Oncol. 2014;**45**:2024–2032. Doi: 10.3892/ijo.2014.2641.

[44] Sun X, Geng X, Zhang J, Zhao H, Liu Y. miR-155 promotes the growth of osteosarcoma in a HBP1-dependent mechanism. Mol Cell Biochem. 2015;**403**:139–147. Doi: 10.1007/s11010-015-2344-z.

[45] Lv H, Guo J, Li S, Jiang D. miR-155 inhibitor reduces the proliferation and migration in osteosarcoma MG-63 cells. Exp Ther Med. 2014;**8**:1575–1580. Doi: 10.3892/etm.2014.1942.

[46] Chen L, Jiang K, Jiang H, Wei P. miR-155 mediates drug resistance in osteosarcoma cells via inducing autophagy. Exp Ther Med. 2014;**8**:527–532. Doi: 10.3892/etm.2014.1752

[47] Liu CJ, Yu KL, Liu GL, Tian DH. MiR-214 promotes osteosarcoma tumor growth and metastasis by decreasing the expression of PTEN. Mol Med Rep. 2015;**12**:6261–6266. Doi: 10.3892/mmr.2015.4197.

[48] Wang X, Sun J, Fu C, Wang D, Bi Z. MicroRNA-214 regulates osteosarcoma survival and growth by directly targeting phosphatase and tensin homolog. Mol Med Rep. 2014;**10**:3073–3079. Doi: 10.3892/mmr.2014.2616.

[49] Xu Z, Wang T. miR-214 promotes the proliferation and invasion of osteosarcoma cells through direct suppression of LZTS1. Biochem Biophys Res Commun. 2014;**449**:190–195. Doi: 10.1016/j.bbrc.2014.04.140.

[50] Tang N, Song WX, Luo J, Haydon RC, He TC. Osteosarcoma development and stem cell differentiation. Clin Orthop Relat Res. 2008;**466**:2114–2130. Doi: 10.1007/s11999-008-0335-z.

[51] Ta HT, Dass CR, Choong PF, Dunstan DE. Osteosarcoma treatment: state of the art. Cancer Metastasis Rev. 2009;**28**:247–263. Doi: 10.1007/s10555-009-9186-7.

[52] Novello C, Pazzaglia L, Conti A, Quattrini I, Pollino S, Perego P, et al. P53-dependent activation of microRNA-34a in response to etoposide-induced DNA damage in osteosarcoma cell lines not impaired by dominant negative p53 expression. PLoS One. 2014;**9**:1–15. Doi: 10.1371/journal.pone.0114757.

[53] Fletcher CDM, Bridge JA, Hogendoorn PCW, Mertens F. WHO Classification of tumours of soft tissue and bone. 2013. Lyon IARC. 2003; pp. 305–10.

[54] Poos K, Smida J, Nathrath M, Maugg D, Baumhoer D, Korsching E. How MicroRNA and transcription factor co-regulatory networks affect osteosarcoma cell proliferation. PLoS Comput Biol. 2013;**9**:e1003210. Doi: 10.1371/journal.pcbi.1003210.

[55] Van Der Deen M, Taipaleenmäki H, Zhang Y, Teplyuk NM, Gupta A, Cinghu S, et al. MicroRNA-34c inversely couples the biological functions of the runt-related transcription factor RUNX2 and the tumor suppressor p53 in osteosarcoma. J Biol Chem. 2013;**288**:21307–21319. Doi: 10.1074/jbc.M112.445890.

[56] Liu B, Ma W, Jha RK, Gurung K. Cancer stem cells in osteosarcoma: Recent progress and perspective. Acta Oncol. 2011;**50**:1142–1150. Doi: 10.3109/0284186X.2011.584553.

[57] Di Fiore R, Drago-Ferrante R, Pentimali F, Di Marzo D, Forte IM, D'anneo A, et al. MicroRNA-29b-1 impairs in vitro cell proliferation, self-renewal and chemoresistance of human osteosarcoma 3AB-OS cancer stem cells. Int J Oncol. 2014;**45**:2013–2023. Doi: 10.3892/ijo.2014.2618.

[58] Xu M, Jin H, Xu CX, Sun B, Song ZG, Bi WZ, et al. miR-382 inhibits osteosarcoma metastasis and relapse by targeting Y box-binding protein 1. Mol Ther. 2015;**23**:89–98. Doi: 10.1038/mt.2014.197.

[59] Zhang Y, Duan G, Feng S. MicroRNA-301a modulates doxorubicin resistance in osteosarcoma cells by targeting AMP-activated protein kinase alpha 1. Biochem Biophys Res Commun. 2015;**459**:367–373. Doi: 10.1016/j.bbrc.2015.02.101.

[60] Chang Z, Huo L, Li K, Wu Y, Hu Z. Blocked autophagy by miR-101 enhances osteosarcoma cell chemosensitivity in vitro. Sci World J. 2014;**2014**:794756. Doi: 10.1155/2014/794756.

[61] Lin BC, Huang D, Yu CQ, Mou Y, Liu YH, Zhang DW, et al. MicroRNA-184 modulates doxorubicin resistance in osteosarcoma cells by targeting BCL2L1. Med Sci Monit. 2016;**22**:1761–1765.

[62] Geng S, Gu L, Ju F, Zhang H, Wang Y, Tang H, et al. MicroRNA-224 promotes the sensitivity of osteosarcoma cells to cisplatin by targeting Rac1. J Cell Mol Med. 2016;**20**:1611–1619. Doi: 10.1111/jcmm.12852.

[63] Zhou Y, Huang Z, Wu S, Zang X, Liu M, Shi J. miR-33a is up-regulated in chemoresistant osteosarcoma and promotes osteosarcoma cell resistance to cisplatin by down-regulating TWIST. J Exp Clin Cancer Res. 2014;**33**:12. Doi: 10.1186/1756-9966-33-12.

[64] Shao X, Miao M, Xue J, Xue J, Ji X, Zhu H. The down-regulation of MicroRNA-497 contributes to cell growth and cisplatin resistance through PI3K/Akt pathway in osteosarcoma. Cell Physiol Biochem. 2015;**36**:2051–2062. Doi: 10.1159/000430172.

[65] Zhu Z, Tang J, Wang J, Duan G, Zhou L, Zhou X. MiR-138 acts as a tumor suppressor by targeting EZH2 and enhances cisplatin-induced apoptosis in osteosarcoma cells. PLoS One. 2016;**11**: e0150026. Doi: 10.1371/journal.pone.0150026.

[66] Jiang L, He A, He X, Tao C. MicroRNA-126 enhances the sensitivity of osteosarcoma cells to cisplatin and methotrexate. Oncol Lett. 2015;**10**:3769–3778.

[67] Song B, Wang Y, Xi Y, Kudo K, Bruheim S, Botchkina GI, et al. Mechanism of chemoresistance mediated by miR-140 in human osteosarcoma and colon cancer cells. Oncogene. 2009;**28**:4065–4074. Doi: 10.1038/onc.2009.274.

[68] Song B, Wang Y, Titmus MA, Botchkina G, Formentini A, Kornmann M, et al. Molecular mechanism of chemoresistance by miR-215 in osteosarcoma and colon cancer cells. Mol Cancer. 2010;**6**:96. Doi: 10.1186/1476-4598-9-96.

[69] Gougelet A, Pissaloux D, Besse A, Perez J, Duc A, Dutour A, et al. Micro-RNA profiles in osteosarcoma as a predictive tool for ifosfamide response. Int J Cancer. 2011;**129**:680–690. Doi: 10.1002/ijc.25715.

[70] Ren HY, Sun LL, Li HY, Ye ZM. Prognostic significance of serum alkaline phosphatase level in osteosarcoma: a meta-analysis of published data. Biomed Res Int. 2015;**2015**:160835. Doi: 10.1155/2015/160835.

[71] Yang Z, Zhang Y, Zhang X, Zhang M, Liu H, Zhang S, et al. Serum microRNA-221 functions as a potential diagnostic and prognostic marker for patients with osteosarcoma. Biomed Pharmacother. 2015;**75**:153–158.

[72] Tang J, Zhao H, Cai H, Wu H. Diagnostic and prognostic potentials of microRNA-27a in osteosarcoma. Biomed Pharmacother. 2015;**71**:222–226. Doi: 10.1016/j.biopha.2015.01.025.

[73] Wang T, Ji F, Dai Z, Xie Y, Yuan D. Increased expression of microRNA-191 as a potential serum biomarker for diagnosis and prognosis in human osteosarcoma. Cancer Biomarkers. 2015;**15**:543–550. Doi: 10.3233/CBM-150493.

[74] Yuan J, Chen L, Chen X, Sun W, Zhou X. Identification of serum microRNA-21 as a biomarker for chemosensitivity and prognosis in human osteosarcoma. J Int Med Res. 2012;**40**:2090–2097.

[75] Ouyang L, Liu P, Yang S, Ye S, Xu W, Liu X. A three-plasma miRNA signature serves as novel biomarkers for osteosarcoma. Med Oncol. 2013;**30**:340. Doi: 10.1007/s12032-012-0340-7.

[76] Zhou G, Lu M, Chen J, Li C, Zhang J, Chen J, et al. Identification of miR-199a-5p in serum as noninvasive biomarkers for detecting and monitoring osteosarcoma. Tumour Biol. 2015;**36**:8845–8852. Doi: 10.1007/s13277-015-3421-3.

[77] Lian F, Cui Y, Zhou C, Gao K, Wu L. Identification of a plasma four-microRNA panel as potential noninvasive biomarker for osteosarcoma. PLoS One. 2015;**10**: e0121499. Doi: 10.1371/journal.pone.0121499.

[78] Zhang C, Yao C, Li H, Wang G, He X. Combined elevation of microRNA-196a and microRNA-196b in sera predicts unfavorable prognosis in patients with osteosarcomas. Int J Mol Sci. 2014;**15**:6544–6555. Doi: 10.3390/ijms15046544.

[79] Dong J, Liu Y, Liao W, Liu R, Shi P, Wang L. miRNA-223 is a potential diagnostic and prognostic marker for osteosarcoma. J Bone Oncol. 2016;**5**:74–79. Doi: 10.1016/j.jbo.2016.05.001.

[80] Cai H, Zhao H, Tang J, Wu H. Serum miR-195 is a diagnostic and prognostic marker for osteosarcoma. J Surg Res. 2015;**194**:505–510. Doi: 10.1016/j.jss.2014.11.025.

[81] Tian Q, Jia J, Ling S, Liu Y, Yang S, Shao Z. A causal role for circulating miR-34b in osteosarcoma. Eur J Surg Oncol. 2014;**40**:67–72. Doi: 10.1016/j.ejso.2013.08.024.

[82] Zhang C, Yao C, Li H, Wang G, He X. Serum levels of microRNA-133b and microRNA-206 expression predict prognosis in patients with osteosarcoma. Int J Clin Exp Pathol. 2014;**7**:4194–4203.

[83] Fei D, Li Y, Zhao D, Zhao K, Dai L, Gao Z. Serum miR-9 as a prognostic biomarker in patients with osteosarcoma. J Int Med Res. 2014;**42**:932–937. Doi: 10.1177/0300060514534643.

[84] Li H, Zhang K, Liu LH, Ouyang Y, Guo HB, Zhang H, et al. MicroRNA screening identifies circulating microRNAs as potential biomarkers for osteosarcoma. Oncol Lett. 2015;**10**:1662–1668. Doi: 10.3892/ol.2015.3378.

Chapter 10

OMICS Approach for Identifying Predictive Biomarkers in Osteosarcoma

Tadashi Kondo

Additional information is available at the end of the chapter

http://dx.doi.org/10.5772/67449

Abstract

Osteosarcoma has a complex genetic background, and the response to treatments varies among patients. Induction chemotherapy has substantially improved the clinical outcome of osteosarcoma. Currently, there is no practical predictive modality in clinical settings, and therefore, uniform chemotherapy is applied for all patients. However, since the response to induction chemotherapy considerably influences the prognosis, the therapeutic strategy should be optimized for each patient before initiating treatments. Therefore, identification and establishment of predictive biomarkers for induction chemotherapy have been a long-standing goal in osteosarcoma research. Because of the complex genetic traits associated with osteosarcoma, adoption of an omics approach for global gene expression is attractive in the search for predictive biomarkers, and omics technologies have recently been applied to the development of predictive biomarkers in malignancies, including osteosarcoma. Global studies have been performed at the genome, transcriptome, and proteome levels in osteosarcoma, and various candidate biomarkers have been reported using clinical specimens. Further investigation of the clinical utilities of these identified predictive biomarkers will be merited through validation and verification studies.

Keywords: osteosarcoma, biomarker, chemotherapy, omics, genome, transcriptome, proteome

1. Introduction

Osteosarcoma is a rare mesenchymal malignancy, accounting for less than 1% of all adult cancers [1]. In contrast, osteosarcoma represents the most frequent type of malignant tumor in children and adolescents, and its incidence has increased over time in younger cases [1, 2]. Mesenchymal malignancies are classified according to the unique molecular background:

those characterized by unique transfusion genes and simple karyotypes, and those without unique genetic characters but complex genetic backgrounds [3]. Osteosarcoma is a typical example of the latter case and is associated with highly complex karyotypes and frequent chromosomal copy number changes [4–11]. The advent of chemotherapy has improved the clinical outcome of patients with nonmetastatic osteosarcoma [12–16]. However, despite the considerable progress in cancer research, no novel therapeutic strategies for osteosarcomas have been established since the 1980s, and the cure rate of osteosarcoma patients has thus reached a plateau [15]. Effective molecular targeting drugs that may inhibit specific molecular aberrations common in certain cancer types are not currently available for osteosarcoma, which is likely attributed to the complex molecular backgrounds. Consequently, uniform induction chemotherapy is performed for all patients with osteosarcoma.

The identification of predictive biomarkers has been a long-standing goal in osteosarcoma research. The response to induction chemotherapy is evaluated by histopathological examination of tumor necrosis. When a tumor responds to the induction chemotherapy, a better prognosis can be expected [17–19]. Studies of the molecular events contributing to the different responses to induction chemotherapy have been undertaken using clinical samples. As osteosarcoma is not associated with typical genetic alterations, a global approach to investigating the molecular backgrounds may be the most promising strategy. With the advent of modern technologies, omics approaches have become increasingly popular in translational research and are starting to be applied in the studies of predictive biomarkers in various types of cancers, including osteosarcoma.

In this article, we review the researches on potential biomarkers for osteosarcoma with the intention to establish predictive biomarkers for induction chemotherapy. Providing an overview of the current status of knowledge on these predictive biomarkers will offer a perspective for further development of osteosarcoma treatments as well as new ideas of what is needed to achieve a better clinical outcome for osteosarcoma patients.

2. Omics studies for predictive biomarkers in osteosarcoma

2.1. Genomic studies

Predictive biomarkers based on genomic knowledge have proven to be clinically beneficial for various types of malignancies. Schwaederle et al. reported the results of a meta-analysis of 570 Phase II studies, including 32,000 patients with various types of malignancies [20]. They reported that the use of predictive genomic biomarkers resulted in a higher treatment response rate and prolonged progression-free survival as well as overall survival. These results should motivate and facilitate the development and use of predictive genomic biomarkers in osteosarcoma.

Smida et al. reported the DNA copy number alterations and allelic imbalances associated with the response to induction chemotherapy using single nucleotide polymorphism (SNP) arrays [21]. They investigated the biopsy samples from 44 patients with osteosarcoma who have a record of the subsequent response to chemotherapy. They reported that patients with a significantly higher frequency of loss of heterozygosity (LOH) often had a poor response to chemotherapy compared to patients with a lower LOH frequency. They also showed that specific chromosomal regions in chromosomes 10 and 11 were associated with the poor response to chemotherapy. Further investigations of these molecules will likely lead to the establishment of novel predictive modalities in osteosarcomas.

Hagleitner et al. investigated 384 SNPs among 54 selected genes in 177 osteosarcoma patients, with the aim of identifying genetic variants associated with survival. The 54 genes included representative candidate genes involved in the cisplatin and doxorubicin pathway, according to the literature and Pharmacogenomics Knowledge Base (https://www.pharmgkb.org/). In addition to SNPs associated with progression-free survival, they found 14 SNPs that were significantly associated with the poor response to chemotherapy [22]. The clinical utility of these 14 SNPs has not yet been evaluated, and thus, further investigation is needed for validation.

2.2. Transcriptomic studies

Technologies for comprehensive analyses of mRNA and microRNA expression became available more than a decade ago and have since been widely used for biomarker development in various malignancies [23–28].

Ochi et al. examined the mRNA expression profiles of biopsied tumor tissues from osteosarcoma patients using a cDNA microarray consisting of 23,040 genes [29]. They compared six responders and seven nonresponders to induction chemotherapy and identified 60 genes whose expression patterns were associated with favorable or poor response to neoadjuvant chemotherapy. Man et al. identified a novel molecular signature of chemoresistance by comparing the profiles of 7 responders and 13 nonresponders using surgically resected tissues after chemotherapy [30]. They hypothesized that the surgically resected tumor tissues of nonresponders were enriched for resistant cells. The identified tissues consisted of 45 unique genes, and their predictive performance was confirmed in 14 biopsied tumor tissues obtained before chemotherapy. Moreover, the expression levels measured by cDNA microarray were confirmed for seven genes using quantitative reverse transcription-polymerase chain reaction (RT-PCR).

Although these three studies had the common goal of identifying predictive biomarkers and used biopsy tumor tissues of osteosarcoma patients, the genes involved in the chemoresistance signatures were quite different. This difference may be attributed to the different age distributions, small sample sizes, different chemotherapy regimens, and different methods used for expression analysis among the studies. Therefore, to establish the clinical utilities of the candidate predictive biomarkers, extensive validation studies as well as functional studies of the identified genes will be required.

Kubota et al. examined the microRNA expression profiles of open-biopsied tumor tissues from osteosarcoma patients using a microarray [31]. They compared four responders and four nonresponders to induction chemotherapy and identified six microRNAs whose expression patterns were associated with favorable or poor response to neoadjuvant chemotherapy. They confirmed the significant association of miR-125b and miR-100 with poor response to chemotherapy by RT-PCR. The association between poor prognosis and the abundance of miR-125b and miR-100 was confirmed in 20 additional osteosarcoma patients. Overexpression of these microRNAs in three osteosarcoma cell lines resulted in the enhanced cell proliferation, invasiveness, and resistance to chemotherapeutic drugs. As the area under the receiver operating curve for these microRNAs were approximately 0.9 ($p < 0.01$), their clinical application is worth challenging. Kubota et al. reported mRNAs whose expression was commonly affected by the transfection of miR-125b and miR-100 in osteosarcomas [31]. Those included sirtuin (silent mating type information regulation 2 homolog 5, SIRT5), which was previously associated with the resistance against therapeutic reagents in nonsmall cell lung cancer [32]. Thus, the expression profiles of miRNAs may be linked to those of mRNAs and provide a clue to understand the multilayer omics data in osteosarcomas.

2.3. Proteomics studies

Proteomics is another promising approach to biomarker discovery because the proteome is the functional translation of the genome, directly regulating the phenotypes of tumors. The modalities of proteomics have been considerably developed and applied to several cancer biomarker studies. Proteomics provides unique data that cannot be obtained with other technologies. This level of analysis is important, given the frequent reports of the discordance between protein and mRNA expression in global expression studies. In particular, proteomics is the only omics modality that can identify the protein status and characteristics such as post-translational modifications, intra- and extracellular localization, complex formation, activity, and degradation. Therefore, adoption of a proteomics approach shows good promise for biomarker development in osteosarcoma.

Arai et al. reported the proteins corresponding to the response to chemotherapy reagents in 11 osteosarcoma cell lines using two-dimensional differential gel electrophoresis (2D-DIGE) [33]. They found a differential response to the drugs between monolayer and spheroid cultured cells. Among the 4762 protein species observed, they reported the upregulation of cathepsin D in spheroid cells that showed resistance to a chemotherapy reagent. Cathepsin D has been implicated in chemoresistance, and its clinical utilities were suggested in various malignancies [33]. Saini et al. also compared monolayer and spheroid culture cells using proteomic, transcriptomic, and immunophenotyping approaches and identified CBX3 and ABCA5 as possible biomarkers for tumor stem cells that showed heterogeneous response to anti-cancer drugs [34]. Moreover, they reported that spheres and monolayers showed different responses to the approved cancer drugs. The applications of spheroidal cells may offer a great opportunity to evaluate the drug effects in preclinical studies, and adoption of an omics approach will be a powerful tool to further develop the biomarkers to predict the response to treatments.

Li et al. reported plasma proteins that may have good predictive performance for osteosarcoma patients [35]. They investigated the proteome of plasma collected from 54 osteosarcoma patients comparing before ($n = 27$) and after ($n = 27$) induction chemotherapy. They developed two classifiers for responsiveness and revealed that both showed 85% accuracy for prediction of response. They also examined the biological backgrounds of serum amyloid protein A and transthyretin, which were included in the classifiers. An extensive list of plasma proteins in osteosarcoma patients was established using a proteomics approach [36], which should serve as a useful dataset for the plasma proteomics of osteosarcoma.

To characterize the proteome backgrounds associated with resistance to induction chemotherapy, Kikuta et al. examined the differential protein expression between patients who showed a favorable response to induction chemotherapy and those who did not [37]. Among the several thousand protein species observed by 2D-DIGE, they focused on peroxiredoxin 2 (PRDX2), an enzyme that catalyzes the free radicals produced by catalase and protects cells from oxidative stress. The patients with primary tumor tissues showing high PRDX2 expression ultimately developed resistance to induction chemotherapy, and vice versa. The results were validated in additional cases of osteosarcoma using the specific antibody for PRDX2. Kikuta et al. examined osteosarcoma patients who received combination therapy with isofomide, cisplatin, and doxorubicin, and in a subsequent study, Kubota et al. used 2D-DIGE to examine the protein expression in the osteosarcoma patients who received different versions of induction chemotherapy: methotorexate, cisplatin, or doxorubicin [38]. Both studies concordantly identified the high expression of PRDX2 in the nonresponders. The functional significance of the high expression of PRDX2 was also investigated in an in vitro experiment; the gene silencing of endogenous PRDX increased the sensitivity of cells to chemotherapy reagents. These results were reproduced using additional osteosarcoma cases receiving the same induction chemotherapy.

3. Future treatments for osteosarcoma patients with poor chemo-response potential

One of the most critical questions in the study of predictive biomarkers is what options to offer patients who are predicted to show an unfavorable response to induction chemotherapy. Due to the lack of predictive biomarkers for chemotherapy response in osteosarcoma, there has been no clinical trial conducted to identify patients with poor response. However, many lines of evidence suggest several possible therapeutic strategies for osteosarcoma patients. Meyers et al. reported that the addition of muramyl tripeptide to chemotherapy improved the overall survival of osteosarcoma patients [39]. Lewis et al. reported the possible application of interleukin-11 receptor alpha as a functional target in osteosarcoma [40]. In addition, there are also several possible immunotherapies for osteosarcoma. Cripe et al. reported the possible application of treatment with a vaccinia virus, pexastimogene devacirepvec, through viral lysis and induction of granulocyte macrophage colony-stimulating factor-driven tumor-specific immunity in osteosarcoma [41]. Tsukahara et al. demonstrated the possibility of peptide therapy in osteosarcoma [42]. Lussier et al. reported that combination immunotherapy with alpha-CTLA-4 and alpha-PD-L1 antibody might be effective for treating metastatic osteosarcoma [43]. Moreover, therapy using a genetically modified T cell line has been under evaluation for osteosarcoma patients [44]. Because these therapeutic approaches may have different modes of action compared with the conventional chemotherapeutic reagents, combinatory treatment of these novel drugs and conventional chemo-agents will promise new therapeutic strategy against osteosarcoma. Clinical trials of the novel treatment strategies are strongly desired to establish predictive biomarkers especially for the patients with potential of resistance to conventional chemotherapy.

4. Perspective of predictive biomarker identification with an omics approach

The advent of omics technology has made it feasible to observe tens of thousands of genes and proteins simultaneously with relative ease. Technologies for omics studies are continuously been developed, with expected improvements in terms of accuracy, comprehensiveness, and cost-effectiveness, which can be applied to osteosarcoma research. Next-generation sequencing (NGS) technologies have made it possible to produce even more detailed omics data. For example, NGS-based methods can be used to obtain the expression data of individual splice variants of mRNAs, which are not possible using conventional DNA microarray systems. Therefore, refined data of mRNA expression can be obtained by applying the novel technologies to previously examined sample sets. Moreover, proteomics was traditionally used to examine only protein expression levels, which do not necessary correlate with protein activity. The recent advent of high-throughput technology allows for the measurement of the actual activities of various specific kinases as well as nuclear receptors across hundreds of samples in only a few hours. All these omics technologies will be useful for advancing the study of predictive biomarkers in osteosarcoma.

One of the major current limitations of current studies for predictive biomarkers in osteosarcoma would be the small number and amount of clinical materials available. Considering the low prevalence of osteosarcoma, it is going to be very difficult to achieve the sufficient sample collection by single institutes and individual efforts alone. Therefore, nation-wide and/or international collaboration studies will be required.

The perspective provided herein on searching for predictive biomarkers in osteosarcoma, a rare malignancy with complex genetic traits, could be applicable to other major malignancies like lung cancers. Indeed, a recent NGS-based analysis revealed that the majority of lung cancers can be grouped into various minor subtypes according to the clinically important genetic aberrations. We believe that innovations developed in rare malignancies like osteosarcoma will not only benefit the patients with those diseases but also make a great impact on the researches for majority of malignancies.

Acknowledgements

This research was supported by the Practical Research for Innovative Cancer Control Program (15ck0106089h0002) from the Japan Agency for Medical Research and Development (AMED), and the National Cancer Center Research Core Facility and National Cancer Center Research and Development Fund (26-A-9).

Conflict of interest

The authors declare that they have no conflicts of interest.

http://dx.doi.org/10.5772/67449

Author details

Tadashi Kondo

Address all correspondence to: takondo@ncc.go.jp

Division of Rare Cancer Research, National Cancer Center Research Institute, Tokyo, Japan

References

[1] Mirabello, L., Troisi, R. J. & Savage, S. A. (2009) Osteosarcoma incidence and survival rates from 1973 to 2004: data from the Surveillance, Epidemiology, and End Results Program, *Cancer*. **115**, 1531–43.

[2] Savage, S. A., Mirabello, L. Using epidemiology and genomics to understand osteosarcoma etiology. *Sarcoma*. 2011:**2011**:548151. PubMed PMID: 21437228; PubMed Central PMCID: PMC3061299. doi:10.1155/2011/548151

[3] Taylor, B. S., Barretina, J., Maki, R. G., Antonescu, C. R., Singer, S. & Ladanyi, M. (2011) Advances in sarcoma genomics and new therapeutic targets, *Nat Rev Cancer*. **11**, 541–57.

[4] Bridge, J. A., Nelson, M., McComb, E., McGuire, M. H., Rosenthal, H., Vergara, G., Maale, G. E., Spanier, S. & Neff, J. R. (1997) Cytogenetic findings in 73 osteosarcoma specimens and a review of the literature, *Cancer Genet Cytogenet*. **95**, 74–87.

[5] Boehm, A. K., Neff, J. R., Squire, J. A., Bayani, J., Nelson, M., Bridge, J. A. Cytogenetic Findings in 36 Osteosarcoma Specimens and a Review of the Literature. Pediatric Pathology & Molecular Medicine. 2000 Issue 5;**19**, 359–376.

[6] Zielenska, M., Bayani, J., Pandita, A., Toledo, S., Marrano, P., Andrade, J., Petrilli, A., Thorner, P., Sorensen, P. & Squire, J. A. (2001) Comparative genomic hybridization analysis identifies gains of 1p35 approximately p36 and chromosome 19 in osteosarcoma, *Cancer Genet Cytogenet*. **130**, 14–21.

[7] Ozaki, T., Schaefer, K. L., Wai, D., Buerger, H., Flege, S., Lindner, N., Kevric, M., Diallo, R., Bankfalvi, A., Brinkschmidt, C., Juergens, H., Winkelmann, W., Dockhorn-Dworniczak, B., Bielack, S. S. & Poremba, C. (2002) Genetic imbalances revealed by comparative genomic hybridization in osteosarcomas, *Int J Cancer*. **102**, 355–65.

[8] Bayani, J., Zielenska, M., Pandita, A., Al-Romaih, K., Karaskova, J., Harrison, K., Bridge, J. A., Sorensen, P., Thorner, P. & Squire, J. A. (2003) Spectral karyotyping identifies recurrent complex rearrangements of chromosomes 8, 17, and 20 in osteosarcomas, *Genes Chromosomes Cancer*. **36**, 7–16.

[9] Al-Romaih, K., Bayani, J., Vorobyova, J., Karaskova, J., Park, P. C., Zielenska, M. & Squire, J. A. (2003) Chromosomal instability in osteosarcoma and its association with centrosome abnormalities, *Cancer Genet Cytogenet*. **144**, 91–9.

[10] Squire, J. A., Pei, J., Marrano, P., Beheshti, B., Bayani, J., Lim, G., Moldovan, L. & Zielenska, M. (2003) High-resolution mapping of amplifications and deletions in pediatric osteosarcoma by use of CGH analysis of cDNA microarrays, *Genes Chromosomes Cancer.* **38**, 215–25.

[11] Man, T. K., Lu, X. Y., Jaeweon, K., Perlaky, L., Harris, C. P., Shah, S., Ladanyi, M., Gorlick, R., Lau, C. C. & Rao, P. H. (2004) Genome-wide array comparative genomic hybridization analysis reveals distinct amplifications in osteosarcoma, *BMC Cancer.* **4**, 45.

[12] Carter, S. K. (1980) The dilemma of adjuvant chemotherapy for osteogenic sarcoma, *Cancer Clin Trials.* **3**, 29–36.

[13] Provisor, A. J., Ettinger, L. J., Nachman, J. B., Krailo, M. D., Makley, J. T., Yunis, E. J., Huvos, A. G., Betcher, D. L., Baum, E. S., Kisker, C. T. & Miser, J. S. (1997) Treatment of nonmetastatic osteosarcoma of the extremity with preoperative and postoperative chemotherapy: a report from the Children's Cancer Group, *J Clin Oncol.* **15**, 76–84.

[14] Bielack, S. S., Kempf-Bielack, B., Delling, G., Exner, G. U., Flege, S., Helmke, K., Kotz, R., Salzer-Kuntschik, M., Werner, M., Winkelmann, W., Zoubek, A., Jurgens, H. & Winkler, K. (2002) Prognostic factors in high-grade osteosarcoma of the extremities or trunk: an analysis of 1,702 patients treated on neoadjuvant cooperative osteosarcoma study group protocols, *J Clin Oncol.* **20**, 776–90.

[15] Hagleitner, M. M., de Bont, E. S. & te Loo, D. M. (2012) Survival trends and long-term toxicity in pediatric patients with osteosarcoma, *Sarcoma.* **2012**, 636405.

[16] Whelan, J. S., Jinks, R. C., McTiernan, A., Sydes, M. R., Hook, J. M., Trani, L., Uscinska, B., Bramwell, V., Lewis, I. J., Nooij, M. A., van Glabbeke, M., Grimer, R. J., Hogendoorn, P. C., Taminiau, A. H. & Gelderblom, H. (2012) Survival from high-grade localised extremity osteosarcoma: combined results and prognostic factors from three European Osteosarcoma Intergroup randomised controlled trials, *Ann Oncol.* **23**, 1607–16.

[17] Rosen, G., Caparros, B., Groshen, S., Nirenberg, A., Cacavio, A., Marcove, R. C., Lane, J. M. & Huvos, A. G. (1984) Primary osteogenic sarcoma of the femur: a model for the use of preoperative chemotherapy in high risk malignant tumors, *Cancer Invest.* **2**, 181–92.

[18] Bacci, G., Avella, M., Brach Del Prevert, A., Capanna, R., Fiorentini, G., Malaguti, C., Picci, P., Rosito, P. & Campanacci, M. (1988) Neoadjuvant chemotherapy for osteosarcoma of the extremities. Good response of the primary tumor after preoperative chemotherapy with high-dose methotrexate followed by cisplatinum and adriamycin. Preliminary results, *Chemioterapia.* **7**, 138–42.

[19] Winkler, K., Beron, G., Delling, G., Heise, U., Kabisch, H., Purfürst, C., Berger, J., Ritter, J., Jurgens, H., Gerein, V. & et al. (1988) Neoadjuvant chemotherapy of osteosarcoma: results of a randomized cooperative trial (COSS-82) with salvage chemotherapy based on histological tumor response, *J Clin Oncol.* **6**, 329–37.

[20] Schwaederle, M., Zhao, M., Lee, J. J., Eggermont, A. M., Schilsky, R. L., Mendelsohn, J., Lazar, V. & Kurzrock, R. (2015) Impact of precision medicine in diverse cancers: a meta-analysis of phase II clinical trials, *J Clin Oncol.* **33**, 3817–25.

[21] Smida, J., Baumhoer, D., Rosemann, M., Walch, A., Bielack, S., Poremba, C., Remberger, K., Korsching, E., Scheurlen, W., Dierkes, C., Burdach, S., Jundt, G., Atkinson, M. J. & Nathrath, M. (2010) Genomic alterations and allelic imbalances are strong prognostic predictors in osteosarcoma, *Clin Cancer Res.* **16**, 4256–67.

[22] Hagleitner, M. M., Coenen, M. J., Gelderblom, H., Makkinje, R. R., Vos, H. I., de Bont, E. S., van der Graaf, W. T., Schreuder, H. W., Flucke, U., van Leeuwen, F. N., Hoogerbrugge, P. M., Guchelaar, H. J. & te Loo, D. M. (2015) A first step toward personalized medicine in osteosarcoma: pharmacogenetics as predictive marker of outcome after chemotherapy-based treatment, *Clin Cancer Res.* **21**, 3436–41.

[23] Masica, D. L. & Karchin, R. (2013) Collections of simultaneously altered genes as biomarkers of cancer cell drug response, *Cancer Res.* **73**, 1699–708.

[24] Puyo, S., Houede, N., Kauffmann, A., Richaud, P., Robert, J. & Pourquier, P. (2012) Gene expression signature predicting high-grade prostate cancer responses to oxaliplatin, *Mol Pharmacol.* **82**, 1205–16.

[25] Kim, M. K., Osada, T., Barry, W. T., Yang, X. Y., Freedman, J. A., Tsamis, K. A., Datto, M., Clary, B. M., Clay, T., Morse, M. A., Febbo, P. G., Lyerly, H. K. & Hsu, D. S. (2012) Characterization of an oxaliplatin sensitivity predictor in a preclinical murine model of colorectal cancer, *Mol Cancer Ther.* **11**, 1500–9.

[26] Dao, P., Wang, K., Collins, C., Ester, M., Lapuk, A. & Sahinalp, S. C. (2011) Optimally discriminative subnetwork markers predict response to chemotherapy, *Bioinformatics.* **27**, i205–13.

[27] Nagji, A. S., Cho, S. H., Liu, Y., Lee, J. K. & Jones, D. R. (2010) Multigene expression-based predictors for sensitivity to Vorinostat and Velcade in non-small cell lung cancer, *Mol Cancer Ther.* **9**, 2834–43.

[28] Dry, J. R., Pavey, S., Pratilas, C. A., Harbron, C., Runswick, S., Hodgson, D., Chresta, C., McCormack, R., Byrne, N., Cockerill, M., Graham, A., Beran, G., Cassidy, A., Haggerty, C., Brown, H., Ellison, G., Dering, J., Taylor, B. S., Stark, M., Bonazzi, V., Ravishankar, S., Packer, L., Xing, F., Solit, D. B., Finn, R. S., Rosen, N., Hayward, N. K., French, T. & Smith, P. D. (2010) Transcriptional pathway signatures predict MEK addiction and response to selumetinib (AZD6244), *Cancer Res.* **70**, 2264–73.

[29] Ochi, K., Daigo, Y., Katagiri, T., Nagayama, S., Tsunoda, T., Myoui, A., Naka, N., Araki, N., Kudawara, I., Ieguchi, M., Toyama, Y., Toguchida, J., Yoshikawa, H. & Nakamura, Y. (2004) Prediction of response to neoadjuvant chemotherapy for osteosarcoma by gene-expression profiles, *Int J Oncol.* **24**, 647–55.

[30] Man, T. K., Chintagumpala, M., Visvanathan, J., Shen, J., Perlaky, L., Hicks, J., Johnson, M., Davino, N., Murray, J., Helman,L., Meyer, W., Triche, T., Wong, K. K. & Lau, C. C. (2005) Expression profiles of osteosarcoma that can predict response to chemotherapy, *Cancer Res.* **65**, 8142–50.

[31] Kubota D, Kosaka N, Fujiwara T, Yoshida A, Arai Y, Qiao Z, Takeshita F, Ochiya T, Kawai A, Kondo T. miR-125b and miR-100 Are Predictive Biomarkers of Response to Induction Chemotherapy in Osteosarcoma. Sarcoma. 2016;2016:1390571. PubMed PMID: 27990096; PubMed Central PMCID: PMC5136640.

[32] Lu, W., Zuo, Y., Feng, Y. & Zhang, M. (2014) SIRT5 facilitates cancer cell growth and drug resistance in non-small cell lung cancer, *Tumour Biol.* **35**, 10699–705.

[33] Arai, K., Sakamoto, R., Kubota, D. & Kondo, T. (2013) Proteomic approach toward molecular backgrounds of drug resistance of osteosarcoma cells in spheroid culture system, *Proteomics.* **13**, 2351–60.

[34] Saini, V., Hose, C. D., Monks, A., Nagashima, K., Han, B., Newton, D. L., Millione, A., Shah, J., Hollingshead, M. G., Hite, K. M., Burkett, M. W., Delosh, R. M., Silvers, T. E., Scudiero, D. A. & Shoemaker, R. H. (2012) Identification of CBX3 and ABCA5 as putative biomarkers for tumor stem cells in osteosarcoma, *PLoS One.* **7**, e41401.

[35] Li, Y., Dang, T. A., Shen, J., Hicks, J., Chintagumpala, M., Lau, C. C. & Man, T. K. (2011) Plasma proteome predicts chemotherapy response in osteosarcoma patients, *Oncol Rep.* **25**, 303–14.

[36] Li, Y., Dang, T. A. & Man, T. K. (2012) Plasma proteomic profiling of pediatric osteosarcoma, *Methods Mol Biol.* **818**, 81–96.

[37] Kikuta, K., Tochigi, N., Saito, S., Shimoda, T., Morioka, H., Toyama, Y., Hosono, A., Suehara, Y., Beppu, Y., Kawai, A., Hirohashi, S. & Kondo, T. (2010) Peroxiredoxin 2 as a chemotherapy responsiveness biomarker candidate in osteosarcoma revealed by proteomics, *Proteomics Clin Appl.* **4**, 560–7.

[38] Kubota, D., Mukaihara, K., Yoshida, A., Tsuda, H., Kawai, A. & Kondo, T. (2013) Proteomics study of open biopsy samples identifies peroxiredoxin 2 as a predictive biomarker of response to induction chemotherapy in osteosarcoma, *J Proteomics.* **91**, 393–404.

[39] Meyers, P. A., Schwartz, C. L., Krailo, M. D., Healey, J. H., Bernstein, M. L., Betcher, D., Ferguson, W. S., Gebhardt, M. C., Goorin, A. M., Harris, M., Kleinerman, E., Link, M. P., Nadel, H., Nieder, M., Siegal, G. P., Weiner, M. A., Wells, R. J., Womer, R. B., Grier, H. E. & Children's Oncology, G. (2008) Osteosarcoma: the addition of muramyl tripeptide to chemotherapy improves overall survival—a report from the Children's Oncology Group, *J Clin Oncol.* **26**, 633–8.

[40] Lewis, V. O., Ozawa, M. G., Deavers, M. T., Wang, G., Shintani, T., Arap, W. & Pasqualini, R. (2009) The interleukin-11 receptor alpha as a candidate ligand-directed target in osteosarcoma: consistent data from cell lines, orthotopic models, and human tumor samples, *Cancer Res.* **69**, 1995–9.

[41] Cripe, T. P., Ngo, M. C., Geller, J. I., Louis, C. U., Currier, M. A., Racadio, J. M., Towbin, A. J., Rooney, C. M., Pelusio, A., Moon, A., Hwang, T. H., Burke, J. M., Bell, J. C., Kirn, D. H. & Breitbach, C. J. (2015) Phase 1 study of intratumoral Pexa-Vec (JX-594), an oncolytic and immunotherapeutic vaccinia virus, in pediatric cancer patients, *Mol Ther.* **23**, 602–8.

[42] Tsukahara, T., Emori, M., Murata, K., Hirano, T., Muroi, N., Kyono, M., Toji, S., Watanabe, K., Torigoe, T., Kochin, V., Asanuma, H., Matsumiya, H., Yamashita, K., Himi, T., Ichimiya, S., Wada, T., Yamashita, T., Hasegawa, T. & Sato, N. (2014) Specific targeting of a naturally presented osteosarcoma antigen, papillomavirus binding factor peptide, using an artificial monoclonal antibody, *J Biol Chem.* **289**, 22035–47.

[43] Lussier, D. M., Johnson, J. L., Hingorani, P. & Blattman, J. N. (2015) Combination immunotherapy with alpha-CTLA-4 and alpha-PD-L1 antibody blockade prevents immune escape and leads to complete control of metastatic osteosarcoma, *J Immunother Cancer.* **3**, 21.

[44] DeRenzo, C. & Gottschalk, S. (2014) Genetically modified T-cell therapy for osteosarcoma, *Adv Exp Med Biol.* **804**, 323–40.

Section 4

Clinical Sciences

Chapter 11

Biological Reconstruction Using Liquid Nitrogen-Treated Tumor Bearing Bone

Norio Yamamoto and Hiroyuki Tsuchiya

Additional information is available at the end of the chapter

http://dx.doi.org/10.5772/67487

Abstract

In general, a tumor prosthesis is used for reconstruction after removal of osteosarcoma. However, the durability of artificial materials becomes a problem in the long term, and many patients inevitably undergo revision due to loose or damaged prostheses. Moreover, preservation of articular surface is the key to maintain better limb function for long duration. Reconstruction of affected limbs using biological materials has been sought to overcome the aforementioned problems. In some countries, it is significantly difficult to obtain allograft as a biological reconstruction material because of socio-religious or cost problem. Thus, a biological reconstruction method has been developed in which the patient's affected bone is treated and used for reconstruction. Especially in recycling treatment for affected autologous bone, liquid nitrogen treatment has several favorable characteristics. There is optimal morphological fit because the treated bone itself is one's own, and bone strength is maintained after treatment. Satisfactory bone union and bone regeneration are expected to be achieved due to good osteoconduction and osteoinduction because proteins and enzymes are preserved in the bone.

Keywords: osteosarcoma, biological reconstruction, liquid nitrogen, frozen autograft, joint preservation

1. Background

Osteosarcoma is the most common primary malignant bone tumor, but the reported incidence is very rare about 1 in 200,000 compared to other malignant neoplasms such as breast and lung cancer [1]. Because it has a predilection for children in the second decade of life, in order to ensure a prognosis that preserves life and limb function as well, treatment must be carried out with the utmost care. Limb-sparing surgery has become the standard surgical treatment for malignant bone tumors including osteosarcoma in recent years, and mega-prosthesis replacement is generally used in reconstruction for limb salvage. Using mega-prosthesis for bone tumors usually results in good limb function in short term but various complications due to deterioration of non-biological materials in longer term. Total joint replacement for osteoarthritis of knee joint showed good functional results for instance, and several designs for total joint replacement have been applied for more rigorous position and alignment in recent years to obtain better functions in contrast to hinge or rotating hinge-type prosthesis. Limitation of the mega-prosthesis for reconstruction of bone tumor resection is much larger than such surface replacement regarding alignment and torsion force. Thus, activities of daily life would be much more restricted, and various problems may occur especially in younger patients with osteosarcoma after mega-prosthetic replacement.

To overcome these problems, so-called biological reconstructions using allogenic bone graft, vascularized or non-vascularized autologous bone graft, autologous bone extension, and sterilized processing autologous bone grafts have been utilized, and those reconstruction methods were more desired than mega-prosthesis in some regions in the world due to sociological and economic reasons. Sterilized autologous bone grafts have been developed by killing cancer cells using irradiation, autoclaving, or pasteurization onto patient's own diseased bone. Each processing methods for sterilization of diseased bone has the problem such as special equipment for irradiation and autoclaving, temperature control for pasteurization and those are sometimes complicated. One of the biggest problems is the quality of processed bone after autoclaving, irradiation, and pasteurization. Therefore, we developed the processing method by freezing using liquid nitrogen (LN2) and confirmed the feasibility of LN2-freezed bone in terms of safety and quality issues [2, 3]. We applied this freezing method to reconstructive surgery for bone tumor including osteosarcoma and obtained the satisfied results up to date [4, 5]. In addition, histological examination revealed good regenerative activity of LN2-processed bone [6–8].

2. Characteristics of liquid nitrogen–treated bone

The characteristics of LN2-treated bone show several advantages compared to other processed methods. That includes simple procedure without any specific equipment and complicated temperature control; strength of treated bone and superior osteo-conductive and osteo-inductive capacity with spared matrix proteins and enzymes; best compatibility of size and form and attachment of soft tissues such as ligaments and tendons [2, 3, 11]. These advantages could lead to more preferable bone regeneration and limb functions.

3. Indication of reconstruction using LN2-treated bone

Bone-forming tumor such as osteosarcoma is the good indication for reconstruction using LN2-treated bone. Thus, we applied this method mainly to the patients with osteosarcoma. However, this method can be applied to the cases of osteolytic-type bone tumors such as bone metastasis with the reinforcement by polymethyl methacrylate. The tumor location, tumor origin (primary or metastatic), will not be a limiting factor for this method. Minimum equipment is a sterile thermos (Dewar) and sufficient amount of LN2 (usually 10–20 L) to immerse the disease-affected bone for freezing (**Figure 1A** and **B**).

http://dx.doi.org/10.5772/67487

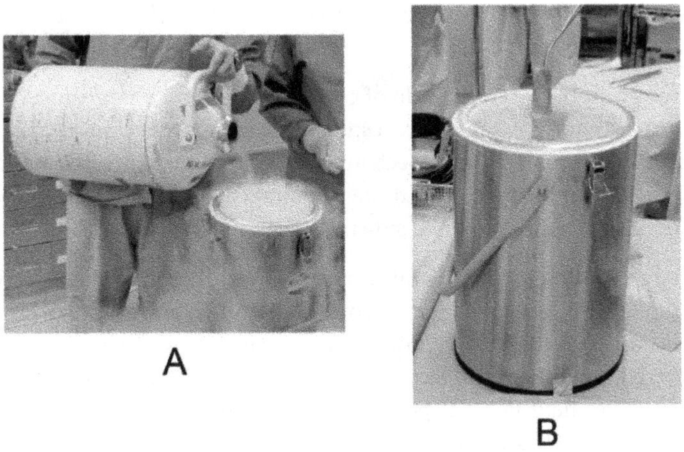

Figure 1. Intraoperative photograph of free-freezing method: (A) pour enough liquid nitrogen into a sterilized thermos (Dewar) such that the affected bone can be completely immersed and (B) allow the diseased bone to be processed in the liquid nitrogen for 20 min.

4. Processing method for LN2 treatment of disease-affected bone

Freezing methods of disease-affected bone can be classified as so-called 'free-freezing' and 'pedicle-freezing' method. The free-freezing method is performed in a way of complete disconnection of disease-affected bone from patient's body, immersion into LN2 and returning into patient's body (**Figure 2I** and **II**) [4]. Pedicle-freezing method is performed in a way of making the distal portion of the limb from the tumor as a pedicle with continuity with the

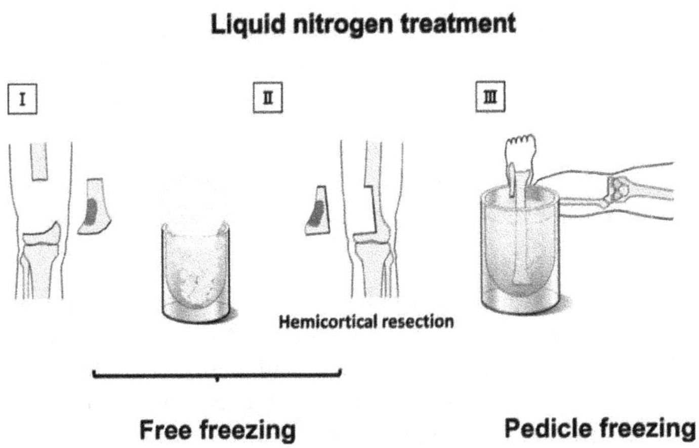

Figure 2. Types of liquid nitrogen treatment methods: for the free-freezing method, a conventional wide resection should be performed. A hemi-cortical resection can be applied to preserve the healthy bone cortex of contralateral side. For the pedicle-freezing method, the process is carried out without any breakage of continuity between the body and the affected bone.

patient's body, inversion of the limb into LN2 to immerse the affected site, then putting back into the patient's body (**Figure 2 III**) [9].

Hemi-cortical resection preserving a side of cortical bone can be performed in free-freezing method if the tumor margin is safe. That results in an increase of contact area between graft and host bone, which secures a high mechanical force and good treated-bone regeneration (**Figure 2 II**). Pedicle-freezing method is more advantageous for processed-bone regeneration because osteotomy site is only proximal side from the tumor [10].

Since the procedure of this method is quite simple, it can be performed everywhere in the world. However, several concerns have been raised, and fracture during LN2 treatment is one of main concerns. Because the expansion coefficients during freezing in LN2 are different among bone matrix, tumor bed, and blood, fracture is sometimes inevitable, such that careful curettage and reinforcement using Kirschner wire would be important to prevent fracture. Therefore, alternative operation plans such as mega-prosthesis replacement should be prepared in case.

5. Reconstruction by free-freezing method

Site and route for biopsy should be placed under the careful consideration of the mode of definitive surgery. Resection of the tumor must secure the wide surgical margin including biopsy route and chevron (V-shaped) osteotomy using micro sagittal saw is recommended to increase the contact area, which reduces torsion force for the reconstruction of osteotomy site. When attempting hemi-cortical resection, fluoroscopy and navigation system in case will help accurate osteotomy to preserve the contralateral cortical bone.

Tumor tissues and other soft tissues excised with the disease-affected bone must be removed before freezing on a workbench separated from the surgical field, then a tunnel through the medullary canal in the affected bone should be created to prevent the fracture during the freezing process (**Figure 3A**).

After LN2 is stabilized in the Dewar, the excised bone tissue will be immersed in LN2 for 20 min, then placed in room temperature for 15 min and thawed in warm distilled water at about 30°C for another 15 min. We sometimes use 1% iodine solution in the distilled water to prevent an infection (**Figure 3B**).

Double-plate fixation or intramedullary nail with plate fixation is strongly recommended to secure the stability at the osteotomy sites (**Figure 3C**). In case of large defect in processed bone, polymethyl methacrylate fulfillment will give strength to the processed bone. Composite graft with allogenic bone can be applied for certain cases too. Soft tissue reconstruction such as insertion of ligaments and tendons can be performed by direct attachment to the processed bone or remaining soft tissues on the processed bone using screws and staples.

http://dx.doi.org/10.5772/67487

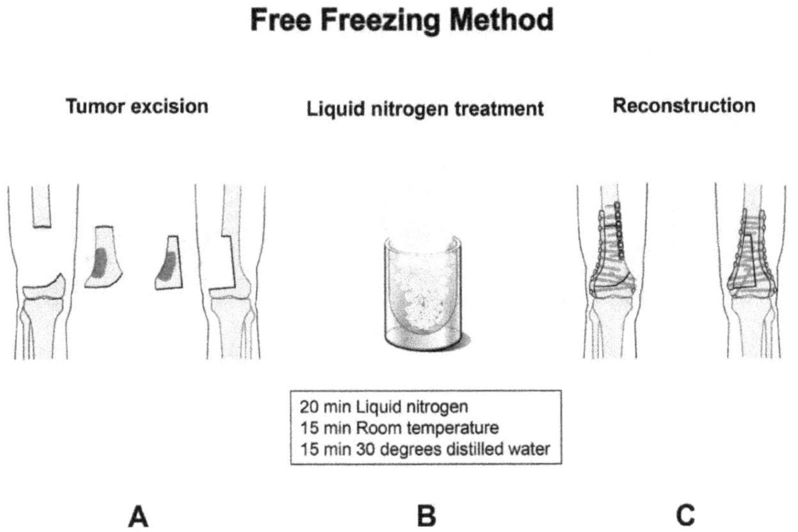

Figure 3. Free-freezing method: (A) perform wide resection of the tumor with or without sparing the contralateral bone cortex; (B) freeze the resected bone in the liquid nitrogen for 20 min; and (C) strong fixation should be done by double plate fixation.

6. Reconstruction by pedicle-freezing method

Basics for the wide resection are as same as the free-freezing method, and chevron (V-shaped) osteotomy should be performed at the proximal side from the tumor with the appropriate surgical margin using a micro-sagittal saw.

Bone with surrounding tissues, which should be excised with a wide margin, can be elevated at the osteotomy site. Unnecessary soft tissues should be detached from the bone at approximately 5-cm distal portion from the planned level for freezing to prevent the unwanted soft tissue damages by LN2 treatment. Marking the position for soaking into LN2 by electrode would be preferable before freezing.

After the detachment of unnecessary soft tissues with wide margin, the bone is elevated, and a tourniquet is applied to the affected limb to prevent bleeding and tumor cell dissemination during the curettage of tumor tissues. Covering the normal soft tissues with cotton and Esmarch lubber bandages and large clean sheets should be applied to prevent the damages by LN2 treatment (**Figure 4A** and **B**).

Tumor tissues must be curetted very carefully as possible without any contamination in the operation field as well as distal portion from the planned freezing site to secure the surgical margins then create a hole in the bone cavity to prevent the fracture during the LN2 treatment. Changing the gloves and scrubs of the operators is required to prevent the contamination with tumor cells (**Figure 5A**).

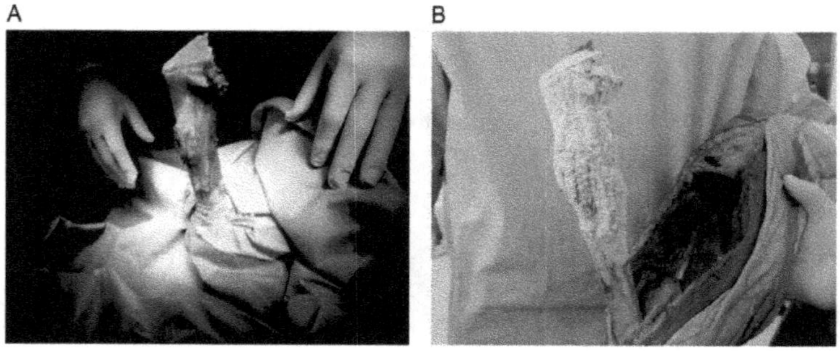

Figure 4. Intraoperative photograph of pedicle-freezing method: (A) secure that no normal soft tissue is frozen during the processing of the affected bone in liquid nitrogen for 20 min and (B) thaw for 15 min at room temperature after freezing.

After curettage, the covering sheets are carefully removed without a contact with the bone. Then, operators firmly hold the elevated affected limb to soak the pedicle bone into LN2. Careful placement of affected bone into LN2 can be secured by controlling the levels of operating table. It is very important to confirm that the bone is properly immersed in LN2 at the level of marking for planned site. The processing will continue in LN2 for 20 min as describe earlier. It is also important to verify that the remaining normal soft tissue is not affected by freezing. At the end of freezing, the operating table is slowly raised to remove the bone from the LN2 (**Figure 5B**).

Thawing in room temperature for 15 min and in the warm distilled water for 15 min will be carried out as same as the free-freezing method. Firm fixation with double plates or intramedullary nailing with plate fixation and supplemental bone grafts if necessary should be performed as described earlier (**Figure 5C**).

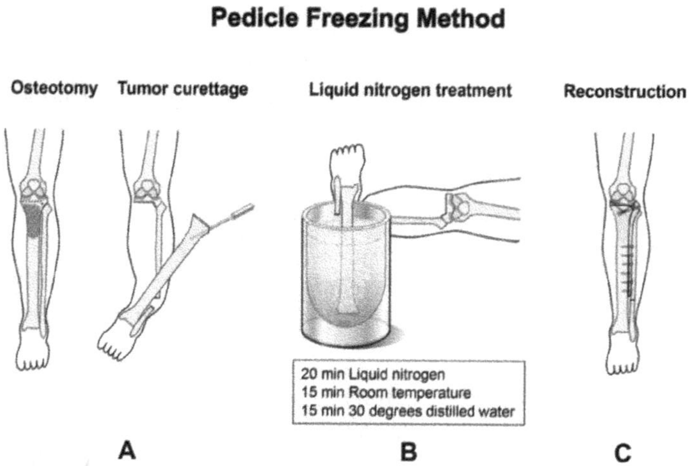

Figure 5. Pedicle-freezing method: (A) make the osteotomy on the proximal side of the tumor location. Careful curettage should be performed and bone tunnels are created to prevent fractures; (B) the distal portion maintains continuity with the body in a pedicle form, and inversion of affected limb and soaking into liquid nitrogen is performed; and (C) strong fixation should be done as same as free-freezing method.

http://dx.doi.org/10.5772/67487

7. Conclusion

The procedure in reconstruction using liquid nitrogen-treated bone is simple. If surgeons learn small skills of this techniques, this procedure can be used in many institutions. When surgeons become familiar with the procedure, bone fractures rarely occur under processing. However, it is important to prepare cable system or tumor prosthesis in case.

Surgical resection of joint surface and prosthetic reconstruction has several disadvantages and is not only option for reconstruction after osteosarcoma resection. Surgeons should keep in mind that joint preservation technique has the advantages for better limb function especially with longer durability. Thus, reconstruction methods including recycled bone technology as describe above might be considered as an alternative rather than prosthetic reconstruction for more precise surgery in osteosarcoma.

Author details

Norio Yamamoto* and Hiroyuki Tsuchiya

*Address all correspondence to: norinori@med.kanazawa-u.ac.jp

Department of Orthopedic Surgery, Graduate School of Medical Sciences, Kanazawa University, Kanazawa, Ishikawa, Japan

References

[1] Souhami RL, Craft AW, Van der Eijken JW, et al: Randomized trial of regimens of chemotherapy in operable osteosarcoma: a study of the European Osteosarcoma Intergroup. Lancet **350**: 911–917, 1997

[2] Yamamoto N. Experimental study for reconstruction using liquid nitrogen treated tumor bearing bone. Juzen Gakkaishi **109**: 193–202, 2000.

[3] Yamamoto N, Tsuchiya H, Tomita K. Effects of liquid nitrogen treatment on the proliferation of osteosarcoma and the biomechanical properties of normal bone. J Orthop Sci **8**: 374–380, 2003.

[4] Tsuchiya H, Wan SL, Sakayama K, et al. Reconstruction using an autograft containing tumour treated by liquid nitrogen. J Bone Joint Surg Br **87**: 218–225, 2005.

[5] Igarashi K, Yamamoto N, Shirai T, et al. The long-term outcome following the use of frozen autograft treated with liquid nitrogen in the management of bone and soft-tissue sarcomas. Bone Joint J **96-B**: 555–561, 2014

[6] Sakayama K, Tsuchiya H, Fujibuchi T, et al. Pathological findings of an autograft containing osteosarcoma treated by liquid nitrogen retrieved 2 years after implantation. J Orthop Sci **11**: 655–656, 2006.

[7] Tanzawa Y, Tsuchiya H, Shirai T, et al. Histological examination of frozen autograft treated by liquid nitrogen removed after implantation. J Orthop Sci **14**: 761–768, 2009.

[8] Yamamoto N, Inatani H, Shirai T, et al. Histological study on liquid nitrogen-treated tumor-bearing bone of the proximal femur excised eight years after transplantation. Low Temp Med **38**: 5–8, 2012.

[9] Tsuchiya H, Nishida H, Srisawat P, Shirai T, Hayashi K, Takeuchi A, Yamamoto N, Tomita K. Pedicle frozen autograft reconstruction in malignant bone tumors. J Orthop Sci **15**: 340–349, 2010.

[10] Shimozaki S, Yamamoto N, Shirai T, et al. Pedicle versus free frozen autograft for reconstruction in malignant bone and soft tissue tumors of the lower extremities. J Orthop Sci **19**: 156–163, 2014.

[11] Takata M, Sugimoto N, Yamamoto N, et al. Activity of bone morphogenetic protein-7 after treatment at various temperatures: freezing vs. pasteurization vs. allograft. Cryobiology **63**: 235–239, 2011.

Chapter 12

Osteosarcoma of the Jaw: Classification, Diagnosis and Treatment

Daris Ferrari, Laura Moneghini, Fabiana Allevi,
Gaetano Bulfamante and Federico Biglioli

Additional information is available at the end of the chapter

http://dx.doi.org/10.5772/67564

Abstract

Osteosarcomas are rare, highly malignant, bone tumors defined by the presence of malignant mesenchymal cells producing osteoid or immature bone. Osteosarcomas of the jaws are extremely rare, representing about 7% of all osteosarcomas and 1% of all head and neck malignancies. An accurate diagnosis, usually facilitated by chemotherapy (CT), MRI and biopsy, is required in order to define the stage of the disease and plane the adequate treatment. Aggressive surgical resection and advanced technique reconstruction are the mainstay of treatment, as the single most important factor for cure is radical resection. Clinical outcomes can be improved by a multimodal strategy combining surgery with neo-adjuvant and adjuvant chemotherapy in selected cases, and adjuvant radiotherapy in the absence of clear margins.

Keywords: jaw osteosarcoma, sarcoma, reconstructive surgery, chemotherapy, radiotherapy

1. Introduction

Osteosarcoma is the most common malignant primary tumor of bone, with an estimated incidence of approximately two cases per million persons per year. It accounts for 40–60% of all primary malignant bone tumors [1–4].

Its peak incidence is in the second to fourth decades and is more frequent in fast growing bones. When the diagnosis of osteosarcoma is made earlier than the second decade or after the cessation of skeletal growth, an association with other osseous abnormalities should be searched. Indeed, osteosarcoma can arise in the context of a genetic predisposition or underlying abnormalities such as Paget disease or fibrous dysplasia. Later in life, it can present in previously irradiated bone [3, 5].

The histopathological characteristic of osteosarcoma is the presence of aggressive malignant mesenchymal cells producing osteoid or immature bone.

Osteosarcoma of the jaw (JOS) is extremely rare, representing about 7% of all osteosarcomas and 1% of all head and neck malignancies [1, 2, 5–9].

The mandible and maxilla are almost equally involved. Unlike long-bone osteosarcoma, JOS is diagnosed more frequently in men than in females and presents about two decades later [5].

Microscopically, approximately 50% of JOS are chondroblastic or osteoblastic. In the first case, a minimal production of osteoid matrix is present which, on the contrary, prevails in the latter [1, 3, 6, 7].

If untreated, the prognosis of JOS is extremely poor. Surgery has a crucial role as the ability to treat a patient rest on a combination of aggressive surgical resection and advanced reconstructive techniques. The single most important factor for definite cure is radical resection [5, 7–23] with particular attention to achieve clear margins, a difficult task in relation to the complex anatomy of the maxillofacial region [13, 14, 20–23].

Many factors affect the prognosis of osteosarcoma. The most studied are histological subtype, grade, tumor size, patient age and response to chemotherapy (CTx) [5, 9–11, 24, 25].

From studies carried out on long bone sarcomas, it is well known that the most important prognostic indicator is the grade of CTx-induced necrosis, classified on the basis of viable tumor found in the surgical sample after resection [10, 11, 25].

Increasing necrosis with neoadjuvant chemotherapy positively correlates with efficacy, but this association has been recently questioned [26] and has to be further assessed in the future.

The clinical and biological behavior of long-bone and jaw osteosarcomas slightly differs. Head and neck osteosarcomas have a tendency to recur locally, and frequent symptoms are swelling at the site of disease, facial dysesthesia and loosening of the teeth. They give rise to distant metastases less frequently than osteosarcomas of the extremities [1, 2, 5, 7, 8, 12], which usually reveal their presence with swelling and pain, but sometimes even with disseminated symptomatic disease.

At present, a multimodal approach consisting of a combination of surgery, CTx and/or radiotherapy (RTx), has gained strong consideration, and the prognosis has progressively improved over the years.

Nonetheless, the role of CTx and RTx is still evolving [13, 14, 19–23, 27].

Considering that micrometastases can be present at diagnosis, perioperative CTx can offer some potential benefit in order to improve loco-regional control and to reduce the occurrence of distant metastases. The degree of histologic response to CTx provides the treatment team with useful information about tumor chemosensitivity. The role of RTx is still not clear in the multimodal strategy. It must be strongly considered in case of positive margins or high-grade tumors [12, 13, 21, 28].

For patients who are not candidates for surgery because of choice or associated comorbidities, RTx is an alternative for local control. Patients with poor performance status or seriously ill should be offered optimal supportive care in order to control symptoms and preserve quality of life.

2. Epidemiology, risk factors and genetics

Osteosarcoma is a disease of childhood and adolescence peaking in the second decade of life. Worldwide, a second smaller peak has been recognized later, in the seventh decade of life. The incidence rates in childhood and adolescent osteosarcoma range between 3 and 4.5 cases/million population/year, whereas the rates in older persons are estimated to be about 1 to 2 cases/million population/year for persons aged 25–59 years and 1.5–4.5 cases/million population/year for persons over the age of 60 [29].

A higher incidence of childhood osteosarcoma has been reported in Italy, Latin America, Sudan and Uganda compared to other populations around the world. In individuals 25–59 years of age, the incidence is greatest in Blacks, whereas over the age of 60, osteosarcoma incidence is greatest in Whites. Higher rates in the elderly have been reported in the United Kingdom and Australia [29, 30].

When considering a wide range of ages, males are affected with osteosarcoma more frequently than females. Bone growth, hormonal changes and growth during puberty may be involved in osteosarcoma etiology, partly explaining the slightly higher overall incidence in males.

Osteosarcoma occurs most frequently in the lower long bones, whereas the jaws are unusual primary sites of disease. Maxilla and mandible osteosarcoma (equally affected) represent about 7% of all osteosarcomas.

In order to find etiological relationships between environmental exposures and rare cancers such as osteosarcoma, a few studies have been carried out, limited by small sample sizes. Indeed, the cohorts to be studied are usually too large to identify significant correlation in a population where the disease is a rare one.

Among risk factors for osteosarcoma, fluoride exposure has been ascribed to contribute to bone cancer etiology, but subsequent studies did not confirm this finding [31].

Data from recent studies provided no evidence that higher levels of fluoride in drinking water lead to greater risk of either osteosarcoma or Ewing sarcoma.

A predisposition has been found in young patients affected by genetic syndromes characterized by somatic or germline mutations. Inherited cancer predisposition syndromes are a heterogeneous group of disorder in which higher rates of cancer in general and osteosarcoma in particular are noted. An increased risk of osteosarcoma has been associated with the Li-Fraumeni syndrome, caused by autosomal dominant germline mutations in TP53, or with retinoblastoma, caused by mutations in the RB1 tumor suppressor gene. A common feature of the genes involved is their crucial role in normal cell growth and development, apoptosis and DNA repair. Mutations of suppressor genes lead to uncontrolled proliferation and malignant transformation. Also, patients with germline mutations in DNA helicase genes have increased rates of bone sarcoma, as demonstrated in the rare Rothmund Thomas syndrome, Werner syndrome and Bloom syndrome [32].

In more advanced age patients, two risk factors have been recognized: radiation therapy and Paget's disease.

Previous irradiation increases the risk of developing osteosarcoma, mainly for patients who received RTx for leukemia/lymphoma, but no correlation has been found with respect to low dose radiation received for medical diagnostic tests.

Paget's disease of bone is a relatively common metabolic bone disorder characterized by uncoupled bone remodeling, depending on abnormalities in osteoblast and osteoclast communication. The incidence of osteosarcoma secondary to Paget's disease is not known, but it is estimated to be about 1% [33].

This association accounts for about half of the osteosarcomas reported in elderly patients.

Despite many efforts, the etiology of osteosarcoma remains largely unknown. Epidemiologic studies have provided many important associations with puberty and height or disorders of bone growth and remodeling, but this bulk of knowledge is mainly confined to long-bone osteosarcomas. Data on JOS are less conclusive, so further research is still needed in order to improve our diagnostic and therapeutic approach.

3. Pathology

Osteosarcoma is a primary malignant bone tumor in which the mesenchymal neoplastic cells produce osteoid or immature bone. Therefore, the observation of osteoid is the key for the diagnosis of osteosarcoma [**Figure 1**].

3.1. Histotypes

Histologically, osteosarcoma is divided into the central (intramedullary) and peripheral (surface) subtypes.

The main type of central osteosarcoma is the conventional osteosarcoma, which is represented by a broad spectrum of morphologies. Besides the production of osteoid and immature bone, histological features are the presence of neoplastic cells showing anaplasia with epithelioid, plasmacytoid or spindle aspects and the growth with a permeative pattern, filling the marrow space surrounding and eroding pre-existing trabeculae [**Figure 2**]. Depending upon the predominant type of extracellular matrix present, conventional osteosarcoma is classified histopathologically into osteoblastic, chondroblastic and fibroblastic subtypes [34].

http://dx.doi.org/10.5772/67564

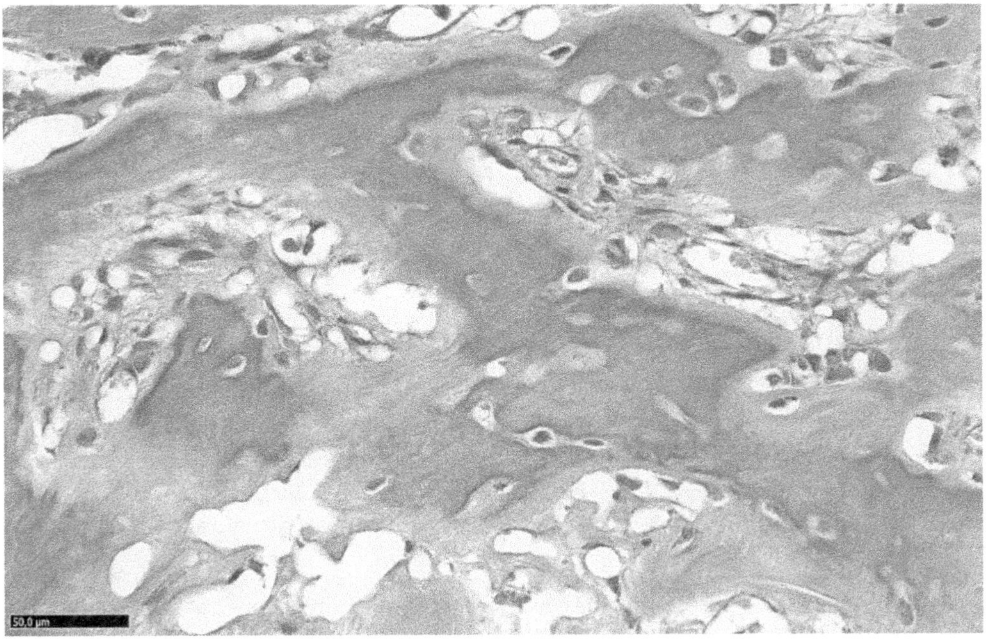

Figure 1. Picture showing osteoid and immature bone in OS.

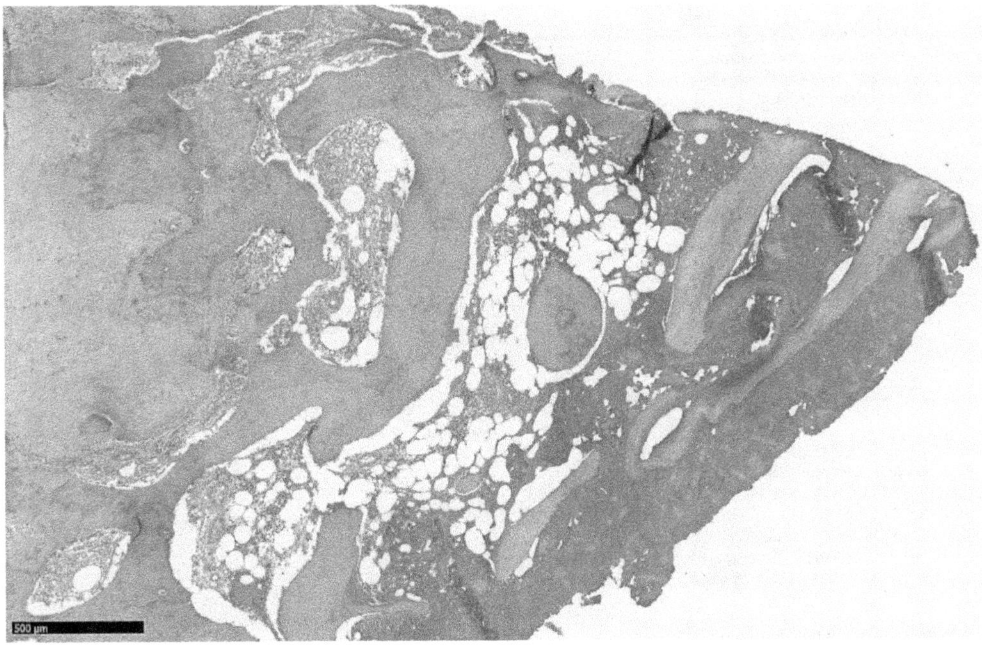

Figure 2. OS with a permeative pattern, filling the marrow space.

The osteoblastic subtype consists of osteoid or immature bone surrounded by haphazardly arranged fibroblast-like or epithelioid cells. The chondroblastic variant shows areas of atypical hyaline chondroid tissue. The cartilage may be the dominant component or scattered throughout the tumor. The fibroblastic subtype shows spindle-shaped neoplastic cells, characteristically arranged in herringbone pattern-like fibrosarcoma. The formation of tumor osteoid differentiates this variant of osteosarcoma from fibrosarcoma.

The World Health Organization (WHO) [35] in 2013 reported other osteosarcoma histotypes such as low-grade, giant cell rich, osteoblastoma and chondroblastoma-like, epithelioid, clear cell types, telangiectasic and small cell (**Table 1**).

The peripheral osteosarcomas are represented by parosteal, periosteal and high-grade surface osteosarcomas.

JOS is relatively rare and the majority of them arise de novo but some of them may develop in bone affected by Paget's disease, fibrous dysplasia, bone infarcts, chronic osteomyelitis, trauma, viral infection, exposure to high-dose radiation, metallic implants, joint prostheses in genetic syndromes such as Li-Fraumeni syndrome, hereditary retinoblastoma and RTx [36].

The JOS histotypes are the same as the conventional ones in long bones but differ from them in predominant differentiation pattern [38].

Most series of JOS report predominantly chondroblastic differentiation subtypes, more often myxoid [**Figure 3**].

Low-grade central osteosarcoma	
Conventional osteosarcoma	Chondroblastic
	Osteoblastic (including sclerosis)
	Fibroblastic
	Giant cell rich
	Osteoblastoma-like
	Chondroblastoma-like
	Epithelioid
	Clear cell
	Secondary
Teleangectasic osteosarcoma	
Small cell osteosarcoma	
Parosteal osteosarcoma	
Periosteal osteosarcoma	
High-grade surface osteosarcoma	

Table 1. Osteosarcoma classification (WHO 2013).

http://dx.doi.org/10.5772/67564

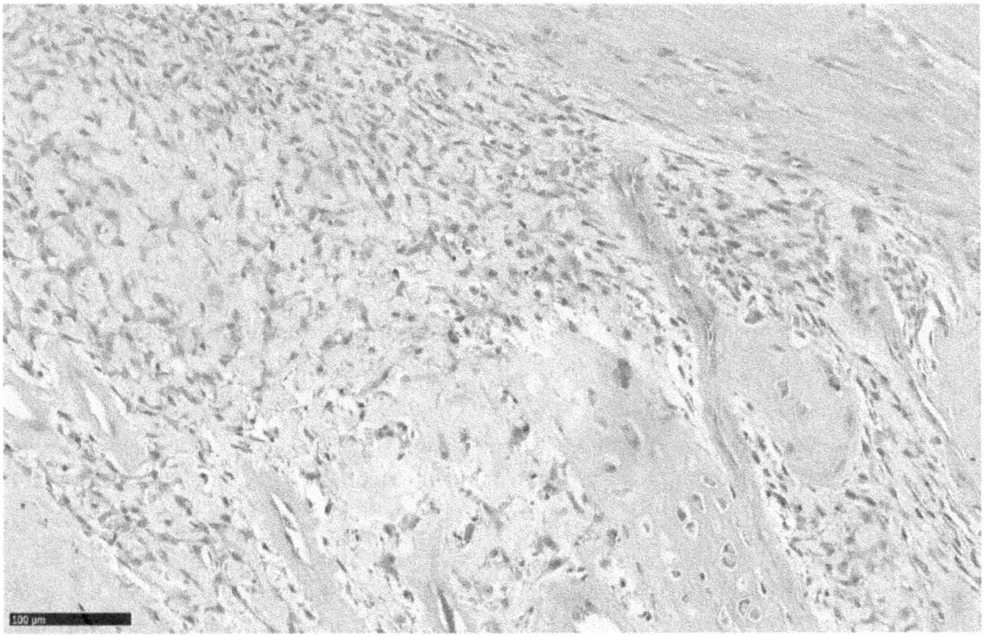

Figure 3. OS with myxoid aspect.

Mardinger et al.—for example—reported the highest prevalence for chondroblastic OS (42%), osteoblastic osteosarcomas being lesser (33%) in JOS [37].

In other series, the osteoblastic pattern was predominant, followed by the chondroblastic pattern [39, 40].

Finally, there is no consensus regarding the main differentiation patterns (osteoblastic and chondroblastic), and more often JOS display a more heterogeneous histotype as Bennett et al. [41] and Nissanka et al. [42] also pointed out.

The histologic heterogeneity of osteosarcoma highlights the need for histology to be supported by clinical and radiographic data for a correct diagnosis [33].

Other less frequent but not less important histological subtype of central JOS is the low-grade central osteosarcoma (LGCO)(1–2% in JOS). This is a well-differentiated osteosarcoma consisting of spindle cell fibroblastic proliferation with low cellularity, no significant atypia, low mitotic figures and a variable osteoid production. The most important feature of LGCO in long bones, and also in the jaw, is its similarities with benign lesions, first of all with fibrous dysplasia. Histological characteristics, including cellularity amount, cellular atypia and mitotic activity rate, are not very helpful, and the interpretation of small biopsies is very difficult, unless there are definite radiographic evidences showing the presence of an aggressive lesion. An excisional biopsy specimen must contain a large and adequate part of the tumor tissue together with surrounding tissue, with tumoral cells infiltrating into the bone marrow, cortical destruction by tumor and tumor invasion into soft tissues. Curettage should not be performed [43].

The peripheral osteosarcomas occasionally affect the jaw. The most frequent is parosteal (or juxtacortical) osteosarcoma which represents less than 5% of all osteosarcomas. It is well differentiated and characterized by spindle cell stroma with minimal atypia and rare mitotic figures separating irregular trabeculae of woven bone, arranged in a parallel manner. With time, the trabeculae often coalesce and form a large mass of solid bone. About 40–50% of parosteal osteosarcomas exhibit foci of cartilage. Approximately 10–25% of parosteal osteosarcomas dedifferentiate into high-grade osteosarcoma with a corresponding worsening of prognosis [34, 44].

3.2. Immunohistochemistry

Immunohistochemical detection of MDM2 and CDK4 may provide useful diagnostic tool [34, 45].

Recently, Yoshida et al. reported that the combination of MDM2 and CDK4 by immunohistochemical analysis shows 100% sensitivity and 97.5% specificity for the diagnosis of low-grade osteosarcoma. They concluded that MDM2 and CDK4 immunostains reliably distinguish low-grade osteosarcoma from benign lesions, and their combination may serve as a useful adjunct in this difficult differential diagnosis [46].

However, Tabareau-Dalanlande et al. noted discordant results, with 33% of ossifying fibromas and 12% of fibrous dysplasias exhibiting MDM2 amplification by qRT-PCR but no cases exhibiting MDM2 overexpression by immunohistochemistry. These investigators also showed amplification of an MDM2 neighbor, RASAL1, in all the fibro-osseous lesions with MDM2 amplification but in none of the low-grade osteosarcomas studied [47].

A recent study illustrated that some high-grade JOS is differentiated/dedifferentiated osteosarcomas harboring overexpression and amplification of MDM2. Juvenile ossifying fibromas can rarely evolve into giant cell-rich high-grade osteosarcomas and are characterized by a RASAL1 amplification [48].

3.3. Grading

Cellularity is the most important criterion used for histological grading. In general, the more cellular a tumor is, the higher is the grade. Irregularity of the nuclear contour, enlargement and hyperchromasia of the nuclei are correlated with grade. Mitotic figures and necrosis are additional features useful in grading. The grade is divided into low grade (G1) and high grade (G2) [34].

The surface osteosarcomas are further divided into parosteal, well-differentiated (low-grade), periosteal low- to intermediate-grade and high-grade surface osteosarcomas [49–51].

Although there have been various attempts to grade histological osteosarcomas, the reproducibility is poor [40].

3.4. Staging

Staging incorporates the degree of differentiation as well as local and distant spread, in order to estimate the prognosis of the patient. The universal Tumor Lymph nodes Metastasis (TNM) staging system is not commonly used for sarcomas because they are unlikely to metastasize in lymph nodes.

http://dx.doi.org/10.5772/67564

The American Joint Committee on Cancer (AJCC) System for bone sarcomas still recognizes four stages: Stage I and II for low grade and high grade without metastasis, respectively, Stage III for "skip metastasis" and Stage IV for metastatic sarcomas.

The system used most often to formally stage bone sarcomas is known as the Musculo-skeletal Tumor Society (MSTS) or Enneking system [52].

It is based on the grade (G) of the tumor, the local extent of the primary tumor (T), and whether or not it has metastasized to regional lymph nodes or other organs (M). The extent of the primary tumor is classified as either intra-compartmental (T1), meaning it has basically remained in place, or extra-compartmental (T2), meaning it has extended into other nearby structures. Tumors that have not spread to the lymph nodes or other organs are considered M0, while those that have spread are M1 [53].

In summary, low-grade tumors are defined as stage I, high-grade tumors as stage II and metastatic tumors (regardless of grade) as stage III.

3.5. Prognosis

Osteosarcoma of the jaw is usually considered clinically as intermediate grade tumors and most authors point to the favorable prognosis of JOS compared with long-bone osteosarcomas. Paget's disease-related JOS is, however, aggressive tumors [40].

The two main prognostic criteria of JOS are tumor size and resectability at presentation [54].

Positive margins are strongly associated with poor prognosis; unfortunately, marginal excision is unavoidable in some JOS due to anatomic difficulties [15].

Complete resection of tumors involving the maxilla can be technically challenging, so local recurrence is more frequent in maxillary than mandibular osteosarcomas and, considering both sites, more common than the occurrence of distant metastases [5, 15, 16].

Death is usually secondary to local tumor extension with neural and vascular infiltration [38].

4. Clinical features

Males are affected by JOS slightly more frequently than females. Median age is between 30 and 40 years. Maxilla and mandible are equally involved, and the prognosis is similar [23].

The duration of symptoms before presentation is typically about 3–6 months. The most common presenting symptoms are swelling at the site of disease, which is almost universally present, and local pain, reported by approximately 70% of the patients. Other complaints are numbness and facial dysesthesia (32%), loosening of the teeth (14%), trismus, limitation of mouth opening, headache and nasal obstruction or bleeding. Patients rarely complain about systemic symptoms like fever, asthenia or weight loss. A few patients have no symptoms at presentation, and their tumors can be discovered incidentally by radiography. Physical examination can demonstrate a painless, firm mass, fixed to the underlying bone covered with normal tissue. Lymph nodes involvement, either cervical, supraclavicular or axillary, is unusual [22].

At first presentation, metastatic disease is present in 5% of the patients. This is less than in patients with appendicular skeleton osteosarcoma. The lungs are the most frequently involved sites.

Plain radiography and CT scan may demonstrate the presence of lytic lesions or mixed lytic and sclerotic lesions. Intraosseous tumors generally present as a poorly defined combination of radiodense and lucent lesions. In some cases, the cortex is invaded and eroded by the tumor, which extends into the soft tissues, frequently eliciting a periosteal reaction. Sometimes, the tumor grows expanding the bone but without violating the cortex. In other cases, the tumor surface is homogeneously radiodense and well demarcated from the soft tissues, resembling an osteoma. In the purely lytic lesions, the diagnosis may be difficult, as osteosarcomas mimicking hollow areas without new bone formation cannot be differentiated from metastatic disease radiographically.

Some laboratory parameters, such as alkaline phosphatase or lactate dehydrogenase (LDH) serum levels, can be increased in a few patients. Although they do not correlate reliably with disease extent, they may have negative prognostic significance [34].

5. Treatment

The prognosis of patients affected by JOS depends on few recognized risk factors. The most important is the achievement of clear margins with surgery. Furthermore, older age is statistically associated with decreased survival [55]. CTx with four or more agents used in a multimodality strategy is associated with a trend toward better disease-free (DFS) and overall survival (OS) [5].

On a multivariate analysis model recently reported, age (hazard ratio [HR], 1.03; 95% CI, 1.02–1.04 [P < 0.001]), surgery (HR, 0.31; 95% CI, 0.16–0.60 [P < 0.001]) and stage at presentation (HR, 1.37; 95% CI, 1.10–1.71 [P = 0.006]) were found to be independent predictors of OS. Moreover, age (HR, 1.03; 95% CI, 1.02–1.05 [P < 0.001]), surgery (HR, 0.22; 95% CI, 0.09–0.56 [P = 0.001]), tumor size (HR, 1.01; 95% CI, 1.00–1.01 [P = 0.003]) and stage at presentation (HR, 1.34; 95% CI, 1.01–1.76 [P = 0.04]) were found to be independent predictors for disease specific survival [56].

Age under 30 years, early stage (IA-IIB), and surgical treatment significantly correlated with a better prognosis.

5.1. Surgery

As it is the case for other skeletal locations, surgery is a mainstay of osteosarcoma treatment also in the head and neck region. The rationale and principles of surgical treatment of JOS depend on the location of the tumor [23, 57].

Obtaining disease-free resection margins is of course imperative, to avoid the risk of local recurrence.

Nevertheless, this goal is even more difficult to reach when dealing with head and neck osteosarcomas, since resecting few millimeters more often means endangering pivotal

http://dx.doi.org/10.5772/67564

functional structures, with a noticeable decrease in the patients' quality of life. While intraoperative determination of resection margins might represent a useful tool in other head and neck malignancies, osteosarcomas do often pose a significant challenge for the surgeon: Intraoperative pathological examination does not indeed allow for the assessment of bone margins. Only soft tissue margins can be assessed through the intraoperative consultation [58].

Because of the anatomical complexity of the region, tumor resections are occasionally incomplete. Local recurrences and intracranial invasion have long been reported as the major causes of treatment failure due to incomplete neoplasm resection [59].

For the head and neck region, appropriate preoperative information is usually derived from the combined study of CT scans and MR imaging, both with contrast [**Figure 4**].

The CT scan allows a better assessment of the bone involvement and extension (better hard tissue definition), whereas the MR imaging aims at defining with considerable accuracy the soft tissue involvement [60].

While whole body bone scintigraphy and chest CT scan area advised for the initial staging [61], there is no general consensus for the routine implementation of whole-body MR and positron emission tomography (PET)/CT or PET/MR, which are under evaluation both for staging and treatment response evaluation [62].

According to the histopathological diagnosis, obtained through the biopsy, and the extension of the neoplasm, the multidisciplinary team indicates the best treatment for the patient [57].

When dealing with high-grade osteosarcomas, the best curative option is represented by a multimodal treatment. Multimodality increases DFS from the disappointing 10–20% of surgery alone to a solid > 60%. On the other hand, the treatment of low-grade central and parosteal osteosarcomas can rely on surgery alone, provided a complete assessment of their metastatic potential [63].

Irrespective of the treatment plan, whether monomodal or multimodal, the principles of surgery remain just the same. Effective treatment requires wide resections, as disease-free margins are associated with lower risk of local recurrence and higher overall survival. Nevertheless, despite the best staging and the most delicate and careful reconstruction techniques, it comes naturally that the 3 cm resection margin usually advocated for sarcomas of other sites (e.g., long bones sarcomas) is unthinkable when dealing with the head and neck structures. If we take into account literature reports, safety margins for head and neck osteosarcoma vary, from the observation of Granados-Garcia, who suggests a resection tailored on tumor size in the head and neck region [64], to the 1 cm minimal resection margin suggested by Ketabchi [65] [**Figure 5**].

As previously anticipated, despite obtaining adequate margins being the first goal of surgery, resection of head and neck osteosarcomas requires a careful balance between effective surgery and function-sparing procedures [25].

Surgical planning and the technical execution should be based on the expectation of performing a functionally effective reconstructive surgery [12, 25].

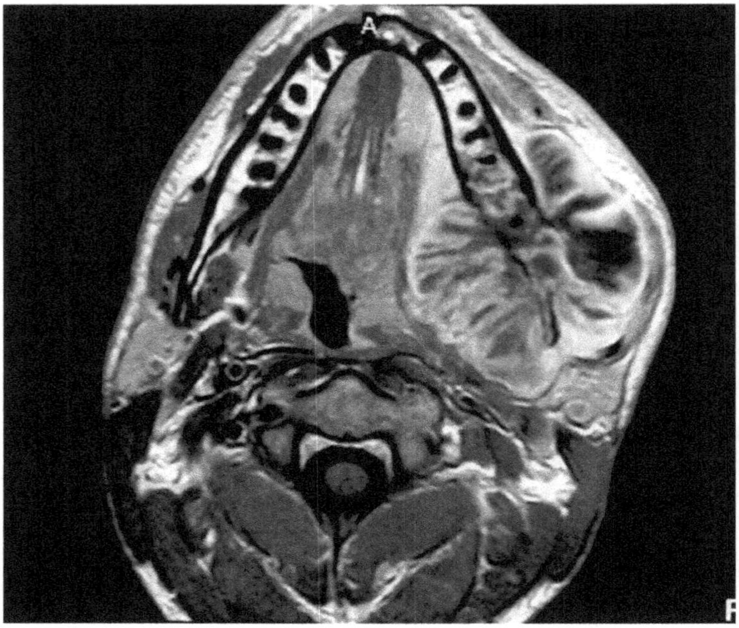

Figure 4. Preoperative MR imaging scan showing the extension of the mandibular neoplasm.

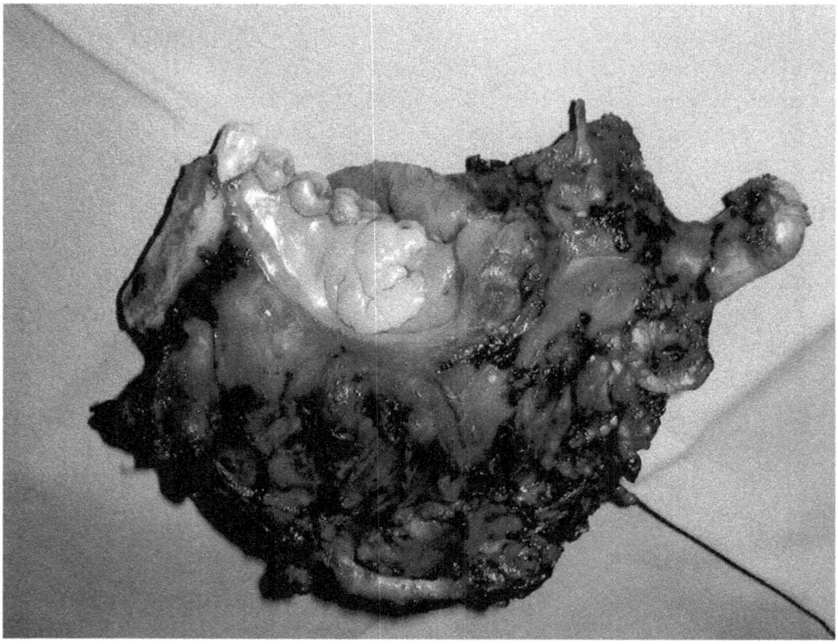

Figure 5. Intraoperative view of the mandibulectomy specimen after resection.

http://dx.doi.org/10.5772/67564

The management of tissue defects in head and neck oncological surgery relies on loco-regional flaps for small deficits or on free microvascular flaps and metal prosthetics plates for large resections. When dealing with JOS, it is of the utmost importance that such free flaps allow also for transposing bony tissues. These technically refined procedures, which are usually performed in tertiary referral centers, enable not only a functional and aesthetic reconstruction but also a better future prosthetic rehabilitation of the patient's dentition, which has a relevant and natural role not only in food processing but also in social relationships [63].

Different flaps have already been proposed including the iliac crest microvascular free flaps [64], radial forearm flap with partial radius inclusion [67] and scapula osteocutaneous flap [68].

Nevertheless, the fibula flap, introduced by Taylor and colleagues [69], has become the most utilized in mandibular reconstruction due to its favorable characteristics (co-harvesting with multiple skin paddles, harvesting as a neurosensory flap, optimal form restoration and acceptable functional results), high rate of success and low rate of complications in both recipient and donor sites [**Figures 6**, **7**].

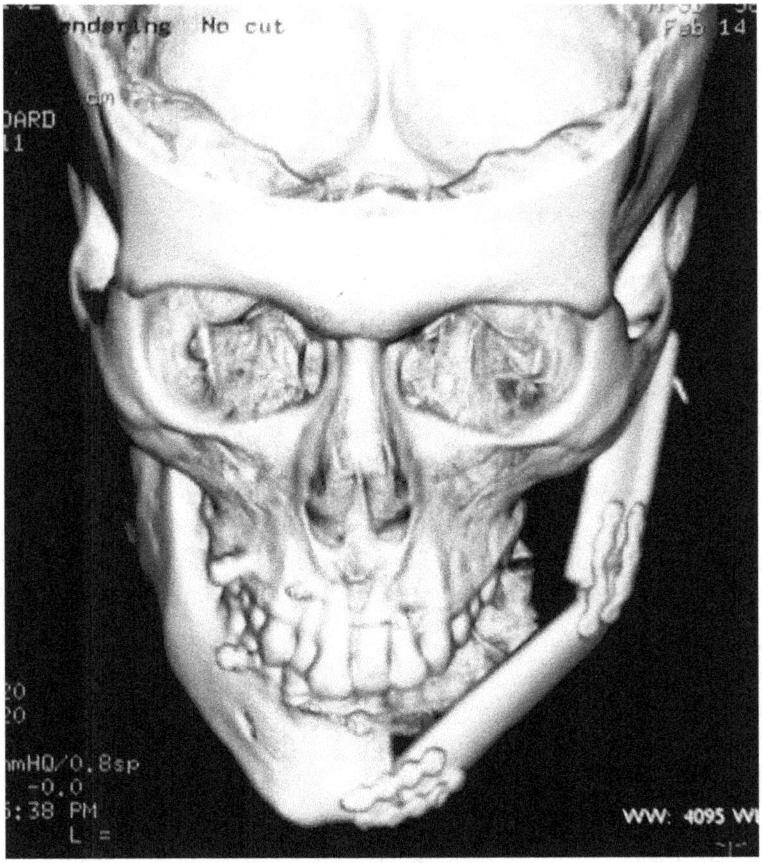

Figure 6. Postoperative 3D CT scan showing mandibular reconstruction with fibula free flap.

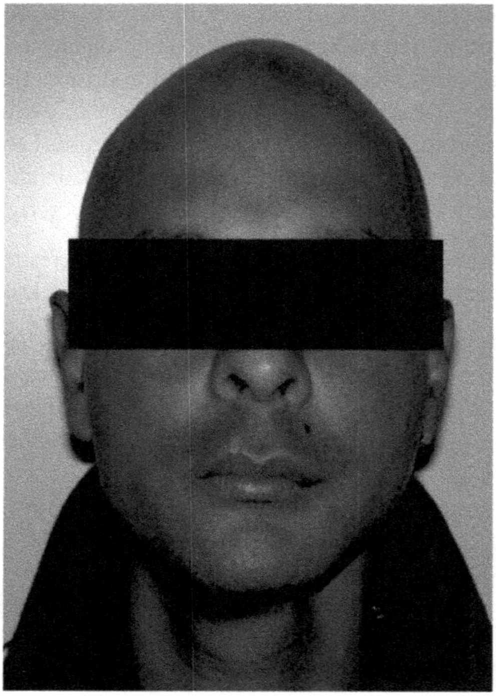

Figure 7. Frontal postoperative picture showing the excellent symmetry of the face.

These impressive reconstructions have been further enhanced by the progressive implementation of techniques such as virtual surgical planning using computer-assisted modeling [70].

This technique allows reconstructing defects with astonishing anatomical faithfulness not only with free flaps but also with custom-made synthetic plates which are the standard reconstruction method in elderly or compromised patients. It has to be noted that reconstruction, despite being almost unavoidable in order to obtain a good quality of life, makes the radiologic follow-up more complex, due to the increased effort required by the specialist in differentiating normal, neoplastic and grafted tissues. These features must be taken into account when planning the procedure and informing the patient, and radiologic follow-up examination should be conducted in specialized structures with dedicated personnel.

Large bone and soft tissue free margins are more easily achievable in osteosarcomas involving the mandible than in sarcoma of the upper jaw, were posterior control of resection and may be extremely difficult. This is particularly true when upper jaw malignancies involve the skull base, either to its osseous portion or the dura. Due to this peculiar feature, mandibular sarcomas are characterized by a better local control and a higher DFS and OS than the facial bones and skull base mesenchymal tumors [71].

In particular, when dealing with malignancies of the upper jaw, new technologies allowing careful three-dimensional tumor resection planning are helpful. Specific software that elaborates

http://dx.doi.org/10.5772/67564

radiological Digital Imaging and COmmunications in Medicine (DICOM) images allows tailored surgical cutting guides to help precise excision of the tumor and high-quality simultaneous reconstruction, equally computer planned and guide-aided [72, 73].

Similarly, optimal margin control can be achieved also using intraoperative image-guided navigation systems that allow the comparison of the anatomical features with the available radiographic reconstructions, with a considerable learning curve [74].

On the other hand, while lower jaw resections are considered technically easier than upper jaw resection, due to more restricted growing patterns of the tumor and the relative lack of other fundamental surrounding structures, mandibular reconstruction is a major challenge for the surgeon. When dealing with defects following extensive mandibular resection, it is mandatory to evaluate which components of the hard and soft tissue are missing in order to select the best reconstruction method (from simple rigid internal fixation to microvascular free tissue transfer). It is also crucial to grant an adequate bone vertical height and to contour clearly the margins of the alveolar bone, in order to achieve both an aesthetically appealing result and to restore mastication to the patient [75, 76].

Furthermore, correctly designing the reconstruction and adequately reproducing the mandibular contour and the consequent occlusion allow for safe and correct implant placement, which restores the functions under a gnatologic and logopedic point of view [66].

While bony tissue reconstruction may pose the most challenging procedural issues, it has to be noted that soft tissue defect repair has a prominent role in preserving the patient's aesthetics. Healthy transposed soft tissue with an adequate height can adequately restore the facial contour, providing correct coverage of the underlying framework reconstruction [64, 76].

On the other hand, inadequately transposed soft tissues may produce poor results, requiring further ancillary procedure to replace the defect [77].

The use of neoadjuvant RTx in cervicofacial osteosarcoma, though not advised, has not been fully abandoned. Therefore, surgery may also follow RTx, which is a recognized major cause of increased surgical complications and free flap reconstruction failure, even with modern stereotactic protocols [78].

Such risk tends to increase proportionally to the RTx dose, since RTx induces definite changes in tissues (inflammation followed by fibrosis and a prothrombotic state with reduced vascular supply) which, in turn, lead to reduced wound healing and increased scar tissue formation [79].

In these patients, surgery can be performed, but both the surgeon and the patient must be aware of the higher complication rate and the postoperative management must be extremely careful. In these regards, it must be noted that the use of microvascular flap offers the best chances of a successful reconstruction, since the harvested tissue bears no microvessel damage due to radiation and is featured by a better overall vitality, given the appropriate blood supply through the anastomoses.

When dealing with head and neck malignancies, it comes naturally to evaluate a possible prognostic/therapeutic role for functional or selective neck dissection [80].

Although there is no general consensus, nodal localization should be treated surgically and should be considered adverse features when evaluating adjuvant treatments. Conversely (this is the major difference when compared to other common malignancies of the head and neck), prophylactic neck dissection is not advised also for high grade or large osteosarcomas of the head and neck region. Although more research would be advisable in these regards, it should be noted that the only, albeit old, data available report that prophylactic nodal dissection has a detrimental effect on patients' OS [81].

5.2. Medical treatment

The role of surgery in the treatment of jaw osteosarcoma is unquestioned [10].

The manuscript by Bertoni et al. [15] reported the Istituto Rizzoli-Beretta experience with JOS. They treated 26 of 28 patients with surgery and two patients with RTx. Adjuvant treatment was offered only to three patients (RTx in two cases and CTx in one): the 5-year OS rate for the whole group was disappointing (23%), as was the recurrence rate (85.7%). Such poor results are likely due to inadequate surgery (50% positive margins) and to the inefficiency of surgery as a single treatment [15].

While the use of preoperative and adjuvant CTx has become the standard of care in long bone osteosarcomas, its role in JOS is still controversial [11, 82, 83].

Adding CTx or RTx to surgery has demonstrated improved survival in locoregionally advanced head and neck cancer. The aim of chemotherapy is to reduce tumor size ameliorating surgical outcome, improve local control and reduce distant metastases. RTx is usually employed in the adjuvant setting and has the fundamental role of decreasing locoregional relapse.

The role of RTx in the multimodal treatment has been studied by Guadagnolo et al. [12]., who evaluated the role of RTx in 119 patients affected by JOS. While 92 patients underwent surgery alone, in 27 cases, surgery was followed by radiotherapy. Stratified analysis by resection margin status demonstrated that the combined use of surgery and radiotherapy was superior to surgery alone and could improve OS (80 vs. 31%) and DFS (80 vs. 35%) in patients with positive or uncertain margins. This high-risk group is inclined to get the best results, while no advantage is expected for patients with negative margins.

Two small retrospective studies on osteosarcoma of the jaws from Link et al. [82] and Doval et al. [84] using different CTx protocols in addition to surgery were the first to demonstrate that CTx could favorably impact on survival, though at a small rate.

The role of CTx (and RTx) has been further addressed in a systematic review on 201 patients from 20 uncontrolled series [14]. Various CTx regimens were given to 60 patients prior to (neo-adjuvant, 18 patients) or after surgery (adjuvant, 42 patients), performed in 180 patients. Surgical resection was complete in 105 cases (58.3%). RTx was used in 69 patients. The 5-year OS and Progression-Free Survival (PFS) in this group of patients undergoing multimodal therapy (surgery and neo-adjuvant and/or adjuvant Chemotherapy (CHT)) were 80 and 75%, respectively. The 5-year OS and DFS in those patients subjected to radical surgery alone were 40 and 33%, respectively. From this review, it was clearly evident that CTx significantly improved survival when combined with radical surgery, while the effect of RTx was insignificant [15].

http://dx.doi.org/10.5772/67564

The analysis of a small series of patients suggested the efficacy of multimodal treatment combining neo-adjuvant CTx, surgery and adjuvant CTx with excellent results in terms of 5-year OS and PFS [22].

A subsequent analysis on patients treated before and after 1991 demonstrated that the 5-year OS was 52% in the former group and 77% in the latter [85], reflecting earlier diagnosis and more aggressive treatment, namely the adoption of neoadjuvant CTx and of better reconstructive options.

According to Ferrari et al. [60], a multimodal approach consisting of radical surgery and CTx, with or without RTx, favorably compares with previous reports, achieving 5-year OS and DFS rates of 77 and 73%, respectively. In line with retrospective reviews stressing the prognostic importance of CTx-induced necrosis for local control [11, 25] also in this study, the rate of necrosis was a statistically significant factor, with poor prognosis correlating with ≤50% necrosis. These data confirm that JOS treated with perioperative CTx and radical surgery maximizes DFS and OS. CTx-related toxicity remains an issue that both oncologists and patients have to deal with. Adjuvant RTx can be useful in selected cases but the most relevant results are clearly related to the completeness of surgery.

Although multimodal treatment can improve clinical outcomes, what could be the best treatment for small, easily operable osteosarcomas remains to be assessed. It is likely that small low-grade lesions (T1) can be definitely eradicated by adequate surgery with no need for neo-adjuvant or adjuvant therapy.

We do not think that we ought to discourage research, but it is reasonable to believe that controlled prospective and randomized trials on this argument are unlikely to be performed.

6. Conclusion

Through the years, the survival of patients with JOS has greatly improved, due to an aggressive systemic approach and to the refined surgical and reconstructive techniques. Today, we can reasonably hope to cure the majority of patients affected by JOS. However, opportunities for clinical and biological research remain. Our knowledge of the pathways involved in sarcomagenesis is lacking, and new insights are eagerly awaited in the perspective of developing an effective target therapy to combine with surgery.

Author details

Daris Ferrari[1*], Laura Moneghini[2], Fabiana Allevi[3], Gaetano Bulfamante[2] and Federico Biglioli[3]

*Address all correspondence to: daris.ferrari@asst-santipaolocarlo.it

1 Medical Oncology, San Paolo Hospital, University of Milan, Milan, Italy

2 Department of Pathology, San Paolo Hospital, University of Milan, Milan, Italy

3 Maxillofacial Department, San Paolo Hospital, University of Milan, Milan, Italy

References

[1] Campanacci M. Bone and soft tissue tumors. Springer-Verlag, Wien, New York; 1999.

[2] Dahlin DC UKK. Osteosarcoma bone tumors. CC Thomas, Springfield; 1986.

[3] Klein MJ, Siegal GP. Osteosarcoma: anatomic and histologic variants. Am J Clin Pathol. 2006;125(4):555–581. doi:10.1177/1066896908319675Epub 2008 Jul 8.

[4] Motamedi M, Jafari SM, Azizi T. Gnathic osteosarcomas: A 10-year multi-center demographic study. Indian J Cancer. 2009;46(3):231–233. doi:10.4103/0019-509X.52958.

[5] August M, Magennis P, Dewitt D. Osteogenic sarcoma of the jaws: factors influencing prognosis. Int J Oral Maxillofac Surg. 1997;26(3):198–204.

[6] Nakayama E, Sugiura K, Kobayashi I, Oobu K, Ishibashi H, Kanda S. The association between the computed tomography findings, histologic features, and outcome of osteosarcoma of the jaw. J Oral Maxillofac Surg. 2005;63(3):311–318. doi:10.1016/j.joms.2004.04.033.

[7] Clark JL, Unni KK, Dahlin DC, Devine KD. Osteosarcoma of the jaw. Cancer. 1983;51(12):2311–2316.

[8] Dahlin DC. Prognostic factors in osteosarcoma. Int J Radiat Oncol Biol Phys. 1980;6(12):1755.

[9] Vadillo RM, Contreras SJS, Canales JOG. Prognostic factors in patients with jaw sarcomas. Braz Oral Res. 2011;25(5):421–426.

[10] Garrington GE, Scofield HH, Cornyn J, Hooker SP. Osteosarcoma of the jaws. Analysis of 56 cases. Cancer. 1967;20(3):377–391.

[11] Rosen G, Caparros B, Huvos AG, Kosloff C, Nirenberg A, Cacavio A, Morcove RC, Lane JM, Mehta B, Urban C. Preoperative chemotherapy for osteogenic sarcoma: selection of postoperative adjuvant chemotherapy based on the response of the primary tumor to preoperative chemotherapy. Cancer. 1982;49(6):1221–1230 .

[12] Guadagnolo BA, Ashleigh Guadagnolo B, Zagars GK, Kevin Raymond A, Benjamin RS, Sturgis EM. Osteosarcoma of the jaw/craniofacial region. Cancer. 2009;115(14):3262–3270.

[13] Jasnau S, Meyer U, Potratz J, Jundt G, Kevric M, Joos UK, Jürgens H, Bielack SS. Craniofacial osteosarcoma experience of the cooperative German-Austrian-Swiss osteosarcoma study group. Oral Oncol. 2008;44(3):286–294. doi:10.1016/j.oraloncology.2007.03.001.

[14] Smeele LE, Kostense PJ, van der Waal I, Snow GB. Effect of chemotherapy on survival of craniofacial osteosarcoma: a systematic review of 201 patients. J Clin Oncol. 1997;15(1):363–367.

[15] Bertoni F, Dallera P, Bacchini P, Marchetti C, Campobassi A. The Istituto Rizzoli-Beretta experience with osteosarcoma of the jaw. Cancer. 1991;68(7):1555–1563.

[16] Canadian Society of Otolaryngology-Head and Neck Surgery Oncology Study Group. Osteogenic sarcoma of the mandible and maxilla: a Canadian review (1980–2000). J Otolaryngol. 2004;33(3):139–144.

[17] Ha PK, Eisele DW, Frassica FJ, Zahurak ML, McCarthy EF. Osteosarcoma of the head and neck: a review of the Johns Hopkins experience. Laryngoscope. 1999;109(6):964–969.

[18] Smeele LE, van der Wal JE, van Diest PJ, van der Waal I, Snow GB. Radical surgical treatment in craniofacial osteosarcoma gives excellent survival. A retrospective cohort study of 14 patients. Eur J Cancer B Oral Oncol. 1994;30B(6):374–376.

[19] Potter BO, Sturgis EM. Sarcomas of the head and neck. Surg Oncol Clin N Am. 2003;12(2):379–417.

[20] Carrle D, Dorothe C, Bielack SS. Current strategies of chemotherapy in osteosarcoma. Int Orthop. 2006;30(6):445–451. doi:10.1007/s00264-006-0192-x.

[21] Fernandes R, Nikitakis NG, Pazoki A, Ord RA. Osteogenic sarcoma of the jaw: a 10-year experience. J Oral Maxillofac Surg. 2007;65(7):1286–1291. doi:10.1016/j.joms.2006.10.030.

[22] Thiele OC, Freier K, Bacon C, Egerer G, Hofele CM. Interdisciplinary combined treatment of craniofacial osteosarcoma with neoadjuvant and adjuvant chemotherapy and excision of the tumour: a retrospective study. Br J Oral Maxillofac Surg. 2008;46(7):533–536. doi:10.1016/j.bjoms.2008.03.010.

[23] Kassir RR, Rassekh CH, Kinsella JB, Segas J, Carrau RL, Hokanson JA. Osteosarcoma of the head and neck: meta-analysis of nonrandomized studies. Laryngoscope. 1997;107(1):56–61.

[24] Coindre JM, Trojani M, Contesso G, David M, Rouesse J, Bui NB, Bodaert A, De Mascarel I, De Mascarel A, Goussot JF. Reproducibility of a histopathologic grading system for adult soft tissue sarcoma. Cancer. 1986;58(2):306–309.

[25] Picci P, Sangiorgi L, Rougraff BT, Neff JR, Casadei R, Campanacci M. Relationship of chemotherapy-induced necrosis and surgical margins to local recurrence in osteosarcoma. J Clin Oncol. 1994;12(12):2699–2705.

[26] Mullen JT1, Hornicek FJ, Harmon DC, Raskin KA, Chen YL, Szymonifka J, Yeap BY, Choy E, DeLaney TF, Nielsen GP. Prognostic significance of treatment-induced pathologic necrosis in extremity and truncal soft tissue sarcoma after neoadjuvant chemoradiotherapy. Cancer. 2014;120(23):3676–3682.

[27] Colville RJ, James Colville R, Fraser C, Kelly CG, Nicoll JJ, McLean NR. Multidisciplinary management of head and neck sarcomas. Head Neck. 2005;27(9):814–824. doi:10.1002/hed.20232.

[28] DeLaney TF, Park L, Goldberg SI, Hug EB, Liebsch NJ, Munzenrider JE, Suit HD. Radiotherapy for local control of osteosarcoma. Int J Radiat Oncol Biol Phys. 2005; 61(2):492–498. doi:10.1016/j.ijrobp.2004.05.051.

[29] Mirabello L, Troisi RJ, Savage SA. International osteosarcoma incidence patterns in children and adolescents, middle ages and elderly persons. Int J Cancer. 2009;125(1):229–234. doi:10.1002/ijc.24320.

[30] Parkin DM, KramárováE, Draper GJ, Masuyer E, Michaelis J, Neglia J, Qureshi S, Stiller CA. International incidence of childhood cancer, Vol. 2. IARC Scientific Publications N°144, Lyon; 1998.

[31] Eyre R, Feltbower RG, Mubwandarikwa E, Eden TO, McNally RJ. Epidemiology of bone tumours in children and young adults. Pediatr Blood Cancer. 2009;53(6):941–952. doi:10.1002/pbc.22194.

[32] Shaikh AB, Li F, Li M, He B, He X, Chen G, Guo B, Li D, Jiang F, Dang L, Zheng S, Liang C, Liu J, Lu C, Liu B, Lu J, Wang L, Lu A, Zhang G. Present advances and future perspectives of molecular targeted therapy for osteosarcoma. Int J Mol Sci. 2016;17(4):506–526. doi:10.3390/ijms17040506.

[33] Herrmann A, Zöller J. Clinical features and treatment of osteogenic sarcoma of the jaws. Dtsch Z Mund Kiefer Gesichtschir. 1990;14(3):180–186.

[34] Chaudhary M, Chaudhary SD. Osteosarcoma of jaws. J Oral Maxillofac Pathol. 2012;16(2):233–238. doi:10.4103/0973-029X.99075.

[35] Fletcher CDM. WHO classification of tumours of soft tissue and bone. World Health Organization; 2013. Geneva.

[36] George A, Mani V. Gnathic osteosarcomas: review of literature and report of two cases in maxilla. J Oral Maxillofac Pathol.2011;15(2):138–143. doi:10.4103/0973-029X.84476.

[37] Paparella ML, Olvi LG, Brandizzi D, Keszler A, Santini-Araujo E, Cabrini RL. Osteosarcoma of the jaw: an analysis of a series of 74 cases. Histopathology. 2013;63(4):551–557. doi: 10.1111/his.12191.

[38] Mardinger O, Givol N, Talmi YP, Taicher S. Osteosarcoma of the jaw. The Chaim Sheba Medical Center experience. Oral Surg Oral Med Oral Pathol Oral Radiol Endod. 2001;91(4):445–451. doi:10.1067/moe.2001.112330.

[39] Argon A, Doğanavşargıl B, ÜnalYıldırım F, Sezak M, Midilli R, Öztop F. Osteosarcomas of jaw: experience of a single centre. J Plast Surg Hand Surg. 2015;49(1):13–18. doi:10.3109/2000656X.2014.909364.

[40] Yildiz FR, Avci A, Dereci O, Erol B, Celasun B, Gunhan O. Gnathic osteosarcomas, experience of four institutions from Turkey. Int J Clin Exp Pathol. 2014;7(6):2800–2808.

[41] Bennett JH, Thomas G, Evans AW, Speight PM. Osteosarcoma of the jaws: a 30-year retrospective review. Oral Surg Oral Med Oral Pathol Oral Radiol Endod. 2000;90(3):323–332.

[42] Nissanka EH, Amaratunge EAPD, Tilakaratne WM. Clinicopathological analysis of osteosarcoma of jaw bones. Oral Dis. 2007;13(1):82–87. doi:10.1111/j.1601-0825.2006.01251.x.

[43] Tabatabaei SH, Jahanshahi G, DehghanMarvasti F. Diagnostic challenges of low-grade central osteosarcoma of jaw: a literature review. J Dent. 2015;16(2):62–67.

[44] Puranik SR, Puranik RS, Ramdurg PK, Choudhary GRC. Parosteal osteosarcoma: report of a rare juxtacortical variant of osteosarcoma affecting the maxilla. J Oral Maxillofac Pathol. 2014;18(3):432–436. doi:10.4103/0973-029X.151340.

[45] Dujardin F, Binh MB, Bouvier C, Gomez-Brouchet A, Larousserie F, Muret Ad, Louis-Brennetot C, Aurias A, Coindre JM, Guillou L, Pedeutour F, Duval H, Collin C, de Pinieux G. MDM2 and CDK4 immunohistochemistry is a valuable tool in the differential diagnosis of low-grade osteosarcomas and other primary fibro-osseous lesions of the bone. Mod Pathol. 2011;24(5):624–637. doi:10.1038/modpathol.2010.229.

[46] Yoshida A, Ushiku T, Motoi T, Beppu Y, Fukayama M, Tsuda H, Shibata T. MDM2 and CDK4 immunohistochemical coexpression in high-grade osteosarcoma: correlation with a dedifferentiated subtype. Am J Surg Pathol. 2012;36(3):423–431. doi:10.1097/PAS.0b013e31824230d0.

[47] Tabareau-Delalande F, Collin C, Gomez-Brouchet A, Bouvier C, Decouvelaere AV, de Muret A, Pagès JC, de Pinieux G. Chromosome 12 long arm rearrangement covering MDM2 and RASAL1 is associated with aggressive craniofacial juvenile ossifying fibroma and extracranial psammomatoid fibro-osseous lesions. Mod Pathol. 2014;28(1):48–56. doi:10.1038/modpathol.2014.80.

[48] Guérin M, Thariat J, Ouali M, Bouvier C, Decouvelaere AV, Cassagnau E, Aubert S, Lepreux S, Coindre JM, Valmary-Degano S, Larousserie F, Meilleroux J, Projetti F, Stock N, Galant C, Marie B, Peyrottes I, de Pinieux G, Gomez-Brouchet A. A new subtype of high-grade mandibular osteosarcoma with RASAL1/MDM2 amplification. Hum Pathol. 2016;50:70–78. doi:10.1016/j.humpath.2015.11.012.

[49] Sorensen DM, Gokden M, El-Naggar A, Byers RM. Quiz case 1. Periosteal osteosarcoma (PO) of the mandible. Arch Otolaryngol Head Neck Surg. 2000;126(4):550–552.

[50] Anithabojan, Christy W, Chanmougananda S, Ashokan K. Osteosarcoma of mandible: a case report and review of literature. J Clin Diagn Res. 2012;6:753–757.

[51] Unni KK, Dahlin DC. Grading of bone tumors. Semin Diagn Pathol. 1984;1(3):165–172.

[52] Enneking WF. A system of staging musculoskeletal neoplasms. Clin Orthop Relat Res.1986;(204):9–24.

[53] TNM–Classification of malignant tumours - UICC - Seventh Edition 2009. John Wiley & Sons Ltd. UK.

[54] Gadwal SR, Gannon FH, Fanburg-Smith JC, Becoskie EM, Thompson LD. Primary osteosarcoma of the head and neck in pediatric patients: a clinicopathologic study of 22 cases with a review of the literature. Cancer. 2001;91(3):598–605.

[55] van den Berg H, Schreuder WH, de Lange J. Osteosarcoma: a comparison of Jaw versus Nonjaw Localizations and review of the literature. Sarcoma. 2013;2013:1–9. doi:10.1155/2013/316123.

[56] Lee RJ, Arshi A, Schwartz HC, Christensen RE. Characteristics and prognostic factors of osteosarcoma of the jaws: a retrospective cohort study. JAMA Otolaryngol Head Neck Surg. 2015;141(5):470–477. doi:10.1001/jamaoto.2015.0340.

[57] Mendenhall WM, Fernandes R, Werning JW, Vaysberg M, Malyapa RS, Mendenhall NP. Head and neck osteosarcoma. Am J Otolaryngol. 2011;32(6):597–600. doi:10.1016/j.amjoto.2010.09.002.

[58] deFries HO, Perlin E, Leibel SA. Treatment of osteogenic sarcoma of the mandible. Arch Otolaryngol Head Neck Surg. 1979;105(6):358–359.

[59] Geopfert H, Raymond AK, Spires JR. Osteosarcoma of the head and neck. Cancer Bull. 1990;42:347–354.

[60] Ferrari D, Codecà C, Battisti N, Broggio F, Crepaldi F, Violati M, Bertuzzi C, Dottorini L, Caldiera S, Luciani A, Moneghini L, Biglioli F, Cassinelli G, Morabito A, Foa P. Multimodality treatment of osteosarcoma of the jaw: a single institution experience. Med Oncol. 2014;31(9):171. doi:10.1007/s12032-014-0171-9.

[61] Picci P, Vanel D, Briccoli A, Talle K, Haakenaasen U, Malaguti C, Monti C, Ferrari C, Bacci G, Saeter G, Alvegard TA Computed tomography of pulmonary metastases from osteosarcoma: the less poor technique. A study of 51 patients with histological correlation. Ann Oncol. 2001;12(11):1601–1604.

[62] Benz MR, Tchekmedyian N, Eilber FC, Federman N, Czernin J, Tap WD. Utilization of positron emission tomography in the management of patients with sarcoma. Curr Opin Oncol. 2009;21(4):345–351. doi:10.1097/CCO.0b013e32832c95e2.

[63] The ESMO/European Sarcoma Network Working Group. Bone sarcomas: ESMO clinical practice guidelines for diagnosis, treatment and follow-up. Ann Oncol. 2012;23: vii100–vii109.

[64] Granados-Garcia M, Luna-Ortiz K, Castillo-Oliva HA, Villavicencio-Valencia V, Herrera-Gómez A, Mosqueda-Taylor A, Aguilar-Ponce JL, Poitevin-Chacón A. Free osseous and soft tissue surgical margins as prognostic factors in mandibular osteosarcoma. Oral Oncol. 2006;42(2):172–176. doi:10.1016/j.oraloncology.2005.06.027.

[65] Ketabchi A, Kalavrezos N, Newman L. Sarcomas of the head and neck: a 10-year retrospective of 25 patients to evaluate treatment modalities, function and survival. Br J Oral Maxillofac Surg. 2011;49(2):116–120. doi:10.1016/j.bjoms.2010.02.012.

[66] Chiapasco M, Biglioli F, Autelitano L, Romeo E, Brusati R. Clinical outcome of dental implants placed in fibula-free flaps used for the reconstruction of maxillo-mandibular defects following ablation for tumors or osteoradionecrosis. Clin Oral Implants Res. 2006;17(2):220–228. doi:10.1111/j.1600-0501.2005.01212.x.

[67] Soutar D, Scheker L, Tanner N, McGregor I. The radial forearm flap: a versatile method for intra-oral reconstruction. Br J Plast Surg. 1983;36(1):1–8.

[68] Swartz WM, Banis JC, Newton ED, Ramasastry SS, Jones NF, Acland R. The osteocutaneous scapular flap for mandibular and maxillary reconstruction. Plast Reconstr Surg. 1986;77(4):530–545.

[69] Taylor GI, Miller GD, Ham FJ. The free vascularized bone graft. A clinical extension of microvascular techniques. Plast Reconstr Surg. 1975;55(5):533–544.

[70] Hirsch DL, Garfein ES, Christensen AM, Weimer KA, Saddeh PB, Levine JP. Use of computer-aided design and computer-aided manufacturing to produce orthognathically ideal surgical outcomes: a paradigm shift in head and neck reconstruction. J Oral Maxillofac Surg. 2009;67(10):2115–2122. doi:10.1016/j.joms.2009.02.007.

[71] Thariat J, Julieron M, Brouchet A, Italiano A, Schouman T, Marcy PY, Odin G, Lacout A, Dassonville O, Peyrottes-Birstwisles I, Miller R, Thyss A, Isambert N. Osteosarcomas of the mandible: are they different from other tumor sites? Crit Rev Oncol Hematol. 2012;82(3):280–295. doi:10.1016/j.critrevonc.2011.07.001.

[72] Bai G, He D, Yang C, Lu C, Huang D, Chen M, Yuan J. Effect of digital template in the assistant of a giant condylar osteochondroma resection. J Craniofac Surg. 2014;25(3):e301–4. doi: 10.1097/SCS.0000000000000745.

[73] Coppen C, Weijs W, BergéSJ, Maal TJ. Oromandibular reconstruction using 3D planned triple template method. J Oral Maxillofac Surg. 2013;71(8):e243–e247. doi:10.1016/j.joms.2013.03.004.

[74] Yu H, Wang X, Zhang S, Zhang L, Xin P, Shen SG. Navigation-guided en bloc resection and defect reconstruction of craniomaxillary bony tumours. Int J Oral Maxillofac Surg. 2013;42(11):1409–1413. doi:10.1016/j.ijom.2013.05.011.

[75] Fernandes RP, Yetzer JG. Reconstruction of acquired oromandibular defects. Oral Maxillofac Surg Clin North Am. 2013;25(2):241–249. doi:10.1016/j.coms.2013.02.003.

[76] Ferreira JJ, Zagalo CM, Oliveira ML, Correia AM, Reis AR. Mandible reconstruction: history, state of the art and persistent problems. Prosthet Orthot Int. 2015;39(3):182–189. doi:10.1177/0309364613520032.

[77] Piombino P, Marenzi G, Dell'AversanaOrabona G, Califano L, Sammartino G. Autologous fat grafting in facial volumetric restoration. J Craniofac Surg. 2015;26(3):756–759. doi: 10.1097/SCS.0000000000001663.

[78] Herle P, Shukla L, Morrison WA, Shayan R. Preoperative radiation and free flap outcomes for head and neck reconstruction: a systematic review and meta-analysis. ANZ J Surg. 2015;85(3):121–127. doi:10.1111/ans.12888.

[79] Paderno A, Piazza C, Bresciani L, Vella R, Nicolai P. Microvascular head and neck reconstruction after (chemo)radiation: facts and prejudices. Curr Opin Otolaryngol Head Neck Surg. 2016;24(2):83–90. doi:10.1097/MOO.0000000000000243.

[80] Thampi S, Matthay KK, Goldsby R, DuBois SG. Adverse impact of regional lymph node involvement in osteosarcoma. Eur J Cancer. 2013;49(16):3471–3476. doi:10.1016/j.ejca.2013.06.023.

[81] Rao RS, Rao DN. Prognostic significance of the regional lymph nodes in osteosarcoma. J SurgOncol. 1977;9(2):123–130.

[82] Link MP, Goorin AM, Horowitz M, Meyer WH, Belasco J, Baker A, Ayala A, Shuster J. Adjuvant chemotherapy of high-grade osteosarcoma of the extremity: updated results of the multi-institutional osteosarcoma study. Clin Orthop Relat Res. 1991;(270):8–14.

[83] Bacci G, Avella M, Capanna R, Boriani S, Dallari D, Galletti S, Giunti A, Madon E, Mancini A, Mercuri M. Neoadjuvant chemotherapy in the treatment of osteosarcoma of the extremities: preliminary results in 131 cases treated preoperatively with methotrexate and cis-diamminoplatinum. Ital J Orthop Traumatol. 1988;14(1):23–39.

[84] Doval DC, Kumar RV, Kannan V, Sabitha KS, Misra S, Vijay Kumar M, Hegde P, Bapsy PP, Mani K, Shenoy AM, Kumarswamy SV. Osteosarcoma of the jaw bones. Br J Oral Maxillofac Surg. 1997;35(5):357–362.

[85] Granowski-LeCornu M, Chuang SK, Kaban LB, August M. Osteosarcoma of the jaws: factors influencing prognosis. J Oral Maxillofac Surg. 2011;69(9):2368–2375. doi:10.1016/j.joms.2010.10.023.

Section 5

Comparative Oncology

Chapter 13

A Dog in the Cancer Fight: Comparative Oncology in Osteosarcoma

Alexander L. Lazarides, Allison B. Putterman,
William C. Eward and Cindy Eward

Additional information is available at the end of the chapter

http://dx.doi.org/10.5772/66847

Abstract

Since the great Rudolf Virchow advised, "Between animal and human medicine there is no dividing line, nor should there be," limited attention has been paid to cancer in animals. This is finally changing thanks to a renewed focus on studying pet dogs with cancer. Unlike the laboratory mice who have been the mainstay of animal models of disease, pet dogs share an environment with their human owners, have an intact immune system, and often develop diseases spontaneously in ways that mimic their human counterparts. Osteosarcoma (OSA) – while uncommon in humans - is a common malignancy in dogs. This comparatively high incidence alone renders pet dogs an ideal "model" to conduct translational and clinical research into OSA. Indeed, there are many similarities between the two species with respect to this disease. However, owing to the shorter life span and accelerated disease progression, treatment effects can be assessed much more rapidly in canines than in humans. Overall, dogs represent a unique model to study OSA; this chapter aims to discuss the ways that comparative oncology between dogs and humans are being used from basic science research, to genetics and mechanisms of disease, to tumor biology and finally to developing novel treatments.

Keywords: canine, osteosarcoma, human, comparative oncology, novel treatments, genomic analysis

1. Introduction

Making meaningful advances in osteosarcoma (OSA) therapy has been hindered by the low incidence of the disease in humans. In contrast to the low incidence in humans, OSA is a common malignancy affecting pet dogs. While there are fewer than 1000 new human OSA diagnoses in the USA each year, there no fewer than 10,000 canine cases of OSA every year, by conservative assessments made several decades ago [1, 2]. This relatively high incidence in dogs provides an ideal "model" for conducting translational research and clinical research and for gaining insight into the biology of OSA. This paradigm depends upon canine OSA having specific parallels with human OSA. Indeed, there are many similarities between the two species with respect to this disease: from location of the primary tumors and patterns of metastasis, to the genetic drivers of disease and response to therapy [1]. Because canine OSA is a naturally occurring condition in pets who live alongside us, it arises among the same environmental, dietary and immunologic factors as human OSA. In addition to the similarities, there are several key differences that allow canine OSA to elucidate new information in shorter periods of time. Canine OSA typically displays a more aggressive biology and a much faster rate of metastasis than in humans, with death often occurring within 6 months and with 96% of canine OSA patients dying from the disease [3]. Because of these differences, treatment effects from novel interventions can be seen much more rapidly, with a fraction of the longevity and cost required of human clinical trials. Such comparative, cross-species trials conducted in dogs are often met with enthusiasm by owners and with fewer regulatory hindrances that would face human patients [4]. This field of cross-species cancer research is known as "comparative oncology." Dogs present to us a unique, powerful and underutilized model to study OSA; this chapter aims to demonstrate and discuss the ways that comparative oncology between dogs and humans with OSA can be used to inform genetics and mechanisms of disease, tumor biology and behavior and the development of novel treatments.

2. Canine osteosarcoma: overview

Osteosarcoma is the most common primary bone tumor in dogs [5–9]. It is estimated to occur in more than 10,000 dogs each year in the USA [1, 10]. This estimate is likely conservative, as the number of pet dogs has increased dramatically since these early studies of the incidence of canine OSA and there are still many dogs who do not receive medical attention. Canine OSA tends to occur in middle-aged to older dogs (median age of 7 years), with a small number of cases presenting between 18 and 24 months of age [11]. Primary rib OSA occurs in younger adult dogs with a mean age of 4.5–5.4 years [12, 13]. Historically, the incidence of OSA in dogs has been considered to be higher in males than females [3, 5–7, 11, 14]; however, more recent data suggest an equal sex distribution [15]. Large and giant breed dogs are predominantly affected. The breeds that are most at risk for OSA are Saint Bernard, Great Dane, Irish setter, Doberman pinscher, Rottweiler, German shepherd and golden retriever. Increased weight and, in particular, height appear to be the most predisposing factors [5–8, 11, 16–19]. Many domestic breeds have narrow genetic diversity due to selective breeding practices, which provides a unique opportunity to more clearly elucidate the hereditary basis of OSA in dogs [15, 20].

Approximately 75% of canine OSA occurs in the appendicular skeleton [6, 13]. Commonly affected sites, in order of frequency, include the distal radius, proximal humerus, distal ulna, distal femur, proximal tibia, distal tibia and diaphyseal ulna [21]. Primary OSA in the axial skeleton has also been well characterized, in order of frequency, in the mandible, maxilla, spine, cranium, ribs, nasal cavity and paranasal sinuses and pelvis [13]. As in humans, OSA of extraskeletal sites is rare but has been reported in the mammary tissue, subcutaneous tissue, spleen, bowel, liver, kidney, testicle, vagina, eye, gastric ligament, synovium, meninges and adrenal gland [22–28].

Dogs with appendicular OSA often present with lameness and swelling at the affected site. There may be a history of mild trauma prior to the onset of lameness and this may cause an acute exacerbation of clinical signs [15, 21]. The signs associated with axial skeletal OSA are site dependent and vary from localized swelling, dysphagia (oral sites), exophthalmos and pain on opening the mouth (caudal mandibular and ocular sites), facial deformity and nasal discharge (sinus and nasal cavity sites) and hyperesthesia with or without neurologic signs (spinal sites) [15]. Dogs with rib OSA often present because of a palpable mass [15].

3. Genetic factors

Development of canine OSA is characterized by the involvement of sporadic and heritable genetic factors. The most thoroughly described gene mutations in dogs are the *p53* and phosphatase and tensin homolog (*PTEN*) tumor suppressor genes and abnormalities in the *Rb* family members, *Rb*, p107 and p130. Approximately 60% of canine OSA cell lines overexpress mutant *p53* mRNA and protein, which correlates with the presence of missense point mutations within the DNA-binding domain [29]. These findings are corroborated by the identification of mutations in *p53* in 41% of spontaneously arisen OSA tumors. The majority of mutations in these cases were point mutations (74%), with a lesser percentage of mutations being deletions (26%). In the absence of a functional *p53* protein, its transcriptional target, *mdm2*, is not present to destabilize the mutant *p53* protein and mutant *p53* protein accumulates within the cell [30]. Studies have suggested that the RB gene signaling pathway is dysregulated in canine OSA. Analysis of OSA samples identified copy number loss in 29% of cases, resulting in correlative reduction or the absence of RB protein expression in 62% of samples tested [31]. These findings suggest that aberrations in the RB gene likely participate in formation and/or progression of OSA. In addition to *p53* and RB gene abnormalities, genomic loss of the phosphatase and tensin homolog (*PTEN*) tumor suppressor gene is suspected to participate in the genetic pathogenesis of canine OSA. In vitro studies with canine OSA cell lines found that 60% of the cell lines had mutations in *PTEN*, resulting in the absence of gene transcription and protein translation [29].

4. Diagnostic work-up: local disease

The diagnostic evaluation for dogs with OSA is similar to that employed in humans. Initial evaluation of the primary site involves radiographs. Lesions are typically characterized by a mixed pattern of cortical lysis and periosteal proliferation; however, the appearance of OSA can be quite variable. Commonly observed features include cortical lysis, soft tissue extension with soft tissue swelling and new bone (tumor or reactive) formation. Primary lesions are typically monostotic. Based on signalment (patient-specific factors such as breed, sex, age, etc.), history, physical examination and radiographic findings, a presumptive diagnosis of OSA may be made. Cytology may support a tentative diagnosis. In most cases, a definitive diagnosis is made via histopathology. Bone biopsy is performed prior to pursuing treatment. Samples can be obtained via open incisional, closed-needle, or trephine biopsy techniques. In some cases, repeated biopsy attempts yield "reactive bone," making it very difficult to obtain the diagnosis preoperatively. Histopathology is performed after tumor removal (amputation or limb sparing) to confirm the preoperative diagnosis. **Figure 1** summarizes the elements of the diagnostic work-up of OSA in canines.

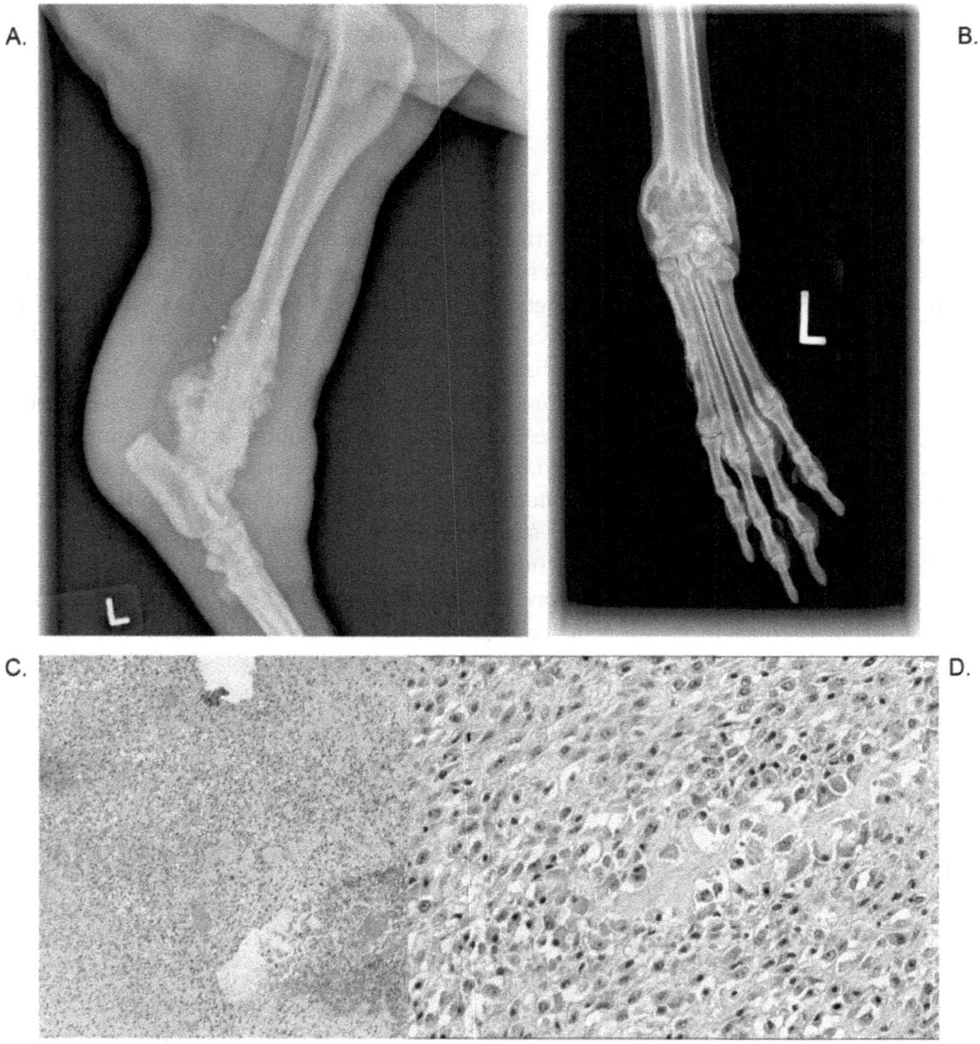

Figure 1. Examples of canine osteosarcoma. (A) and (B) Typical radiographic findings including ill-defined lesions with aggressive periosteal reaction and tumor matrix ossification. (C) and (D) High-grade, highly pleomorphic cells with surrounding osteoid.

http://dx.doi.org/10.5772/66847

5. Diagnostic work-up: metastatic disease

Approximately 10% of dogs will have gross evidence of metastatic disease at diagnosis. Fewer than 15% of cases have detectable pulmonary metastasis and less than 8% have metastasis to other musculoskeletal sites. Three view thoracic radiographs are recommended to evaluate for pulmonary metastasis; however, metastases cannot be detected radiographically until the nodules are 6–8 mm in diameter. This underscores the belief that in dogs, as with humans, the presence of metastatic disease on presentation is likely underappreciated. Advanced imaging (e.g., CT, MRI, PET/CT) may be used for patient staging [32, 33]. A thorough orthopedic examination with palpation of long bones and the accessible axial skeleton is necessary to evaluate for sites of bony metastasis. Bone survey radiographs, including lateral views of all bones in the body and a ventrodorsal projection of the pelvis, have been useful in detecting second skeletal sites of OSA [34]. Whereas whole-body bone scans are standard in human medicine, there are conflicting reports on the utility of nuclear scintigraphy for clinical staging of dogs with OSA [35–39]. It can be useful for detection and localization of bone metastasis in dogs presenting for vague lameness or signs of back pain. Although it is a very sensitive imaging modality, it is not specific for identifying skeletal tumors.

6. Prognostic factors

Tumor size, determined as an actual tumor volume or the percentage of bone length affected by tumor, has been found to be a prognostic indicator in dogs. Large tumors have been found to have a poorer prognosis [11, 27, 40, 41]. Tumor location is also a prognostic factor. In general, tumors of the mandible and scapula carry the most favorable prognosis. Other than the mandible and scapula, tumors of the axial skeleton carry a poor prognosis with survival times often less than 6 months. Tumors of the appendicular skeleton are intermediate in prognosis. Specifically, tumors of the appendicular skeleton (radius, ulna, humerus, femur and tibia) are associated with a median survival time of 1 year when treated with aggressive surgery and chemotherapy [21]. Median disease-free intervals (DFIs) and disease- free survival (DFS) times for skull OSA are 191 days and 204 days, respectively. In one study, dogs with mandibular OSA treated with mandibulectomy alone had a 1-year survival rate of 71% [18]. Dogs with maxillary OSA have been found to have a median survival time of 5 months following maxillectomy [42, 43]. A study of orbital OSA reported long-term survival following complete surgical excision [44]. Median survival time for dogs with rib OSA is reported to be 3 months for cases treated with rib resection alone and 8 months for cases treated with resection and adjuvant chemotherapy [45–48]. DFI and median survival time in dogs with scapula OSA was 210 days and 246 days, respectively, with the use of adjuvant chemotherapy increasing DFI and survival time [49]. Survival time of dogs with OSA distal to the antebrachiocarpal (equivalent of human wrist) or tarsocrural joints (human ankle) has a median survival time of 466 days, which is longer than the survival time of dogs with OSA of more common appendicular sites. However, OSA of these sites is aggressive, with a high potential for metastasis [50]. Extraskeletal OSA has an aggressive systemic behavior with a high metastatic rate, with short median survival times ranging from 1 month to 5 months [27, 28].

As in humans, elevated alkaline phosphatase (ALP) has been associated with a poorer prognosis for dogs with appendicular OSA [27, 51–54]. A preoperative elevation of either serum ALP or the bone isoenzyme of ALP (>110 U/L or 23 U/L, respectively) is associated with a shorter disease-free interval and survival. Dogs that have elevated preoperative values that do not return to normal within 40 days following surgical removal of the primary tumor also develop earlier metastasis. At least one study has suggested that tumor grade, characterized by degree of necrosis, mitotic rate and cell differentiation, is also highly prognostic, with higher grade tumors having shorter survival times and disease-free intervals [55].

7. Treatment

Cure is achieved in fewer than 15% of dogs diagnosed with OSA. For the most effective management, multimodality therapy is required to address both local and systemic disease. Amputation, limb-sparing surgeries, as well as nonsurgical techniques, such as stereotactic radiation therapy (SRT), are highly effective for management of local disease (contrary to management of OSA in humans, in which radiation therapy is rarely used). Amputation is the standard local treatment for appendicular OSA and readily allows for adequate surgical margins. It is well tolerated in dogs and offers significant improvement in pain relief and survival relative to palliative treatment. Pelvic tumors are treated with amputation and hemipelvectomy and these patients generally have good levels of function. Rib tumors are treated with thoracic wall resection; mandibular tumors are treated with hemimandibulectomy and maxillary tumors are treated with partial maxillectomy and/or orbitectomy. Limb salvage surgery, most commonly using bone allografts or metal endoprostheses, can be performed in some dogs with appendicular OSA. The most suitable patients for limb salvage are dogs with tumors in the distal radius or ulna [15], but tumors of the scapula, diaphyseal radius and ulna, metacarpus, metatarsus, diaphyseal humerus, femur and tibia and distal tibia have also been treated with limb salvage surgery [21]. Limb function following limb salvage surgery is found to be good to excellent in most dogs and survival is not adversely affected by removing the primary tumor with marginal resection. Intraoperative radiation therapy and extracorporeal intraoperative RT (IORT) have also been utilized in a small number of canine OSA patients. Stereotactic radiation therapy (SRT) is a nonsurgical alternative method which is used on an increasingly common basis for facilitating canine limb salvage. This technique can provide adequate local control of disease in the context of a life expectancy for dogs that is almost always shorter than 2 years, even with systemic therapy.

Although amputation and limb-sparing surgeries, as well as nonsurgical techniques such as SRT, have proved highly effective for management of local disease, the ability to control the progression of OSA metastases remains a clinical challenge. Systemic chemotherapy is the essential component for management of OSA metastases. Protocols that have shown significant improvement in survival include doxorubicin, cisplatin and carboplatin, with medial survival times of approximately 1 year [18, 40, 56, 57]. Lobaplatin has also been used but provides a median survival time of 7 months [21]. No survival advantage has been found when using combination chemotherapy. Despite the aggressive treatment approach, more than 50%

of dogs do not live beyond 1 year postamputation and 90% die of disease by 2 years [15]. Further research is needed for discovering effective new combination therapies for improving the long-term prognosis of canine OSA.

8. The dog as a "model" of osteosarcoma

A number of animal models of OSA exist; however, the reliance upon mouse models of OSA has limitations. The canine "model" of spontaneously occurring OSA offers several advantages over non-spontaneous models. It is often described as a "model" (emphasis on quotation marks) because for these patients and their owners; it is not a model at all—they are being treated for a pathologic condition. Naturally occurring OSA in dogs better represents the biological complexity and heterogeneity of the disease than traditional rodent models and, as such, shares a wide variety of epidemiologic and clinical features with human OSA [58]. Genetically, there are far more similarities between dogs and humans than between rodents and humans [59]. Pet dogs share a living environment with humans and are subsequently exposed to many of the same environmental risk factors that contribute to the occurrence of solid tumors in humans. Additionally, tumors in canines occur in the context of intact immune systems, allowing for a better representation of immunologic influence on cancer progression and spread [4]. These tumors are further characterized by high levels of heterogeneity between individuals and between tumors; this heterogeneity is often lacking in traditional models. They also demonstrate the capacity for the development of local recurrence, resistance to treatment and distant metastases, typically to the lungs, just as these tumors do in human patients. **Table 1** summarizes the key similarities and differences between human and canine osteosarcoma. **Figure 2** summarizes the diagnostic work-up for human osteosarcoma.

An important power nestled in the study of canine OSA lies in the concept of linkage disequilibrium and the breed structure of canines [61]. Approximately two centuries ago, the practice of selecting canines for certain morphological and behavioral traits grew in popularity, paving the path for modern dog breeds. An unforeseen side effect of breeding was the selection of certain "founder" mutations linked to certain breed-specific traits and diseases. This is seen today in the form of certain breed showing a predilection for species-specific diseases, with the practical result of this "founder" effect being an overall loss of heterogeneity among genes and diseases. Linkage equilibrium is present to a significantly higher degree in canines as compared to humans, making individual breed analysis a strong tool for broad-spectrum genetic mapping [61, 62]. When comparing similar traits between breeds, fine mapping may also be performed, thus making canine models of spontaneously occurring OSA a powerful model for identifying the genetic origins of this disease.

Perhaps, the greatest shortcoming from studying human OSA is the relatively low incidence of the disease. Therapeutics must be evaluated over the course of several years and studies face the challenge of reaching statistically significant power. A solution to this particular challenge is available in the form of cross-species analysis of canine OSA. Canine OSA has an incidence on the order of at least tenfold greater than human OSA [62]. In addition to this significantly larger patient population, dogs also have a shorter life span with faster progression of disease and a shorter period of survival relative to humans [1]. Thus, the collection of data and the evaluation of novel treatments may be carried out more rapidly in dogs than in humans. Although the more rapid life course in dogs is not surprising, as life spans generally decrease along with species size, the reason for poorer outcomes in dogs with OSA is more puzzling. Whether this represents a fundamental difference in treatment (systemic therapy in dogs is relatively less aggressive on a dosage basis) or in disease, biology is not known. Whatever the reason for the difference in survival, the combination of increased patient numbers, time-compressed progression of disease, genetic similarities and spontaneous tumor origin within a natural environmental and immunologic background renders canine OSA an ideal model in which to study the disease.

Variable	Canine	Human
Incidence	>10,000 cases per year	<1000 cases per year
Median age of onset	Middle-aged to older dogs Peak onset 7–9 years Second small peak at 18–24 months	Bimodal disease with peak onset 10–14 years Second peak at >65 years
Race/breed	Large or giant breed Increased height and weight Increased risk in Saint Bernard, Great Dane, Irish setter, Doberman pinscher, Rottweiler, German shepherd, golden retriever	Slightly more common in African Americans and Hispanics
Primary site	75% appendicular skeleton Metaphyseal region of long bones Distal radius > proximal humerus > distal ulna > distal femur > proximal tibia > distal tibia > diaphyseal ulna	90% appendicular skeleton Metaphyseal region of long bones Distal femur > proximal tibia > proximal humerus
Metastatic sites	10% of cases with metastasis at diagnosis Lung > bone > soft tissues	20% of cases with metastasis at diagnosis Lung > bone > soft tissues
Molecular and genetic players	*p53* *Rb* *PTEN* *RTK* *MET* *STAT3*	*p53* *Rb* *PTEN* *RTK* *MET* *STAT3*
Treatment	Amputation Limb-sparing techniques Adjuvant chemotherapy	Neoadjuvant chemotherapy Limb-sparing techniques Amputation (rare)
Survival	~50% survival at 1 year with chemotherapy, 10% at 2 years	60–80% survival at 5 years with chemotherapy
Prognostic factors	Tumor size Tumor location (distal more favorable than proximal) Proximal humeral location Metastasis at diagnosis Serum alkaline phosphatase Response to chemotherapy	Tumor size Tumor location (distal more favorable than proximal) Proximal humeral location Metastasis at diagnosis Serum alkaline phosphatase Serum lactate dehydrogenase Response to chemotherapy

Table 1. Comparison of human and canine osteosarcoma.

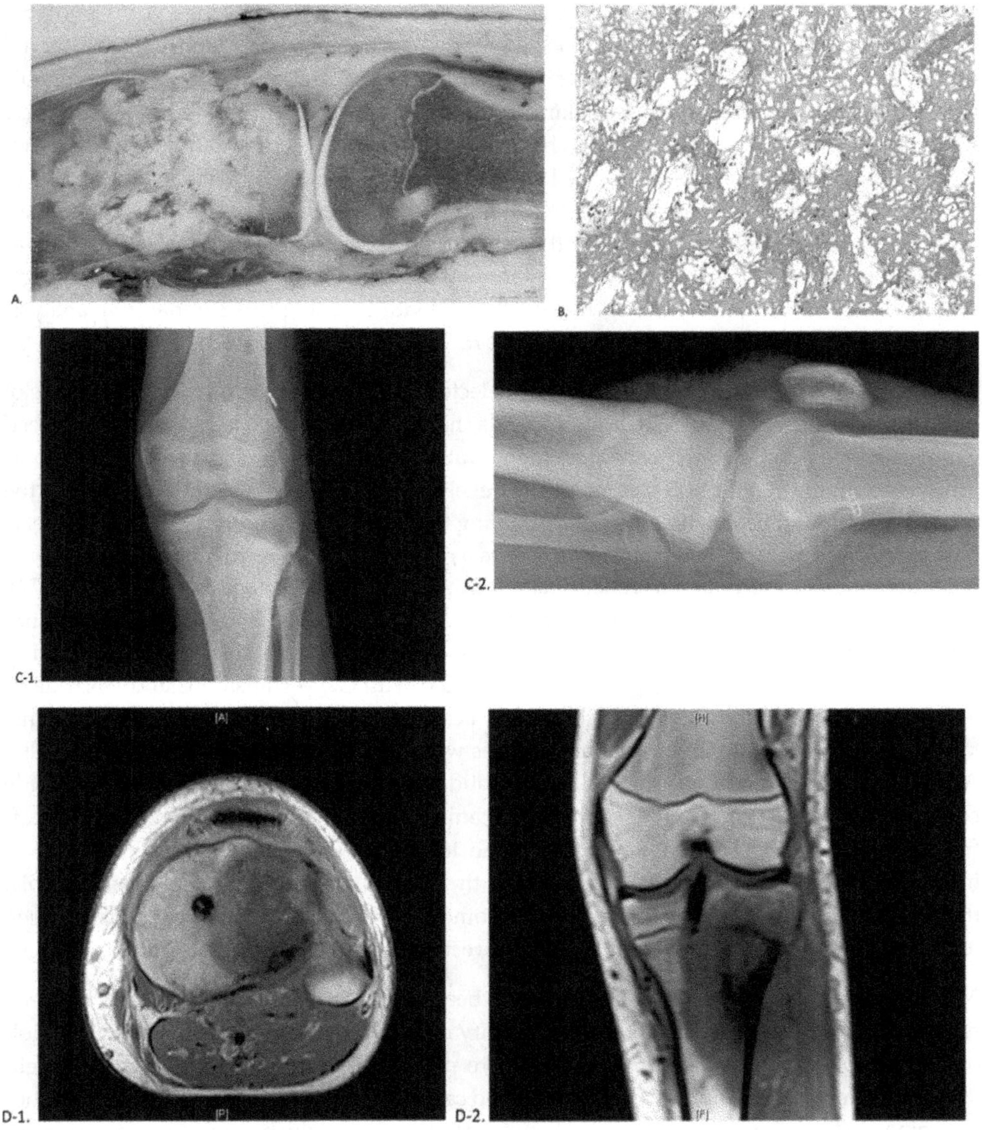

Figure 2. (A) Gross histology demonstrating a destructive osseous lesion with an associated soft tissue mass, (B) high-grade cellular lesion with a trabecular pattern and osteoid production, (C) radiographic findings demonstrating increased sclerosis, with a large periosteal reaction, and (D) MRI images demonstrating cortical destruction and a large soft tissue mass (images collected with permission) [60].

9. Elucidating the genetic origins of osteosarcoma

The genetic and molecular origins of OSA remain poorly understood. Any given tumor may demonstrate tremendous genetic variation and complexity, characterized by abnormal genetic structural and copy number changes, irregular karyotypes and gross aneuploidy, making elucidation of common pathways more difficult [31, 63, 64]. Dogs with spontaneously occurring OSA present a unique alternative to humans for identifying conserved genetic drivers of OSA. The dog genome was mapped a decade ago and is publicly accessible via the CanFam genome browser, making genetic comparisons with the humans relatively simple [59, 65, 66]. Early genetic studies have demonstrated that canine and human OSAs are virtually indistinguishable. A study by Paoloni et al. used parallel oligonucleotide arrays to compare OSA expression signatures between human and canine samples; interestingly, hierarchical clustering could not segregate the samples by species of origin [67]. Studies such as this demonstrate the tremendous capacity for genomic analysis using comparative oncology; a number of shared molecular targets have been identified using this comparative analysis between canines and humans, including *RTK MET*, *STAT3* and others [68–72].

The breeding of dogs has created artificially selected and refined gene pools. Some breeds of dog, such as Rottweilers and Irish wolfhounds, have also developed a reduced intra-breed genetic diversity and disproportionately higher rates of OSA [17, 73]. This presents an opportunity to examine genetic risk factors for the development of OSA. One study examining the Scottish deerhound used whole-genome mapping to find a linkage for the OSA phenotype. A novel locus was identified on chromosome 34 in a region homologous to human chromosome 3q26, demonstrating a potential genetic basis for the disease in both canines and humans [74]. Another study examined the molecular profiles of dogs with OSA in order to identify subtypes and stratify this disease based on gene expression profiling and its biological behavior. This study was able to identify groupings associated with G2/M transitions and DNA damage checkpoints that correlated with biological activity; additionally, these groupings translated to orthologous human molecular subtypes with similar biological activity [75]. Finally, Angstadt et al. used high-resolution oligonucleotide assays to identify common genome-wide copy number aberrations in both human and canine samples of OSA [76]. Their study reaffirmed a number of known aberrant genes and identified several new genes in regions of instability pointing toward possible players in the genetic origin of OSA. Taken as a whole, these studies demonstrate the capacity for genome-wide analysis and comparisons between dogs and humans to identify possible genetic precursors and drivers of OSA.

Numerous somatic genetic similarities have been identified as a commonality between human and canine OSA, which may help identify new and important insights into OSA biology. *p53* and *RB1*, tumor suppressor genes, are possibly two of the best-known and well-described genetic aberrations in both human and canine OSA. With *p53*, genetic abnormalities in canine OSA are typically the result of missense mutations, which result in an overexpression of this gene and are present in 41–67% of primary OSA tumors [29, 30, 77]. While *p53* is often mutated in primary cases of human OSA, it is found at a much lower rate, with only about 20% of cases showing this abnormality [78]; unlike canine OSA, mutations in the *p53* gene in humans are often point mutations [30]. *RB1* is a genetic abnormality that is common in human forms of OSA, estimated to be present in 30–75% of cases [79]. While initial studies questioned the putative role of *RB1*, more recent studies indicate that mutations of this gene are present in 29% of cases of OSA, typically resulting in a reduction or complete absence of the gene product [31, 80]. *PTEN* is another tumor suppressor gene that has been implicated in both human and canine OSA. Early findings in canine OSA cell lines implicated *PTEN* deletions and a reduction in gene expression in the development of this cancer [29]; this was confirmed using a comparative genomic hybridization (CGH) genomic analysis in primary canine OSA, which found that *PTEN* mutations were present in 30–42% of tumors examined [31, 76]. Human studies have similarly identified *PTEN* as a common mutation present in primary cases of OSA [81].

10. Advances in surgical technique and adjunct therapy

10.1. Surgical and medical therapy for canine osteosarcoma parallels human therapy

There are a number of similarities in systemic therapy and surgical management between human and canine OSA. In both patient populations, en bloc surgical resection, in combination with chemotherapy, is the mainstay of treatment; the addition of either neoadjuvant or adjuvant chemotherapy has further improved survival rates and is now also considered a part of standard of care. Most dogs are treated with adjuvant—rather than neoadjuvant—chemotherapy, as there is less data in dogs regarding the prognostic value of histopathologic response to therapy.

Pioneering of limb-sparing techniques in the surgical treatment of OSA was initially conducted in dogs. One of the early studies of the potential role of limb salvage in canine patients with OSA was conducted by LaRue et al. [82]. This study found that limb salvage in addition to multimodality therapy could represent a viable alternative to amputation in the management of certain patients. A subsequent study by Withrow et al. [83] similarly studied the role of limb salvage surgery as an option in the management of OSA. Forty-nine dogs with limb-sparing resection for OSA of the extremity were followed and stratified by the addition of chemotherapy or chemotherapy with radiation therapy. As in humans, outcomes were significantly linked to percent necrosis, which was improved by a combination of chemotherapy with radiation therapy. Higher rates of tumor necrosis resulted in higher overall survival and better outcomes. The breadth of this data is not as extensive in dogs as it is in humans and the paradigm of chemotherapy/surgery/chemotherapy has not become normative in dogs. Despite similarities in overall survival between amputation and limb-sparing surgery, a significant issue with limb salvage in both canines and humans has been the inadequacy of functional outcomes and the prevalence of postoperative complications. A study by Kuntz et al. [84] examined 17 patients with OSA of the proximal humerus undergoing limb salvage surgery using frozen humeral allografts. As expected, completeness of margins significantly impacted the overall rates of survival, with incomplete margins resulting in an eightfold higher rate of distant metastases. As in humans, when comparing limb salvage with amputation, there was no statistically significant difference in overall survival. However, postoperative functional outcomes and rates of complications were deemed to be unacceptable. Only 12% of patients had good or excellent outcomes with many of the dogs treated with limb salvage suffering from biomechanical failure of their mechanical constructs and 41% of patients receiving limb salvage surgery required conversion to amputation. A retrospective study of human OSA by Rougraff et al. found limb salvage demonstrated similar outcomes with respect to disease-free survival and overall survival when local control via limb salvage is compared to local control via amputation [85]. This has similarly been borne out in canine OSA [18].

The addition of chemotherapy to the management of OSA has dramatically improved outcomes and become a mainstay of treatment for both dogs and humans with OSA. The overall survival of dogs treated with amputation is significantly improved by the addition of chemotherapy. In addition to the previously mentioned studies conducted by LaRue et al. and Withrow et al. [82, 83], 30 dogs with appendicular OSA were evaluated in a study evaluating overall survival rates when treated with and without the addition of cisplatin [86]. Mean survival time was 190 days for patients treated with amputation alone; mean survival time improved to 315 days with the addition of cisplatin. Similar results were found in a study by Berg et al. [56], which examined 22 dogs with appendicular OSA treated with surgical resection with and without the addition of cisplatin. They found a statistically significant increase in survival with the addition cisplatin to surgical management. Interestingly, there was no survival difference between chemotherapy in addition to amputation and limb-sparing surgery, though the cohort numbers were likely too low to draw significant results in this regard. Thesis parallels in the medical and surgical management of OSA across species contribute to canine OSA being particularly well suited in comparison with humans undergoing similar treatment [87–89].

10.2. Novel therapeutics and immunotherapies

Canine models have been an important avenue by which to examine novel therapeutic strategies for OSA. With the advent of intra-arterial chemotherapy, randomized control trials were conducted in dogs with spontaneously occurring OSA to evaluate the safety, efficacy and feasibility of this method of delivery in the treatment of OSA [82]. With the advent of intra-arterial chemotherapy, randomized control trials were conducted in canines with spontaneously occurring OSA to evaluate the safety, efficacy and feasibility of this method of delivery in the treatment of OSA [83]. Similarly, dose escalation studies conducted in canines with OSA have allowed for optimization of chemotherapeutic drug delivery in humans. In a study by Paoloni et al., a phase I dose-escalation study was conducted with rapamycin delivery in canines with the simultaneous collection of multiple pre- and posttreatment biopsies and whole blood sampling to establish efficacy and ideal drug pharmacokinetic time points, data that would have been more challenging to collect in human patients [90]. These insights were translated into a human clinical trial of rapamycin, allowing for a better understanding of dosing and efficacy of the drug [91, 92]. These studies allowed optimization of the dose and delivery of chemotherapy in humans with OSA while allowing for earlier screening of treatments that may have a less than favorable therapeutic index before being tested in humans [93, 94]. Beyond cytotoxicity and optimization studies, canines with OSA have also served as the ideal models for identifying and evaluating novel therapeutics.

Early insights into the role of the immune system in OSA disease progression came about by happenstance while studying canine OSA. While studying outcomes in canines undergoing the combination of limb salvage and chemotherapy, Lascelles et al. found that postoperative infection significantly improved survival [95]. These findings were also recapitulated in humans, as a study by Jeys et al. demonstrated; humans with deep infection following limb salvage for OSA experienced a 35% increase in overall survival rate [96, 97]. These survival benefits were hypothesized to be related to an upregulation in the natural antitumoral activity of the host immune system. This has inspired new investigations into the specific role of the immune system in OSA and the ways in which cancer suppresses the natural immune response. Analysis of canines with and without OSA has identified myeloid-derived suppressor cells (MDSCs) and regulatory T cells (Tregs) that may play a role in suppression of the natural antitumor response of the host [98, 99]. These cells normally function to prevent the antitumoral response from overaction and resultant autoimmunity. Suppressing these cells has been hypothesized as a means of promoting the antitumoral response to improve outcomes in OSA. Although some have associated increased ratios of Tregs with poorer outcomes in canine OSA [100], there remain questions as to whether Treg levels are actually different from healthy controls [99]. MDSCs have also been found to be overrepresented in canine OSA, as demonstrated in two studies by Sherger et al. and Goulart et al. [101, 102]. Similar to Tregs, the role of MDSCs in OSA remains unclear, though increased monocyte counts have been associated with worse outcomes and decreased rates of DFS [103, 104]. Despite the ambiguity surrounding their potential role in OSA progression, Tregs and MDSCs highlight the potential for immune targets in the treatment of OSA.

Immunotherapy for sarcoma is an exciting new field of cancer treatment currently being investigated in both humans and canines. One such agent, liposomal muramyl tripeptide phosphatidylethanolamine (L-MTP-PE), had its first success demonstrated in dogs with spontaneously occurring OSA. This synthetic molecule is an analog of a bacterial cell wall component and a potent activator of monocytes/macrophages. It can be incorporated into liposomes and has been shown to selectively induce monocytes to kill tumor cells [105]. In a study of 40 dogs receiving standard therapy with surgery and cisplatin, canines were randomized to receive the addition of either L-MTP-PE or a placebo. Patients receiving L-MTP-PE had significantly better rates of overall survival as compared to placebo [106]. This study has translated to human pediatric patients with OSA as well, with results indicating L-MTP-PE as a possible adjunct in the repertoire of treatments available for OSA [107, 108].

While immunotherapy is an exciting realm of novel therapeutics in canines with OSA, the canine model is equally beneficial in evaluating the safety and efficacy of a variety of novel therapeutics and novel applications of existing therapies [109]. One such application is the use of aerosolized delivery of chemotherapeutics for pulmonary metastases, which has made significant progress thanks to research conducted in dogs with OSA. A translational study by Rodriguez et al. examined the effect of aerosol delivery of gemcitabine to pulmonary metastasis in dogs with OSA [110]. This study demonstrated an increased in Fas expression and increased rates of apoptosis in pulmonary metastases. Cross-species drug development using canines as a model for human OSA has also been suggested for targets including genetic abnormalities (*TP53* and murine double minute-2), growth factors (c-MET and mTOR), angiogenesis (VEGF and HIF-1a) and metastasis (membrane-type-1 matrix metalloproteinase) [23, 54, 90, 111–116].

11. Conclusion: challenges and limitations

OSA remains a challenging diagnosis with little change in the prognosis for several decades. Recognizing the utility of studying animals with diseases shared by humans, Rudolf Virchow stated in the mid-nineteenth century, "Between animal and human medicine there is no dividing line, nor should there be." Yet despite a desperate need to investigate OSA in greater numbers and scope, dogs with naturally occurring OSA were not seriously studied until the late twentieth century. Man's best friend provides us an opportunity to study one of our most dreaded diagnoses in larger numbers than we could ever hope to study in humans alone. With similar disease features and treatment algorithms, research may be carried out in dogs in a more facile manner than in humans. Continuing to expand our understanding and awareness of canine, OSA will be a critical step in developing novel and better therapeutic strategies.

Several challenges do remain [93]. While canine models show an accelerated disease progression as compared to humans, this timeline is still significantly longer than murine models. While funding for mouse models of cancer is widespread, funding for the investigation of canine cancer remains sparse. Some novel therapies, such as species-specific antibodies and proteins, may not translate from canines to humans and vice versa. Finally, regulatory oversight and ethical care mandate that some study designs are simply not feasible in pets. Despite these limitations, this review demonstrates that canines are an ideal—and underutilized—model to deepen our understanding of osteosarcoma and to translate exciting developments from the laboratory into the clinic.

Author details

Alexander L. Lazarides[1*], Allison B. Putterman[2], William C. Eward[1,3] and Cindy Eward DVM[4]

*Address all correspondence to: alexander.lazarides@duke.edu

1 Department of Orthopaedic Surgery, Duke University Medical Center, Durham, NC, USA

2 Veterinary Specialty Hospital of the Carolinas, NC, USA

3 College of Veterinary Medicine, North Carolina State University, NC, USA

4 Triangle Veterinary Referral Hospital, Durham, NC, USA

References

[1] Withrow SJ, Powers BE, Straw RC, Wilkins RM. Comparative aspects of osteosarcoma. Dog versus man. Clin Orthop Relat Res. 1991(270):159-68.

[2] Mirabello L, Troisi RJ, Savage SA. Osteosarcoma incidence and survival rates from 1973 to 2004: data from the Surveillance, Epidemiology, and End Results Program. Cancer. 2009;115(7):1531-43.

[3] Spodnick GJ, Berg J, Rand WM, Schelling SH, Couto G, Harvey HJ, et al. Prognosis for dogs with appendicular osteosarcoma treated by amputation alone: 162 cases (1978–1988). J Am Vet Med Assoc. 1992;200(7):995-9.

[4] Khanna C, Lindblad-Toh K, Vail D, London C, Bergman P, Barber L, et al. The dog as a cancer model. Nature Biotechnol. 2006;24(9):1065-6.

[5] Brodey RS, Mc GJ, Reynolds H. A clinical and radiological study of canine bone neoplasms. I. J Am Vet Med Assoc. 1959;134(2):53-71.

[6] Brodey RS, Riser WH. Canine osteosarcoma. A clinicopathologic study of 194 cases. Clin Orthop Relat Res. 1969;62:54-64.

[7] Brodey RS, Sauer RM, Medway W. Canine bone neoplasms. J Am Vet Med Assoc. 1963;143:471-95.

[8] Dorfman SK, Hurvitz AI, Patnaik AK. Primary and secondary bone tumours in the dog. J Small Anim Pract. 1977;18(5):313-26.

[9] Ling G, Morgan J, Pool R. Primary bone rumors in the dog: a combined clinical, radiographic, and histologic approach to early diagnosis. J Am Vet Med Assoc. 1974;165(1):55.

[10] Priester WA, McKay FW. The occurrence of tumors in domestic animals. Natl Cancer Inst Monogr. 1980(54):1-210.

[11] Misdorp W, Hart A. Some prognostic and epidemiologic factors in canine osteosarcoma. J Natl Cancer Inst. 1979;62(3):537-45.

[12] Feeney DA, Johnston GR, Grindem CB, Toombs JP, Caywood DD, Hanlon GF. Malignant neoplasia of canine ribs: clinical, radiographic, and pathologic findings. J Am Vet Med Assoc. 1982;180(8):927-33.

[13] Heyman SJ, Diefenderfer DL, Goldschmidt MH, Newton CD. Canine axial skeletal osteosarcoma. A retrospective study of 116 cases (1986 to 1989). Vet Surg. 1992;21(4):304-10.

[14] Misdorp W. Skeletal osteosarcoma. Animal model: canine osteosarcoma. Am J Pathol. 1980;98(1):285-8.

[15] Ehrhart NP, Ryan SD, Fan TM. Tumors of the skeletal system. Small Anim Clin Oncol, 5th ed. 2013:463-503.

[16] Alexander JW, Patton CS. Primary tumors of the skeletal system. Vet Clin North Am Small Anim Pract. 1983;13(1):181-95.

[17] Ru G, Terracini B, Glickman LT. Host related risk factors for canine osteosarcoma. Vet J. 1998;156(1):31-9.

[18] Straw RC, Withrow SJ. Limb-sparing surgery versus amputation for dogs with bone tumors. Vet Clin North Am Small Anim Pract. 1996;26(1):135-43.

[19] Wolke RE, Nielsen SW. Site incidence of canine osteosarcoma. J Small Anim Pract. 1966;7(7):489-92.

[20] Fenger JM, London CA, Kisseberth WC. Canine osteosarcoma: a naturally occurring disease to inform pediatric oncology. ILAR J. 2014;55(1):69-85.

[21] Kuntz CA. Appendix B: canine osteosarcoma, In: Malawer MM and Sugarbaker PH (eds). Muscoloskeletal cancer surgery – treatment of sarcomas and allied diseases. Springer Publishers. 2001:603-7.

[22] Patnaik AK. Canine extraskeletal osteosarcoma and chondrosarcoma: a clinicopathologic study of 14 cases. Vet Pathol. 1990;27(1):46-55.

[23] Thamm DH, O'Brien MG, Vail DM. Serum vascular endothelial growth factor concentrations and postsurgical outcome in dogs with osteosarcoma. Vet Comp Oncol. 2008;6(2):126-32.

[24] Salm R, Mayes SE. Retroperitoneal osteosarcoma in a dog. Vet Rec. 1969;85(23):651-3.

[25] Ringenberg MA, Neitzel LE, Zachary JF. Meningeal osteosarcoma in a dog. Vet Pathol. 2000;37(6):653-5.

[26] Bech-Nielsen S, Haskins ME, Reif JS, Brodey RS, Patterson DF, Spielman R. Frequency of osteosarcoma among first-degree relatives of St. Bernard dogs. J Natl Cancer Inst. 1978;60(2):349-53.

[27] Kuntz CA, Dernell WS, Powers BE, Withrow S. Extraskeletal osteosarcomas in dogs: 14 cases. J Am Anim Hosp Assoc. 1998;34(1):26-30.

[28] Langenbach A, Anderson M, Dambach D, Sorenmo K, Shofer F. Extraskeletal osteosarcomas in dogs: a retrospective study of 169 cases (1986–1996). J Am Anim Hosp Assoc. 1998;34(2):113-20.

[29] Levine RA, Fleischli MA. Inactivation of *p53* and retinoblastoma family pathways in canine osteosarcoma cell lines. Vet Pathol. 2000;37(1):54-61.

[30] Kirpensteijn J, Kik M, Teske E, Rutteman GR. TP53 gene mutations in canine osteosarcoma. Vet Surg. 2008;37(5):454-60.

[31] Thomas R, Wang HJ, Tsai PC, Langford CF, Fosmire SP, Jubala CM, et al. Influence of genetic background on tumor karyotypes: evidence for breed-associated cytogenetic aberrations in canine appendicular osteosarcoma. Chromosome Res. 2009;17(3):365-77.

[32] Picci P, Vanel D, Briccoli A, Talle K, Haakenaasen U, Malaguti C, et al. Computed tomography of pulmonary metastases from osteosarcoma: the less poor technique. A study of 51 patients with histological correlation. Ann Oncol. 2001;12(11):1601-4.

[33] Waters DJ, Coakley FV, Cohen MD, Davis MM, Karmazyn B, Gonin R, et al. The detection of pulmonary metastases by helical CT: a clinicopathologic study in dogs. J Comput Assist Tomogr. 1998;22(2):235-40.

[34] LaRue SM, Withrow SJ, Wrigley RH. Radiographic bone surveys in the evaluation of primary bone tumors in dogs. J Am Vet Med Assoc. 1986;188(5):514-6.

[35] Berg J, Lamb CR, O'Callaghan MW. Bone scintigraphy in the initial evaluation of dogs with primary bone tumors. J Am Vet Med Assoc. 1990;196(6):917-20.

[36] Hahn KA, Hurd C, Cantwell HD. Single-phase methylene diphosphate bone scintigraphy in the diagnostic evaluation of dogs with osteosarcoma. J Am Vet Med Assoc. 1990;196(9):1483-6.

[37] Jankowski M, Steyn P, Lana S, Dernell W, Blom C, Uhrig J, et al. Nuclear scanning with 99mTc-HDP for the initial evaluation of osseous metastasis in canine osteosarcoma. Vet Comp Oncol. 2003;1(3):152-8.

[38] Lamb C. Bone scintigraphy in small animals. J Am Vet Med Assoc. 1987;191(12):1616.

[39] Parchman MB, Flanders JA, Erb HN, Wallace R, Kallfelz FA. Nuclear medical bone imaging and targeted radiography for evaluation of skeletal neoplasms in 23 dogs. Vet Surg. 1990;18(6):454-8.

[40] Bergman PJ, MacEwen EG, Kurzman ID, Henry CJ, Hammer AS, Knapp DW, et al. Amputation and carboplatin for treatment of dogs with osteosarcoma: 48 cases (1991 to 1993). J Vet Intern Med. 1996;10(2):76-81.

[41] Cho WH, Song WS, Jeon D-G, Kong C-B, Kim MS, Lee JA, et al. Differential presentations, clinical courses, and survivals of osteosarcomas of the proximal humerus over other extremity locations. Annal Surg Oncol. 2010;17(3):702-8.

[42] Schwarz P, Withrow S, Curtis C, Powers B, Straw R. Partial maxillary resection as a treatment for oral cancer in 61 dogs. J Am Anim Hosp Assoc (USA). 1991.

[43] Wallace J, Matthiesen DT, Patnaik AK. Hemimaxillectomy for the treatment of oral tumors in 69 dogs. Vet Surg. 1992;21(5):337-41.

[44] Hendrix D, Gelatt K. Diagnosis, treatment and outcome of orbital neoplasia in dogs: a retrospective study of 44 cases. J Small Anim Pract. 2000;41(3):105-8.

[45] Baines SJ, Lewis S, White RA. Primary thoracic wall tumours of mesenchymal origin in dogs: a retrospective study of 46 cases. Vet Rec. 2002;150(11):335-9.

[46] Matthiesen DT, Clark GN, Orsher RJ, Pardo AO, Glennon J, Patnaik AK. En bloc resection of primary rib tumors in 40 dogs. Vet Surg. 1992;21(3):201-4.

[47] Montgomery R, Henderson R, Powers R, Withrow S, Straw R, Freund J, et al. Retrospective study of 26 primary tumors of the osseous thoracic wall in dogs. J Am Anim Hosp Assoc (USA). 1993: (29) 68–72.

[48] Pirkey-Ehrhart N, Withrow SJ, Straw RC, Ehrhart EJ, Page RL, Hottinger HL, et al. Primary rib tumors in 54 dogs. J Am Anim Hosp Assoc. 1994;31(1):65-9.

[49] Montinaro V, Boston SE, Buracco P, Culp WT, Romanelli G, Straw R, et al. Clinical outcome of 42 dogs with scapular tumors treated by scapulectomy: A Veterinary Society of Surgical Oncology (VSSO) retrospective study (1995–2010). Vet Surg. 2013;42(8):943-50.

[50] Gamblin RM, Straw RC, Powers BE, Park RD, Bunge MM, Withrow SJ. Primary osteosarcoma distal to the antebrachiocarpal and tarsocrural joints in nine dogs (1980–1992). J Am Anim Hosp Assoc. 1994;31(1):86-91.

[51] Ehrhart N, Dernell W, Hoffmann W, Weigel R, Powers B, Withrow S. Prognostic importance of alkaline phosphatase activity in serum from dogs with appendicular osteosarcoma: 75 cases (1990–1996). J Am Vet Med Assoc. 1998;213(7):1002-6.

[52] Hillers KR, Dernell WS, Lafferty MH, Withrow SJ, Lana SE. Incidence and prognostic importance of lymph node metastases in dogs with appendicular osteosarcoma: 228 cases (1986–2003). J Am Vet Med Assoc. 2005;226(8):1364-7.

[53] Garzotto CK, Berg J, Hoffmann WE, Rand WM. Prognostic significance of serum alkaline phosphatase activity in canine appendicular osteosarcoma. J Vet Intern Med. 2000;14(6):587-92.

[54] Moore AS, Dernell WS, Ogilvie GK, Kristal O, Elmslie R, Kitchell B, et al. Doxorubicin and BAY 12-9566 for the treatment of osteosarcoma in dogs: a randomized, double-blind, placebo-controlled study. J Vet Intern Med. 2007;21(4):783-90.

[55] Kirpensteijn J, Kik M, Rutteman G, Teske E. Prognostic significance of a new histologic grading system for canine osteosarcoma. Vet Pathol Online. 2002;39(2):240-6.

[56] Berg J, Weinstein MJ, Schelling SH, Rand WM. Treatment of dogs with osteosarcoma by administration of cisplatin after amputation or limb-sparing surgery: 22 cases (1987–1990). J Am Vet Med Assoc. 1992;200(12):2005-8.

[57] Maulding G, Matus R, Withrow S, Patnaik A. Canine osteosarcoma. Treatment by amputation and adjuvant chemotherapy using doxorubicin and cisplatin. J Vet Inter Med. 1988;2(4):177-80.

[58] Pinho SS, Carvalho S, Cabral J, Reis CA, Gartner F. Canine tumors: a spontaneous animal model of human carcinogenesis. Transl Res. 2012;159(3):165-72.

[59] Lindblad-Toh K, Wade CM, Mikkelsen TS, Karlsson EK, Jaffe DB, Kamal M, et al. Genome sequence, comparative analysis and haplotype structure of the domestic dog. Nature. 2005;438(7069):803-19.

[60] Lazarides A, Erdmann D, Powers D, Eward W. Custom facial reconstruction for osteosarcoma of the jaw. J Oral Maxillofac Surg. 2014;72(11):2375 e1-10.

[61] Parker HG, Shearin AL, Ostrander EA. Man's best friend becomes biology's best in show: genome analyses in the domestic dog. Annu Rev Genet. 2010;44:309-36.

[62] Rowell JL, McCarthy DO, Alvarez CE. Dog models of naturally occurring cancer. Trends Mol Med. 2011;17(7):380-8.

[63] Maeda J, Yurkon CR, Fujisawa H, Kaneko M, Genet SC, Roybal EJ, et al. Genomic instability and telomere fusion of canine osteosarcoma cells. PLoS One. 2012;7(8):e43355.

[64] Selvarajah S, Yoshimoto M, Ludkovski O, Park PC, Bayani J, Thorner P, et al. Genomic signatures of chromosomal instability and osteosarcoma progression detected by high resolution array CGH and interphase FISH. Cytogenet Genome Res. 2008;122(1):5-15.

[65] Sutter NB, Ostrander EA. Dog star rising: the canine genetic system. Nat Rev Genet. 2004;5(12):900-10.

[66] Ostrander EA, Comstock KE. The domestic dog genome. Curr Biol. 2004;14(3):R98-9.

[67] Paoloni M, Davis S, Lana S, Withrow S, Sangiorgi L, Picci P, et al. Canine tumor cross-species genomics uncovers targets linked to osteosarcoma progression. BMC Genom. 2009;10:625.

[68] Mintz MB, Sowers R, Brown KM, Hilmer SC, Mazza B, Huvos AG, et al. An expression signature classifies chemotherapy-resistant pediatric osteosarcoma. Cancer Res. 2005;65(5):1748-54.

[69] Fossey SL, Liao AT, McCleese JK, Bear MD, Lin J, Li PK, et al. Characterization of STAT3 activation and expression in canine and human osteosarcoma. BMC Cancer. 2009;9:81.

[70] Liao AT, McMahon M, London C. Characterization, expression and function of c-Met in canine spontaneous cancers. Vet Comp Oncol. 2005;3(2):61-72.

[71] MacEwen EG, Kutzke J, Carew J, Pastor J, Schmidt JA, Tsan R, et al. c-Met tyrosine kinase receptor expression and function in human and canine osteosarcoma cells. Clin Exp Metastasis. 2003;20(5):421-30.

[72] Ryu K, Choy E, Yang C, Susa M, Hornicek FJ, Mankin H, et al. Activation of signal transducer and activator of transcription 3 (Stat3) pathway in osteosarcoma cells and overexpression of phosphorylated-Stat3 correlates with poor prognosis. J Orthop Res. 2010;28(7):971-8.

[73] Rosenberger JA, Pablo NV, Crawford PC. Prevalence of and intrinsic risk factors for appendicular osteosarcoma in dogs: 179 cases (1996–2005). J Am Vet Med Assoc. 2007;231(7):1076-80.

[74] Phillips JC, Lembcke L, Chamberlin T. A novel locus for canine osteosarcoma (OSA1) maps to CFA34, the canine orthologue of human 3q26. Genomics. 2010;96(4):220-7.

[75] Scott MC, Sarver AL, Gavin KJ, Thayanithy V, Getzy DM, Newman RA, et al. Molecular subtypes of osteosarcoma identified by reducing tumor heterogeneity through an interspecies comparative approach. Bone. 2011;49(3):356-67.

[76] Angstadt AY, Thayanithy V, Subramanian S, Modiano JF, Breen M. A genome-wide approach to comparative oncology: high-resolution oligonucleotide aCGH of canine and human osteosarcoma pinpoints shared microaberrations. Cancer Genet. 2012;205(11):572-87.

[77] Loukopoulos P, Thornton JR, Robinson WF. Clinical and pathologic relevance of p53 index in canine osseous tumors. Vet Pathol. 2003;40(3):237-48.

[78] Wunder JS, Gokgoz N, Parkes R, Bull SB, Eskandarian S, Davis AM, et al. TP53 mutations and outcome in osteosarcoma: a prospective, multicenter study. J Clin Oncol. 2005;23(7):1483-90.

[79] Ottaviani G, Jaffe N. The epidemiology of osteosarcoma. Cancer Treat Res. 2009;152:3-13.

[80] Mendoza S, Konishi T, Dernell WS, Withrow SJ, Miller CW. Status of the p53, Rb and MDM2 genes in canine osteosarcoma. Anticancer Res. 1998;18(6A):4449-53.

[81] Freeman SS, Allen SW, Ganti R, Wu J, Ma J, Su X, et al. Copy number gains in EGFR and copy number losses in PTEN are common events in osteosarcoma tumors. Cancer. 2008;113(6):1453-61.

[82] LaRue SM, Withrow SJ, Powers BE, Wrigley RH, Gillette EL, Schwarz PD, et al. Limb-sparing treatment for osteosarcoma in dogs. J Am Vet Med Assoc. 1989;195(12):1734-44.

[83] Withrow SJ, Thrall DE, Straw RC, Powers BE, Wrigley RH, Larue SM, et al. Intra-arterial cisplatin with or without radiation in limb-sparing for canine osteosarcoma. Cancer. 1993;71(8):2484-90.

[84] Kuntz CA, Asselin TL, Dernell WS, Powers BE, Straw RC, Withrow SJ. Limb salvage surgery for osteosarcoma of the proximal humerus: outcome in 17 dogs. Vet Surg. 1998;27(5):417-22.

[85] Rougraff BT, Simon MA, Kneisl JS, Greenberg DB, Mankin HJ. Limb salvage compared with amputation for osteosarcoma of the distal end of the femur. A long-term oncological, functional, and quality-of-life study. J Bone Joint Surg Am. 1994;76(5):649-56.

[86] Thompson JP, Fugent MJ. Evaluation of survival times after limb amputation, with and without subsequent administration of cisplatin, for treatment of appendicular osteosarcoma in dogs: 30 cases (1979–1990). J Am Vet Med Assoc. 1992;200(4):531-3.

[87] Eilber F, Giuliano A, Eckardt J, Patterson K, Moseley S, Goodnight J. Adjuvant chemotherapy for osteosarcoma: a randomized prospective trial. J Clin Oncol. 1987;5(1):21-6.

[88] Link MP, Goorin AM, Miser AW, Green AA, Pratt CB, Belasco JB, et al. The effect of adjuvant chemotherapy on relapse-free survival in patients with osteosarcoma of the extremity. N Engl J Med. 1986;314(25):1600-6.

[89] Link MP, Goorin AM, Horowitz M, Meyer WH, Belasco J, Baker A, et al. Adjuvant chemotherapy of high-grade osteosarcoma of the extremity. Updated results of the Multi-Institutional Osteosarcoma Study. Clin Orthop Relat Res. 1991(270):8-14.

[90] Paoloni MC, Mazcko C, Fox E, Fan T, Lana S, Kisseberth W, et al. Rapamycin pharmacokinetic and pharmacodynamic relationships in osteosarcoma: a comparative oncology study in dogs. PLoS One. 2010;5(6):e11013.

[91] Chawla SP, Staddon AP, Baker LH, Schuetze SM, Tolcher AW, D'Amato GZ, et al. Phase II study of the mammalian target of rapamycin inhibitor ridaforolimus in patients with advanced bone and soft tissue sarcomas. J Clin Oncol. 2012;30(1):78-84.

[92] Demetri GD, Chawla SP, Ray-Coquard I, Le Cesne A, Staddon AP, Milhem MM, et al. Results of an international randomized phase III trial of the mammalian target of rapamycin inhibitor ridaforolimus versus placebo to control metastatic sarcomas in patients after benefit from prior chemotherapy. J Clin Oncol. 2013;31(19):2485-92.

[93] Gordon I, Paoloni M, Mazcko C, Khanna C. The Comparative Oncology Trials Consortium: using spontaneously occurring cancers in dogs to inform the cancer drug development pathway. PLoS Med. 2009;6(10):e1000161.

[94] Gordon IK, Khanna C. Modeling opportunities in comparative oncology for drug development. ILAR J. 2010;51(3):214-20.

[95] Lascelles BD, Dernell WS, Correa MT, Lafferty M, Devitt CM, Kuntz CA, et al. Improved survival associated with postoperative wound infection in dogs treated with limb-salvage surgery for osteosarcoma. Ann Surg Oncol. 2005;12(12):1073-83.

[96] Jeys LM, Grimer RJ, Carter SR, Tillman RM, Abudu A. Post operative infection and increased survival in osteosarcoma patients: are they associated? Ann Surg Oncol. 2007;14(10):2887-95.

[97] Wycislo KL, Fan TM. The immunotherapy of canine osteosarcoma: a historical and systematic review. J Vet Intern Med. 2015;29(3):759-69.

[98] Biller BJ, Elmslie RE, Burnett RC, Avery AC, Dow SW. Use of FoxP3 expression to identify regulatory T cells in healthy dogs and dogs with cancer. Vet Immunol Immunopathol. 2007;116(1-2):69-78.

[99] Rissetto KC, Rindt H, Selting KA, Villamil JA, Henry CJ, Reinero CR. Cloning and expression of canine CD25 for validation of an anti-human CD25 antibody to compare T regulatory lymphocytes in healthy dogs and dogs with osteosarcoma. Vet Immunol Immunopathol. 2010;135(1-2):137-45.

[100] Biller BJ, Guth A, Burton JH, Dow SW. Decreased ratio of CD8+ T cells to regulatory T cells associated with decreased survival in dogs with osteosarcoma. J Vet Intern Med. 2010;24(5):1118-23.

[101] Sherger M, Kisseberth W, London C, Olivo-Marston S, Papenfuss TL. Identification of myeloid derived suppressor cells in the peripheral blood of tumor bearing dogs. BMC Vet Res. 2012;8:209.

[102] Goulart MR, Pluhar GE, Ohlfest JR. Identification of myeloid derived suppressor cells in dogs with naturally occurring cancer. PLoS One. 2012;7(3):e33274.

[103] Selmic LE, Lafferty MH, Kamstock DA, Garner A, Ehrhart NP, Worley DR, et al. Outcome and prognostic factors for osteosarcoma of the maxilla, mandible, or calvarium in dogs: 183 cases (1986–2012). J Am Vet Med Assoc. 2014;245(8):930-8.

[104] Sottnik JL, Rao S, Lafferty MH, Thamm DH, Morley PS, Withrow SJ, et al. Association of blood monocyte and lymphocyte count and disease-free interval in dogs with osteosarcoma. J Vet Intern Med. 2010;24(6):1439-44.

[105] Kleinerman ES, Maeda M, Jaffe N. Liposome-encapsulated muramyl tripeptide: a new biologic response modifier for the treatment of osteosarcoma. Cancer Treat Res 1993;62:101-7.

[106] Kurzman ID, MacEwen EG, Rosenthal RC, Fox LE, Keller ET, Helfand SC, et al. Adjuvant therapy for osteosarcoma in dogs: results of randomized clinical trials using combined liposome-encapsulated muramyl tripeptide and cisplatin. Clin Cancer Res. 1995;1(12):1595-601.

[107] Meyers PA, Schwartz CL, Krailo MD, Healey JH, Bernstein ML, Betcher D, et al. Osteosarcoma: the addition of muramyl tripeptide to chemotherapy improves overall survival--a report from the Children's Oncology Group. J Clin Oncol. 2008;26(4):633-8.

[108] Daw NC, Neel MD, Rao BN, Billups CA, Wu J, Jenkins JJ, et al. Frontline treatment of localized osteosarcoma without methotrexate: results of the St. Jude Children's Research Hospital OS99 trial. Cancer. 2011;117(12):2770-8.

[109] Paoloni M, Khanna C. Translation of new cancer treatments from pet dogs to humans. Nat Rev Cancer. 2008;8(2):147-56.

[110] Rodriguez CO, Jr., Crabbs TA, Wilson DW, Cannan VA, Skorupski KA, Gordon N, et al. Aerosol gemcitabine: preclinical safety and in vivo antitumor activity in osteosarcoma-bearing dogs. J Aerosol Med Pulm Drug Deliv. 2010;23(4):197-206.

[111] Zhang J, Chen X, Kent MS, Rodriguez CO, Chen X. Establishment of a dog model for the p53 family pathway and identification of a novel isoform of p21 cyclin-dependent kinase inhibitor. Mol Cancer Res. 2009;7(1):67-78.

[112] Hardcastle IR, Liu J, Valeur E, Watson A, Ahmed SU, Blackburn TJ, et al. Isoindolinone inhibitors of the murine double minute 2 (MDM2)-p53 protein-protein interaction: structure-activity studies leading to improved potency. J Med Chem. 2011;54(5):1233-43.

[113] Rankin KS, Starkey M, Lunec J, Gerrand CH, Murphy S, Biswas S. Of dogs and men: comparative biology as a tool for the discovery of novel biomarkers and drug development targets in osteosarcoma. Pediatr Blood Cancer. 2012;58(3):327-33.

[114] Fieten H, Spee B, Ijzer J, Kik MJ, Penning LC, Kirpensteijn J. Expression of hepatocyte growth factor and the proto-oncogenic receptor c-Met in canine osteosarcoma. Vet Pathol. 2009;46(5):869-77.

[115] Atkinson JM, Falconer RA, Edwards DR, Pennington CJ, Siller CS, Shnyder SD, et al. Development of a novel tumor-targeted vascular disrupting agent activated by membrane-type matrix metalloproteinases. Cancer Res. 2010;70(17):6902-12.

[116] Eisenach PA, Roghi C, Fogarasi M, Murphy G, English WR. MT1-MMP regulates VEGF-A expression through a complex with VEGFR-2 and Src. J Cell Sci. 2010;123(23):4182-93.

www.ingramcontent.com/pod-product-compliance
Lightning Source LLC
Chambersburg PA
CBHW081000290326
41945CB00008B/2000